The Jossey-Bass/AHA Press Series translates the latest ideas on health care management into practical and actionable terms. Together, Jossey-Bass and the American Hospital Association offer these essential resources for the health care leaders of today.

Handbook for the New Health Care Manager

Practical Strategies for the Real World

Second Edition

Donald N. Lombardi

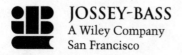

JOSSEY-BASS
A Wiley Company
San Francisco

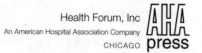

Health Forum, Inc
An American Hospital Association Company
CHICAGO

Library of Congress Cataloging-in-Publication Data
Lombardi, Donald N., 1956–
   Handbook for the new health care manager : practical strategies for the real world / Donald N. Lombardi.— 2nd ed.
     p. ; cm. — (The Jossey-Bass/AHA press series)
Includes bibliographical references and index.
   ISBN 0-7879-5560-4 (alk. paper)
1. Health facilities—Personnel management—Handbooks, manuals, etc. 2. Health services administration—Handbooks, manuals, etc.

   [DNLM: 1. Health Facilities—organization & administration—United States. 2. Delivery of Health Care—organization & administration—United States. 3. Health Facility Administrators—United States. 4. Organizational Case Studies—United States. 5. Personnel Management—methods—United States. WX 159 L842h 2001]   I. Title. II. Series.
   RA971.35 .L65 2001
   362.1'068'3—dc21   2001000637

SECOND EDITION
PB Printing 10 9 8 7 6 5 4 3 2 1

Contents

Preface

When the first edition of this book was written nearly a decade ago, the principal intention of the text was to provide the new health care manager with practical insights, strategies, and tools relative to the most demanding tenets of this challenging role. The modifier *new* in this case meant both the newly appointed leader as well as the already experienced leader who was indeed operating in an emergent environment of managed care, competition, and shrinking resources. By providing field-proven approaches and readily useful strategies in critical leadership and management areas, the first edition was received well throughout the field and seemingly fulfilled its overall objective.

The health care environment has changed dramatically over the past ten years, and the essential accountabilities of the health care manager at every level and of every experience range have expanded widely. On any given day, the health care manager leads and educates, administers and sometimes ministers, negotiates and plans, all the while attending meetings, handling patient complaints, and balancing (hopefully) the semblance of a personal life. The quality of life for a health care manager can often be dependent on the quality of the manager's work life. It is for the enrichment of this latter facet—quality of work life for the health care manager—that this second edition is intended.

Readers of the first edition will recognize several topics and subjects that were covered in the first book. These topics have been revisited with an intent to update, enhance, and enrich the original pretext of those subjects, as new material has been discovered and innovative strategies have been validated through field use at many of our health care organizational clients. In some cases, time-honored maxims have been redefined; in all cases through this book, new axioms and approaches are delineated in the interest of providing the reader with the most effective strategies available in the essential responsibilities of a health care manager.

Additionally, several new chapters have been added and new chapter sections have been introduced, addressing new critical areas of responsibility for the health care manager. The need for the health care manager to negotiate issues, introduce change effectively, and handle the resistance and nonperformance of marginal staff performers are just a few of the new topic areas that this second edition embraces and on which it seeks to provide realistic counsel and elucidation. In a similar vein, the resource section of the text and interspersed practicums contain numerous "how-to," "by-the-numbers" information for immediate utilization in essential areas such as behavioral interviewing, strategic planning, mentoring, and conflict resolution.

This text is a practical guidebook for anyone who enjoys passionately the responsibilities and satisfaction of health care leadership and management, which demands the dedication of the full extent of one's abilities toward achieving excellence in the interest of aiding fellow community members who are in pain and need. It is unlikely that there is a more value-driven profession existent.

Part One of the book, the Health Care Leadership Imperatives, covers the essential issues of leadership intrinsic to the new health care manager's role. Many tomes have dissected and analyzed the differences between management and leadership, but this text claims to make no clear distinction between leadership and management. Rather, *leadership* heads the section of chapters and accountabilities that are related to high-visibility roles and responsibilities regarding crisis, change and character, while the second section, on *management* issues, delves into ongoing, yet important, daily responsibilities.

In the leadership section, I begin with an overview and some "first steps" in understanding and undertaking the role of health care manager. Chapter One provides specific insight into the role and its possibilities, its potentials, and avoidance of initial pitfalls, concluding with a set of detailed "first moves." Chapter Two continues in the provision of guidance for making the transition to management, with a focus on moving from a staff position to that of supervisory responsibilities, and a candid discussion of the nuances inherent with making this transition smoothly and with the best likelihood of long-term success. The establishment of a progressive work environment is fully explored in Chapter Three with pragmatic exposition of how to set the right tone, communication channels, and initial expectations to staff, peers, and hierarchy. Chapter Four covers a topic that has been extremely relevant in the past five years in health care management: the resolution, redirection, and in some cases removal of "nonplayers." This chapter defines the characteristics of the chronic poor performers and dissenters; more importantly, it provides very detailed instruction on minimizing the negative impact of the nonplayers by employing a spectrum of logical tactics for resolution and performance recalibration.

Relatedly, Chapter Five brings a fresh perspective on leading through change, conflict, and crisis, which will likely be one of the first organizational dynamics confronting the new health care manager. Chapter Six gives the reader both the breadth of the practical theory of team building and team progressive action as well as the depth of "real-world" approaches to commanding group action and progress. The strategic planning and decision-making responsibility of a health care leader is a skill that is a requisite for success throughout the entirety of a practitioner's career, and Chapter Seven accordingly covers the topic and presents delineated processes that will lead to the all-important product of positive outcomes producing patient-beneficial action. Chapter Eight covers leadership substance and style and presents exemplars that can be customized comfortably to the natural tendencies of the reader in their leadership roles. The leadership section concludes with a case study in Chapter Nine that provides a practical application summary of the preceding chapters as well as the introduction of additional strategies relevant to leadership strategy.

The second part of the book, Management Strategies, is founded on a triadic confluence of management strategies that were validated in the field as effective from the first edition, new strategies that I have implemented in several leading health care organizations in my consulting practice over the past ten years, and some of the practicum of the vaunted Seton Hall University Master's Degree Program in Strategic Communication and

Leadership. The result is a series of eight chapters that are direct in scope, logically pragmatic in foundation, and user-friendly in their presentation.

Chapter Ten discusses creativity in the health care workplace by demonstrating the implementation of a system that encourages participation by staff members and guidance to successful implementation through artful management. The critical management accountability of selecting and hiring stellar new staff members is covered comprehensively in Chapter Eleven, with discourse on not only interviewing conduct but also the entire sequential range of setting standards and employing a targeted selection system. Performance evaluation is also dealt with practically in Chapter Twelve, and the mysteries of criterion-based evaluation and the complexities of composing and delivering a meaningful evaluation are fully explored and detailed. Chapter Thirteen provides instruction on negotiation skills, replete with examples and a set of progressive guidelines that lend a how-to semblance to gaining outcomes that benefit all, especially the customer-patient. Chapter Fourteen explores several "self-management" topics, such as stress, time, and life-balance issues.

The vital education and development of staff is discussed in Chapter Fifteen, with an emphasis on delegation and other daily opportunities for valuable training and development. Chapter Sixteen moves the topic of management communication past the cliches and into the realistic sphere of influence of the new health care manager, and Chapter Seventeen summarizes and introduces new management techniques in a case study fashion.

Part Three contains three resource appendices, which augment the main text with management tools. Appendix A contains two strategic planning and decision-making tools. Appendix B features a structured selection and behavioral interviewing system of over seventy-five key questions and interpretive clues that have been used by more than two hundred health care organizations as a standard system. Appendix C is a set of fifty guideline sheets that can be used as both mentoring guides and templates for action in a wide array of management areas.

In summary, this text has been specifically written to be a true handbook and guide. It is my greatest hope that it is valuable as you undertake a noble, ever-rewarding vocation.

Acknowledgments

The other day, someone said that the completion of this text, my ninth book, was an "extraordinary accomplishment." Although I appreciate the compliment, I believe the people and places who made this book a reality are really extraordinary.

The home I grew up in was extraordinary, as I am blessed to be part of one of the most loving, compassionate clans to ever grace America with Irish wit and Italian passion. My family continues to grow and amaze on a daily basis, and any specific mentioning of any member would be great fodder for humor, particularly among my nieces, nephews, and godchildren, so allow me a collective word of thanks to all for everything.

Seton Hall University is a very special place. The Virtual Setonia Classroom and the hallowed environs of places like Corrigan Hall are always inhabited by students who are nothing less than inspirational. Two Setonians, Debra LaBarbera and Renee Cicchino, lent their textual and graphic talents, respectively and exemplarily, to this text. My colleagues are second to none in their dedication, drive, and commitment to excellence, to each other, and to our wondrous students.

The United States Marine Corps and the health care professionals I've worked with over the past twenty years have educated me beyond any expectations.

And my wife exceeds all humanly expectations as a friend, colleague, and partner.

To Deborah Ann

The Author

Donald N. Lombardi is the principal partner of CHR/InterVista, a health care management consulting firm based in Mt. Arlington, New Jersey, and an associate academic director of Seton Hall University, where he has taught since 1989. He attended Fordham University and received his bachelor's degree in English (1976) from Florida International University, his master's degree in management (1978) from Pepperdine University, his Ph.D. in industrial psychology from the University of Missouri at St. Louis (1983), and he completed his postdoctoral work (1984) at the University of Pennsylvania.

Dr. Lombardi has been a regular faculty member for the American College of Healthcare Executives since 1985 and has written six of that organization's accreditation courses. He has designed and implemented management systems and reorganizational programs at over 150 health care organizations in all fifty states and ten foreign countries. Prior to his consulting work, he held top human resource positions at American Hospital Supply Corporation and Bristol-Myers, where he was instrumental in implementing organizational systems in American, European, and Caribbean operations.

As an officer in the United States Marine Corps, Lombardi instituted numerous educational and organizational systems that were lauded by both military and civilian experts. He holds more than fifty U.S. copyrights on organizational planning, management, and development systems; has written nine books; and is the author of over sixty journal articles. He is also a senior fellow of the Governance Institute and has acted as a health care advisor to several members of Congress.

Part One

Health Care Leadership Imperatives

Chapter One

Understanding and Undertaking the Role of Health Care Manager

As a new health care manager, you have undertaken a critical role in one of the most essential endeavors in a humane society—the delivery of health care services. You have entered this very demanding, challenging, and rewarding field at a time of great change and active growth. In its desire to rise to the challenges of this field, your organization has many expectations of you. Perhaps the expectation that is most encouraging to you personally is that the organization wants you to succeed. The organization looks good when a new manager succeeds, as success is an attestation to the institution's good judgment, its collective expertise, and its ability to develop talent and maintain organizational integrity. Conversely, when a manager fails, morale and organizational credibility are put at risk. Therefore, your organization has a vested interest in your success and will do everything possible to ensure that your term as a manager is productive.

The organization has many methods of supporting you and helping you attain success as a health care manager. First, it has an informal support system in place and ready for your use. This support system includes your own manager, who will be your primary mentor and advisor as you enter the management field. It also includes your colleagues, your peers on the management team who for the most part will encourage your efforts and provide the benefit of their health care management expertise. The organization will provide you with support in the form of positive role models who will offer you a perspective on what works successfully in management and a frame of reference that you can draw from and apply to your own management responsibilities. By their words and actions, leaders within the organization will guide you to develop your own management approaches and leadership style. Your organization also should have a formal support system of management development programs and leadership education that should assist your initial efforts as a health care manager.

But in absorbing the advice of colleagues and trainers, as well as the advice in this book, do not assume that your efforts to succeed will culminate in finding one particular style of leadership or one set of management applications that will suit all circumstances and situations—nothing could be further from the truth. You will create your own style of leadership, develop sound, comfortable, and effective management strategies, and be prepared to react positively to changing circumstances or particular nuances of your management position. Many of your first-year experiences as a health care manager will provide the insight and framework you need to develop your own leadership style and management strategies. In facing these experiences with the same desire and professional interest that enabled you to attain a management position, you'll benefit practically in developing a progressive approach that will work well for you.

Throughout this book, I present a wide range of management strategies and leadership applications that are immediately adaptable and applicable to your management role. I do not offer magical solutions or present secret formulas for health care management. Rather, I describe a number of effective methods and approaches used by health care managers that have been refined through the process of trial and error. By understanding the material, adopting the strategies that seem most appropriate to your situation, and applying them to your everyday managerial responsibilities, you will take the first step toward successful health care management.

A logical starting point is to examine the health care environment and provide an overview of essential dynamics that will bear on your everyday responsibilities. Within this context, I discuss some basic characteristics needed by a successful health care manager in responding to customer demand and other forces for change. I then shift to the key elements that facilitate the transition from health care professional to health care manager. Because this transition may be difficult for many new health care managers, I provide a positive, progressive orientation to the management field and identify four shifts in perspective and critical skills that new managers must bring to their roles.

The Environmental Context of Health Care Management

The new health care manager must deal with a wide range of expectations from the external environment of the customer-patient community and the internal environment of the health care organization. Both environments impose pressing demands on the health care delivery system, thereby directly and indirectly affecting not only the health care manager's performance but also that of the manager's professional staff. It is important first to understand how these environmental dynamics affect your management activities and, second, to appreciate the increasing intensity of these dynamics as they impact you and your organization.

Effective health care organizations recognize that the customer-patient now has a wider choice of service options and pays more proportionately for those services. The customer-patient must be the organization's top priority and, by extension, your own first concern as a health care manager. However, organizations that consider customer-patient needs secondary to internal dynamics ("business-as-usual" practices) and egocentric institutional politics are destined for failure and closure.

Responding to Public Scrutiny, Customer Expectation, and Demand

Three critical dynamics figure prominently in the changing external environment of health care organizations: public scrutiny, customer expectation, and customer demand. Public scrutiny of health care institutions is at an all-time high. Because individual customer-patients pay a larger portion of their health care bill (for example, a greater share of premiums that formerly were paid by employers, higher deductibles, and escalating, perplexing HMO costs) and because the media, insurance companies, and government regulators focus more attention on cost-quality issues, health care consumers are increasingly aware of the quality of services they receive as well as certain quantity indicators, such as time and expense. As a result, consumers pay closer attention to their local health care providers and the services they provide. In your role as health care manager, therefore, you must be acutely aware of this scrutiny and how your organization is perceived by its paying public. Furthermore, you must be aware that customer-patients' scrutiny extends to your department and your area of responsibility.

As has been emphasized in political circles and the media, modern health care is a public trust, and access to appropriate health care is an inalienable American right. These assertions, combined with the reality that most Americans do pay for their health care, demand that the two Big Es—expectation and effort—be at the forefront of your thinking and your staff's thinking at all times. Customer-patients expect more, and when they are in your care, they are unquestionably the highest priority. The amount and quality of effort demonstrated by you and your staff, as perceived by the customer-patient, is the most critical indicator of whether you are upholding your organization's charter as a public trust. This environmental dynamic applies to any health care department in any institution, regardless of financial structure, geographic location, or delivery orientation.

As a manager, recognize the importance of always maintaining a service-oriented image and realize that the customer-patient drives the organization, not vice versa. Set an example of strong commitment to each customer-patient and establish this commitment as a criterion of service for all staff members. Try to use a stress-positive approach to being customer-patient-oriented. For example, when reading the newspaper or watching the evening news, note any new indicators of increasing public awareness of health care, and ask yourself how they might affect your institution and your department. Rather than allowing these indicators to become a source of negative stress or distress, use this information to educate your staff on the importance of recognizing the customer-patient's needs and directing all their efforts to meeting those needs in a superlative fashion.

Today's health care customer-patient also demands a broader range of newer technologies and services. As a health care manager, be aware of this demand and constantly determine how your department might contribute to your organization's goal of satisfying these new consumer expectations. One reason for the rising demand for innovative delivery is the number of new diseases and maladies. Another reason is that with the advances in medical technology, everything is "curable" in the eyes of the customer-patient: Individuals expect "miracles" from their health care providers. This expectation is reinforced by the move on the part of many health care organizations toward providing extended outpatient services and one-day surgical procedures as a mainstay of their service provision.

Whatever your department's area of specialization might be, each customer-patient expects top services and stellar results. This expectation puts a certain amount of pressure on your department, which you should recognize and educate your staff about immediately. Ensure that your staff take the time to realize that although many procedures seem routine to them, this is not the case with a customer-patient, who looks to your department for care, wellness, and reassurance.

To meet customer-patient needs and fulfill expectations and demand, health care providers are diversifying their delivery systems. In the 1970s, it would have been unique for a community hospital to have a drug awareness program or a rehabilitation program. Today, it would be unusual for a large community hospital not to have both. The spectrum of product and service offerings that have emerged since the 1980s alone can fill an entire book. In your new role as health care manager, you can contribute to this demand for organizational diversity by seeking out opportunities for your department to provide new and better services. In great organizations, great ideas are generated from the bottom up— particularly in health care organizations, where the entire facility relies on individual expertise and business acumen for creative ideas and new solutions. Creativity, innovation, and progressive teamwork will be addressed in later chapters, but for now you should recognize your responsibility and potential to contribute to your organization and the community it serves.

As mentioned earlier, change and growth are the hallmarks of today's health care field. Institutions will continue to evolve, as new care provisions become realities in the health care marketplace. For example, the number of homes for the aging has grown dramatically as the national population and life expectancy combine to create a phenomenon commonly called the Age Wave. Unfortunately, the rise in drug abuse and the preponderance of illegal drugs in our society has spurred growth exponentially in every area of rehabilitation. You must be aware of this type of growth and understand its impact on your department. In particular, recognize that the increased demands on all providers have not been matched by the number of individuals entering the field as potential new employees. Therefore, you must develop expertise in recruitment and selection of new personnel while also recognizing the unique abilities and innate talent of the available pool of candidates for employment. It is essential at the beginning of your management tenure to begin considering not only the types of individuals you will employ, but also potential areas for recruitment and staff development (a later chapter will discuss in detail how to recruit, select, and orient new employees).

Responding Positively to Forces for Change

If you were a professional health care staff member prior to your promotion to management, you are no doubt aware of the transformations that have taken place in health care since you first entered the field. Various regulatory changes and changes in the customer-patient base, how health care services are delivered, and in the financial structure that fiscally supports the health care industry are only a few of the innovations you must address. Although change is not necessarily negative, we often perceive it in a negative light because it confronts us with the unknown, requires us to change our daily routines and readjust our work goals, demands extra effort, and dislodges us from our comfort zones.

As a new health care manager, accept the need for positive change as a progressive growth dynamic within a health care organization. As a health care professional, you might have had occasion to be somewhat resistive to change and certainly have had to work with individuals who were resistive to change. As a health care *man-*

ager, however, be a proponent of positive change. Explain the need for change to your subordinates, facilitate the change dynamic, and ensure that positive results ensue from the implementation of change. For now, I suggest that you simply accept this responsibility and understand your role as an agent for change. In later chapters of this book, I'll provide you with more specific advice on how to make change a positive factor in your particular work area.

A reasonable expectation of a health care organization is that all its managers—regardless of their individual degree of managerial expertise—be able to react positively to change and enlist the support of their respective departments in responding positively to change. If you (1) understand and accept the rationale for a prescribed change and in turn (2) can convey the reasoning to your staff, (3) encourage them to suggest ways to best handle the change dynamic, and then (4) progressively follow a practical plan for action, you can make change a positive dynamic rather than a negative one in your management applications. Again, getting the support of all key members of your organization and gaining the benefit of their insight and experience in managing change can be most constructive in your own change-management efforts.

In addition to public scrutiny, customer expectation, and customer demand, two additional external dynamics in the current health care environment might affect your staff and your responsibilities as a manager. One of these additional dynamics is shrinking financial resources. This means the cliché of "having to do more with less" will continue to apply to health care. Familiarize yourself with the fiscal resources available in your organization and balance those against your department's needs. This task is best accomplished with the help of your manager.

The second additional dynamic is government intervention, and it may have an impact on your new role. With the advent of federal government intervention in health care, along with state and local regulatory agencies, you must be keenly aware of regulatory compliance requirements and policy administration. Make a concerted effort to understand all regulatory issues and government intervention activities as they affect your organization and, what is more important, share pertinent information with your manager and your staff about the extent that legislative and regulatory compliance affects your department.

Seeing Challenges, Not Threats

Many health care managers, particularly those new to health care or those new to management, are overwhelmed by the responsibility inherent in a health care management position. This is a natural reaction, but it should not be a major part of your overall outlook. Although the external dynamics discussed so far might appear daunting, they are not threatening to the point that you should take on a "doom and gloom" outlook in your new job. Rather, they are unique challenges you can meet with the help of your colleagues and others in the organization.

The Transition from Professional to Manager

Perhaps the most critical period in your career as a health care manager is the *transition* from health care professional to manager. Your initial efforts as a manager will set precedents and establish the basic style whereby you will manage and supervise your new staff. Furthermore, in changing your orientation from that of skilled professional to manager, not only must you make the transition from one job to a very different one but you must also shift your attitude.

Shifting Attitude and Work Orientation

Orienting yourself to the management role immediately is essential. Furthermore, in the interest of being as effective as possible in your initial management efforts, avoid making common "rookie mistakes." To accomplish these objectives, you must first understand the transition factors at play as you undertake your new role and orient yourself to the fundamental aspects of health care management. Figure 1.1 shows the four basic transition factors or shifts you will experience as you assume your management responsibilities.

Shift One: From Self-Direction to Selfless Service

Consider your former role as a health professional. Basically, you were in a position that was clearly self-directed. Your job description reflected a range of activities that you pretty much controlled and that required your mastery of a technical discipline. That is,

Figure 1.1. Transition Factors.

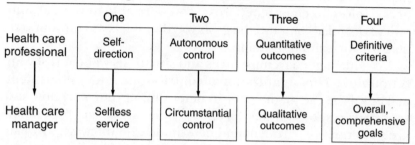

	One	Two	Three	Four
Health care professional	Self-direction	Autonomous control	Quantitative outcomes	Definitive criteria
Health care manager	Selfless service	Circumstantial control	Qualitative outcomes	Overall, comprehensive goals

you made technical judgments without undue reliance on others, and external and internal organizational dynamics had little, if any, impact on your daily activities. In essence, you were responsible only for your own performance. Having total control over your own performance, you were the key-determining factor in ascertaining what quality output you would generate and what contribution you would make to the organization.

Now that you have reached the level of management, however, you are in an area of selfless service. Contrary to your role as a professional centered on self-performance, you now supervise the activities of others, and you will find that you have a great degree of control over and responsibility for their activities. However, your own work role will be constantly interrupted by people problems, organizational mandates, and change in work direction generated by upper management. Furthermore, your first responsibility is to the individuals you supervise, not to yourself. This means that your priorities and interests must take a backseat. Your time is now governed by the work activities and needs of your reporting staff as well as the needs of your organization. Hence, your work activity will be predicated on factors outside your own professional needs and desires.

Shift Two: From Autonomy to Circumstantial Control

In your role as a health care professional, you had autonomous control over your work responsibilities. In many cases, your work activity was primarily governed by a job description, and you performed your tasks almost automatically. You knew what deadlines you had to meet, what work had to get done, and in what sequence. Your workflow depended on routine and proven practices. Unless an emergency arose, you were able to work at your own pace and accomplish the goals you desired, based on your own performance and motivation.

As a manager, circumstances and situations will control your action flow. The organizational contribution your department makes will be the main factor in determining your workflow and your daily responsibilities. As emergencies arise, you must mobilize you entire department and determine who will work to attain specific objectives. Flexibility will become a key factor in your success, whereas a set structure and daily routine defined your former role. This shift in control requires not only a change in work approach, but also in attitude, for you must be positively reactive, adaptable, flexible, and versatile in undertaking your management responsibilities.

Shift Three: From Quantitative to Qualitative Outcomes

Your previous role probably led to a variety of quantitative outcomes. For example, if you were a lab technician, you conducted analysis and assays, which produced numerical (quantitative) outcomes. If you were a staff pharmacist, you were charged with filling a set amount of prescriptions on a daily basis. If you were a plant engineer or a staff nurse, you had a certain number of procedures and activities that, if successfully undertaken, would dictate whether you had a good day. Your performance was assessed based on meeting these quantitative outcomes on a regular basis, and you probably earned exceptional performance ratings because you were able to exceed these key numbers.

As a manager, you will now deal largely in qualitative outcomes. This means that it will be difficult for you to measure your success because fundamentally you are dealing with personalities and perceptions. Even the most important indicator of successful health care management performance—customer-patient satisfaction— is very difficult to measure numerically and is definitely qualitative in scope. On some days, it will be difficult to determine whether you had a good day. (Some managers maintain that getting through a day without a major disaster is indeed a good day!) Immediate gratification and clear measurement of stellar performance will largely become elements of your professional past.

Shift Four: From Focus on Definitive Criteria to Overall, Comprehensive Goals

Finally, as a professional, you dealt with definite outcomes—you either completed the lab analysis or not; filled a prescription correctly or failed to note contraindications. Having clear-cut criteria led to a great degree of satisfaction by enabling you to recognize clearly the contribution you made toward providing stellar health care. Furthermore, this clarity of outcome provided you with a building block sequence, whereby you could improve your performance each day and compare it with a previous level of goal attainment.

Your professional realm having changed, you now work in a health care management capacity, which offers no black-and-white performance criteria. Instead, you have entered an area that nearly all health care executives and managers agree can best be described as "gray." When you consider the impact of all of the dynamics of change and expectations cited at the outset of this chapter, you can appreciate that it will be very difficult to measure performance, clearly identify key performance criteria, and establish reliable goals for optimum performance. As a result, you must adapt your thinking to look more at the breadth of activity, as opposed to the depth of activity. This means looking at the big picture as it relates to all of your department's activities, establishing overall, comprehensive goals, and closely monitoring performance with an open mind—all without ever losing sight of the objective of providing excellent health care.

Honing Your People Skills and Meeting Expectations

Another reality of the health care environment is that it is very people-intensive. An ongoing debate in health policy classrooms and other forums is whether the health care profession is a business or a service. It is both. Even though as a business it must be profitable, it first and foremost is a service dedicated to helping those in pain and in dire health circumstances. The people-intensive nature of health care delivery separates it from almost all other American businesses and is the single most defining factor that makes this business unique.

In this people-intensive environment, it is essential that you hone your people skills as much as possible. This means recognizing that management is a process, the success of which is predicated on the manager's ability to relate to a wide spectrum of people, recognize attitudes, and blend diverse talents into one cohesive team. My intent is that this book will provide you with insight on how to accomplish that end. From the outset of your responsibilities as a manager, strive to learn as much as possible about the individuals who report to you, have a working knowledge of the work personality of each one, and quickly identify telling attitudes (such as adaptability, assertiveness, defensiveness, or openness) of both your employees and your organization's customer-patients. A lack of understanding or empathy for either the patient or the staff member is the quickest route to managerial failure.

Your organization now expects you to be a leader as well as a manager. As a leader, you will be expected to set policy, have exemplary conduct, and promote your organization's vision of success and optimum health care service delivery to customer-patients. As a manager, you will be expected to maintain a hands-on approach toward merging organizational mission and vision with organizational success.

As an interesting aside, the Latin word from which *leader* is derived is also the root for the words *legislate* and *legitimate*. Also, the Latin word from which *manager* is drawn is the word from which the English word *hand* is derived. In essence, a leader sets policy ("lays down the law") for his or her area of responsibility. As noted above, a manager uses a "hands-on" approach to making progressive performance a daily objective. The new health care manager is to fulfill both of these accountabilities. This book will guide you in meeting both of these important expectations; a later chapter, for instance, explores applying proven concepts of leadership.

One of your people-related responsibilities as a new health care manager is the morale of your department. In spite of individual personalities, attitudes, or foibles among your new reporting staff, you will be expected to develop a well-motivated work group. Though easier said than done, this is an achievable and realistic expectation held by your organization. As a manager, you have the advantage of working with a clean slate and are not accountable for the "sins" of the previous manager. Accordingly, you can set your own policies and establish your own relationships with members of your department. The performance of your work group ultimately is what will define your success as a manager.

In addition to building and maintaining morale, your organization will also expect you to contribute to the education and training of your work group, conduct segments of new employee orientation, ensure staff commitment to new organizational programs, and provide leadership among other dynamics that might affect your department's daily activities. Furthermore, the organization will expect your own continued development as a manager and as a leader. This can be achieved by furthering your education—attending professional seminars and workshops, learning from your experiences, and remaining receptive to other practical educational opportunities.

Finally, you will be expected to use your technical expertise in new ways. New health care managers are appointed primarily because of their past technical achievements and contributions, and health care organizations will expect increased technical contributions from their new manager—for example, giving more attention to regulatory compliance, technological innovations, and enhanced training for members of the department. Consider what contributions you can make from a technical perspective and make this consideration part of your initial discussions with the manager to whom you report.

Integrating Your Team Approach into the Organizational Climate

A new health care manager is a team member as well as a team leader. As the newest member of your organization's management team, you are expected to cooperate with all organizational efforts and provide support and expertise to other managers as needed. This charge mandates your participation in meetings and other communication activities with other managers and in an assortment of other organizational efforts. Your contribution is vital to the organization's success, and it should increase proportionately to the amount of time you spend in the management role and the familiarity you gain with organizational activities, objectives, and plans.

In assessing your role as a team member and team leader, acknowledge that the health care business operates in a hyperactive environment. Emergencies must be handled quickly; new ideas and approaches must be adapted efficiently, effectively, and as quickly as possible; and new programs must be instituted successfully, with optimal results and the shortest possible turnaround time. Consequently, your decisions must be as accurate, proactive, and progressive as possible.

Your initial strategy toward meeting these mandates is to realize that time is of the essence in all your activities. Although it is important to deliberate prior to making a decision, decisions must be made in a timely and productive fashion so that action can take place. Furthermore, keep in mind that in any health care business—whether a hospital, long-term facility, or other provider—all departments are interdependent. In many cases, the work of one department cannot be achieved without the participation of another department. Remembering this fact will help you absorb more readily the decision-making and judgment-execution strategies that I discuss later in this book.

Your team approach will come into play in tandem with the organizational expectation of long-term growth. Essentially, your department will be expected to grow as a strategic business unit within the facility. This could mean finding ways for your department to provide new services or develop new technologies that adhere to the imperative of serving the patient population while doing more with less. If your staff members are developing their individual expertise and growing on the job, the natural synergism among the entire work group will become stronger and more progressive, thus contributing to the organization's long-term growth. As an initial strategy, list your own expectations for your department. Then, after you have had time to learn the relative strengths and weaknesses of individual team members (three months, for example), set down your expectations for each member of your staff.

As already stated, a new health care manager's stellar performance is an overriding organizational expectation. In cases where the new manager is perceived a superstar from another organization that is well regarded in the health care industry, or she was an expert technician or high-quality performer in a professional role at the current organization, it is logical that this expectation be heightened. However, although stellar performance should be your primary goal as you undertake your new role, stellar effort is the key to stellar performance, as effort is one of the two Big Es (expectation and effort) referred to earlier. In some situations, perhaps in a department that has had notable success in the past, your efforts will result in success more easily. In other situations, such as a department with a poor performance history, you'll have to work harder to gain results. Your particular situation and the circumstantial dynamics that direct your managerial approach are equal in importance and both will influence your desires and expectations for success. Recognize this reality, deal with it pragmatically, and never compromise your commitment to make your department—and your contribution as a health care manager— the best it can be.

Managing Your Time From Day One

Another critical transition factor is the amount of time you spend on management activities. Without a set shift or nine-to-five routine, your time no longer will be your own. The amount of time you spend on your job largely will be dictated by the organization's needs and those of your department members. Some managers new to their roles overact to the time demands, assuming that the only way to meet their new objectives is to spend eighteen hours a day at work while virtually forgoing a personal life. This quickly results in burnout and failure in the management role. It is essential that during your transition you immediately recognize this fact.

A critical yet often overlooked distinction is the amount of time you spend in your new management responsibilities versus how you spend it. If you consider time allocation in your former role as a health care professional, a typical day probably meant more than 80 percent of time spent in professional activities— conducting laboratory work, treating patients, filling prescriptions, or repairing equipment. As a health care manager, you will find that this quotient will shift drastically.

Figure 1.2 is a pie-chart construction of representative time quotients for an average health care manager. This pie chart is based on input from numerous health care managers who participated in the research conducted for this book. As you can see, almost 65 percent of your time—two-thirds of your working day—involves people-management activities (motivating employees, setting work objectives, dealing with employee performance problems, assisting employees in accomplishing their work goals). This category also includes handling customer-patient requests and complaints, working with peers, and engaging in other people-intensive activities. This time allocation probably differs significantly from your previous role as a health care professional.

Fifteen percent of your time will be absorbed by management activities, including what perhaps is the largest new demand on your time—meetings. Meetings are a necessity as the business itself

Figure 1.2. Management Responsibilities.

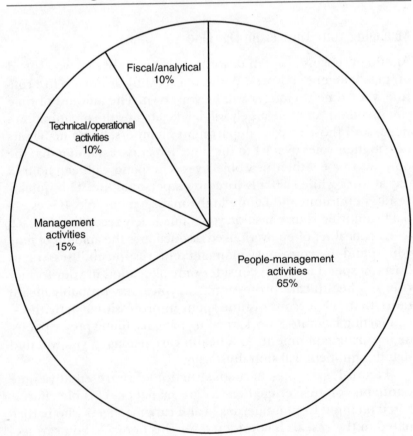

changes and new objectives are established. Other management activities might include employee training and development, participation on councils and committees, and other pursuits that involve your working with colleagues and upper managers.

The remaining 20 percent of the chart is divided equally between fiscal-analytical responsibilities and technical-operational responsibilities. Fiscal-analytical responsibilities might include budgeting processes, financial paperwork, and cost-benefit analyses. In some management roles, this 10 percent quotation can easily be replaced or supplemented with *administrivia,* a popular term that relates to the weighty paperwork attendant to organizational administration (for example, compliance reports and organizational inventories). Technical-operational activities include participation in conferences related to your department's specific area of technical expertise or participation in educational activities aimed at improving your technical proficiency.

Implementing Three Key Strategies

To apply the transition strategies discussed so far successfully, it is essential first to master three keys not only to a healthy transition but also to ongoing successful management. These keys, which are emphasized throughout this book, are being able to communicate, maintaining a sense of perspective, and maintaining a high level of industry in your department.

Communication

As shown in Figure 1.3, management skills are predicated on three basic strengths. Communication is at the apex of the pyramid. Strong communication skills are an absolute prerequisite for developing good people skills. If you cannot communicate effectively, you cannot motivate others, recruit and retain top employees, conduct performance evaluations, or mobilize your staff to work as a team. Furthermore, you cannot successfully express needs and desires for your department, participate in organizational management activities, or deal successfully with customer-patients. Communication skills, though often innate, can also be learned and developed. Most of the strategies presented in this book are communication-driven, but they are also soundly rooted in industrial psychology. Because communication is the key to performance and human behavior, the techniques in this book not only will assist you in the transition into management, but they will also sustain you throughout your management career in your interactions with key players.

A Sense of Perspective

Perspective means the ability to keep a balanced view of things; that is, not succumbing to the temptation to make big things out of little things or to trivialize major events. Keeping a good perspective is an essential managerial requirement, for managers who lose perspective are doomed to a cycle of stress, negative attitude, and ultimate failure in their roles.

Perceptiveness is the cornerstone of a sound perspective. A truly perceptive manager can listen effectively to information, process it, and incorporate it into the proper context. This skill encompasses the ability to pick up on vital clues about performance and communication, to understand the *why, who,* and *what* of communication, and, what is most important, to react proactively and positively to oral or written information. Like communication skills, a sense of perspective is an innate skill that can be honed and developed into a strong management asset—to do so is one of the major objectives of this book.

Industriousness

During your transition into health care management, you must create and maintain a high level of industry within your department

Figure 1.3. Essential Factors of Management.

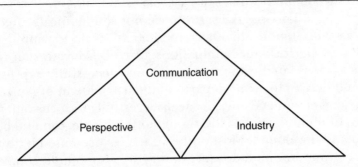

as well as in your own work activities. This means maintaining a sound drive and dedication toward all work objectives and maximizing motivation and performance among all your staff. Without a high level of industry as part of your work ethic and professional outlook, you would have never progressed to the rank of manager.

Stepping into the Spotlight

As a new health care manager, you have relinquished your low profile, as you are no longer part of the rank and file but a group leader. Former colleagues and work buddies are now members of your staff. Individuals who in your former professional role might have looked to you for technical guidance and assistance in a key area of specialization now will look to you for leadership and management.

In your new capacity, your staff will monitor all your activities closely for clues as to what the new work relationship will be. These clues will be derived from your words and actions, your fair treatment of employees, and your demonstrated commitment to accomplishing goals. Furthermore, your peers will look at your initial performance to determine what type of colleague you will be. Family and friends naturally will be concerned about whether your new role will impose drastic changes to the relationship they enjoy with you.

Being in the spotlight is part of the responsibility of management, something you will either enjoy or not enjoy. Your ability to manage high visibility was probably a consideration your organization weighed prior to appointing you to the position. Moreover, in accepting the job you knew that handling the spotlight would be an important part of your responsibilities. I will offer numerous strategies for withstanding criticism and presenting the presence needed to successfully perform your job throughout this book.

In formulating your new relationships with staff, first determine what strategies work for individual staff members or groups of staff. For example, three general classes of employees might make up your department:

- Superstars, who are highly motivated, enjoy their work, and act as positive role models for the whole group

- Steadies, who are best typified as dependable performers who do a solid job but are not particularly motivated to excel or exceed performance expectations on a regular basis
- Nonplayers, who lack motivation and in some cases may even be counterproductive, subversive, and detrimental to the entire work group

One strategic tool for addressing these differences is the performance evaluation. This appraisal tool reinforces positive contribution, pinpoints problem areas (and problem employees), and ultimately clarifies your relationship with your staff. In the next chapter, I provide a comprehensive guide to managing all three of these performance categories, commencing on your first day as a manager.

A Survival Guide to the First Ninety Days

Your first ninety days as a health care manager are critical as you establish your plans for departmental achievement, orient yourself realistically to the role of manager, and fully assume leadership responsibilities. Here are some practical suggestions that will assist you in this important period.

Clarifying Organizational Expectations

The organization has certain expectations of you and your management productivity. To begin with, many new health care managers enter situations that require immediate turnaround, for example, due to poor department performance or lack of employee motivation. Even in a department that has been successful or perhaps has a manager who was promoted to a higher position, the organization may be setting new departmental expectations in terms of increased productivity, absorption of new services, or greater resource management responsibility. As a new manager, you should discover what the expectations are of your department by asking your immediate manager and other involved directors and executives.

All new health care managers are charged with gaining short-term results. Again, ask your supervising manager or others in the chain of command what their expectations are for short-term performance in your department. *Short-term* in this context may be defined as quarterly, the first two quarters, or the initial six months of assumption of your management responsibility. Try to delineate five or seven goals and major objectives for your department to achieve in the agreed-on time frame. These goals should be arrived at jointly by your senior manager and yourself, and they should be attainable give the resources available in your department.

One event your organization will not expect is a major problem or major escalation of an existing problem. Although you are sure to encounter a certain number of crises and changes early on in your new position, the organization will frown on those dynamics becoming formidable, permanent obstacles to organizational achievement. Therefore, be sure to enlist the assistance of senior managers, peers, and other support to deal with any problem expeditiously and effectively. Get into the habit of using your organizational resources early—this is your best insurance policy for learning and avoiding the pitfalls of unwarranted negative performance.

Determining Immediate Action Steps

As you consider the role of a health care manager as depicted in this chapter, turn your attention to some specific transition strategies you can apply immediately. Your first priority should be your new staff. Two general observations will help you in this regard:

1. There are no absolutes in dealing with people. Because there is no set pattern of uniform individual work behavior, there is no set formula for managing people.
2. No one really expects you to change his or her life. Motivated staff members are looking basically for a fair wage, clear work direction, respect, and recognition for their level of performance. For the most part, they seek neither a personal relationship with you nor psychological validation from a you.

With these observations in mind, your first transition strategy is to learn as much as possible about each employee. Within your first month, schedule a day to work with each employee on an individual basis. This entails your sitting at their desk with them or working in their area to observe what they do throughout a typical day and asking as many questions as possible. As you will see throughout the text, a large part of managerial success turns on the ability to ask the right questions. Ask your employees about their primary responsibilities, what resources they need to accomplish their jobs, and what their professional aspirations might be. Most important, ask what they require from you as a manager and how you can best assist them in meeting their professional aspirations. As you spend a day with each employee, deal with his or her personality as a separate issue. For example, it is likely that you know several of the individuals in your department and perhaps are friends with some of them. Even so, apply a universal standard but a customized approach for each employee. In essence, tell employees that you are there to support them, that you take an interest in their work progress, and that you are guided by the adage that nobody wins unless we all win. Prior to sitting with employees, you might hold a departmental meeting to explain your intent to learn what their jobs entail. This way, they can be prepared to answer direct questions tailored to more specific dynamics. For example, if the individual is a personal acquaintance or former colleague, you might underscore the person's interest in developing further skills, while at the same time stating your belief that he expects no special treatment and expressing your hope that you can still remain friends outside the workplace. Even though this effort can become a complex and intricate dynamic, setting relationship parameters is a logical starting point.

Also during the first ninety days as manager, supplement the orientation process described above with five basic communication-based strategies:

1. Listen
2. Observe
3. Ask questions
4. Record information
5. Plan

Listen to as much information as you can possibly absorb. This includes the advice of other managers whom you respect in the organization, the input of all of your employees, and certainly the opinions and viewpoints of your own manager. Maintain your sense of perspective to sort out the value of the information and establish a frame of reference for how the information fits in the context of your new responsibilities.

Observe as much as possible. Study staff activities not only in the interest of learning their jobs, but also to get a feel for their work habits. Watch their interactions with others, their nonverbal behavior, and the level of job interest they display by their actions, pace of activity, and fundamental attitude in the workplace. Another group dynamic is very important in this regard: Observe whether cliques are apparent. *Cliques* can be defined as groups of employees who seem drawn to each other socially or by virtue of their job. Cliques can be unnecessary burdens to new managers if they are negatively motivated, but positively motivated cliques also require special handling.

The importance of *asking questions,* though previously mentioned, bears repeating. Whether in a management meeting or after observing a particular segment of performance, trust your instinct and natural curiosity in this regard if you think your question(s) will provide you with information. All members of your work environment—superiors, peers, and staff—know that you are in a learning phase during your first ninety days on the job and therefore expect you to ask questions.

Record as much information as possible and as needed to establish your frame of reference. Use a notebook or personal computer to record your observations and note significant information. Using a notebook in a meeting or taking notes while spending the day with an employee demonstrates your commitment to learning as much as possible about the employee's responsibilities and overall work life. The staff will conclude that you are truly interested in them as professionals and seek to influence the health care provision process positively.

Plan activities as much as possible, because after your first ninety days, your time will not be your own. Organizational demands, staff demands, change, and other dynamics will define your daily plan for you. Schedule meetings with peers, as appropriate, to learn more about their function, including spending a day in other departments that interact with your own. By all means, schedule meetings with employees on a regular basis, and establish a schedule for departmental meetings—perhaps the first Friday of every other month. Finally, ensure that you get into the habit of scheduling much of your time proactively, as well as your staff's upcoming week's activities. This not only gives you clear direction during the transition, but it also gets you into the healthy pattern of planning your activities progressively.

Avoiding Common Pitfalls

In the interest of helping you avoid common mistakes made by new health care managers, here's a list of pitfalls to avoid during the transition:

- *Never discount any information or experience.* All the experiences and information you collect in your first ninety days probably have potential merit. Although all information is not uniformly useful, never dismiss anything out of hand without first considering its value.
- *Do not assume that you know it all.* By presenting yourself as someone who has all the answers, you will fail to build credibility among staff and peers. Let it be known that you are learning in your initial phase as a manager, and that you need everyone's help in making a successful transition. This is not a sign of weakness but a clear demonstration that you are in touch with reality.
- *Do not assume that you know nothing.* Exercise your native instincts and the technical ability that helped you earn your promotion into management.
- *Do not try to do it all.* Refrain from setting unrealistic expectations for yourself in these first days as well as throughout your management career. Your goal in this phase is to learn as much as possible and to implement some of the management strategies delineated throughout this book.
- *Do not playact or project—be yourself.* At the end of each day, your biggest success lies in knowing you remained true to yourself and to your own comfort zone. Many individuals new to the ranks of management make the mistake of believing they must

assume a new persona. Your staff won't be fooled and will label you a phony. Individuals who make an issue of your personality are probably poor performers—nonplayers—anyway.

- *Do not establish reckless, unhealthy habits.* As noted earlier, avoid a pattern of working eighteen-hour days, putting unrealistic deadlines on yourself, or imposing unrealistic performance goals for your staff. Despite inevitable crises during this period, try to establish healthy norms for yourself, which in turn will send out a positive message to your staff.

Toward the end of the ninety-day transition period, review these points:

- *The majority of people (peers, staff, supervisors) will support you.* They want you to succeed. Their lives will be easier if you succeed than if they have to contend with all the attendant problems if you fail. Conversely, some individuals will test you early in your management tenure—usually these are poor performers who will "make a move" on a new manager. Be guided by your peers and particularly your superiors in dealing with these individuals. Learn as much as possible from the experience.
- *Acknowledge that you are by no means perfect.* You need the assistance of others in your initial activities and are basically in a learning mode. Try to use and be comfortable with the strategies described in this chapter and throughout the book. Always seek the feedback of your staff, peers, and boss in your management efforts, and constantly strive to upgrade your effort.
- *Use your support system to help during the transition.* Not only is your support system a source of feedback, it can also assist you in the trial-and-error process, which is the foundation of health care management development. Have the fortitude to try new approaches as you continue to learn, grow into your responsibilities, and resist the temptation to become impatient or frustrated. By all means, maintain your focus, which is to become a manager who is a catalyst in providing optimal health care service.

You have entered a very challenging profession and undertaken a role of great responsibility and diversity. The transition into this role is critical, and your first objective is to establish a leadership identity with which you are comfortable and that will afford maximum effectiveness in your new role.

Conclusion

Your transition from health care professional staff to health care manager begins with a change in your attitude. No longer are you concerned solely with your own performance and motivation, now you have responsibility for motivating others' performance and attitudes.

This chapter has led you through four specific shifts in attitude (from self-direction to selfless service, from autonomy to being directed by circumstances, from being quantity-focused to being quality-focused, and from having specific parameters to follow to having to define the parameters yourself). The chapter has also presented suggestions for ways to sharpen your people skills, design a team that is compatible with organizational goals, and manage your time effectively. It has also described three key strategies—communicating effectively, maintaining a balanced perspective, and incorporating a sense of industry among your work group.

Along with your new role come the pressures of being in the spotlight (as opposed to your former relative anonymity). A ninety-day survival guide poses ways to cope with this change, as well as clarify your (and your organization's) objectives in your new role, determine what your first actions should be, and avoid common pitfalls suffered by new health care managers. With this preparation, you're ready to initiate your role in perhaps the most rewarding of all human service leadership capacities—health care management.

Chapter Two

Making the Transition

As a new manager, you must orient yourself to becoming a strong team player, group contributor, and resource within the management group. In this chapter I discuss managing the dynamics that will help you make the transition into management. I also describe the process of orientation in terms of your new membership in the management team (rather than as team leader to your staff), including getting to know your management colleagues, learning how to consult and collaborate, and asking for assistance from colleagues. I'll explore two key relationships that affect your new role:

1. The relationship between you and your supervisor
2. The relationship between you and your peers

I also discuss communication within the framework of your management orientation activities, particularly as they relate to the information exchange circuit, including various modes of communication, and suggest how to make your communication more efficient as you transmit and receive information within the management sphere. I examine issues relating to leadership, focusing on your role as a leader within the management team, as well as the group leadership dynamics essential to an organization's success. Finally, I enumerate networking methods that can be used to build a base of professional contacts that will assist you in your ongoing management responsibilities.

I make every effort to provide you with concrete, specific information you can apply immediately, as throughout the book.

Remember, your objective is to provide support to the management team and maximum productivity and performance from your own management role. Try to determine which of the techniques in this chapter you'll be comfortable with and that seem to have the most potential to help you in your specific management role.

Incoming and Outgoing Communication in Your New Role

Exchange of two types of communication will be important as you become established as part of the management team. Incoming communication ranges from directives and mandates to direction and guidance, to support and pride, to feedback and questions, to consultation and advice, and to demands and expectations. Outgoing communication runs the gamut from compliance and professional development to action and growth, to support and team insight, to direction and leadership, to contribution and expertise, and finally to satisfaction and expectation fulfillment. There are six points of contact (sources) along this exchange circuit:

1. The organization
2. Your supervisor
3. Your family and friends
4. Your staff
5. Peers and colleagues
6. Customer-patients

Figure 2.1 depicts the incoming channel (from the six sources to you), and Figure 2.2 shows the outgoing channel (from you to the six sources). Each source, along with its respective scope of communication, is discussed in the following subsections.

The Organization

The health care organization will generate a certain number of directives to you regarding how to manage your staff and your technical activities and the quality of contribution the organization expects from you and your staff. These directives might be presented in written or oral form, and the information might be

Figure 2.1. Incoming Communication for the New Health Care Manager.

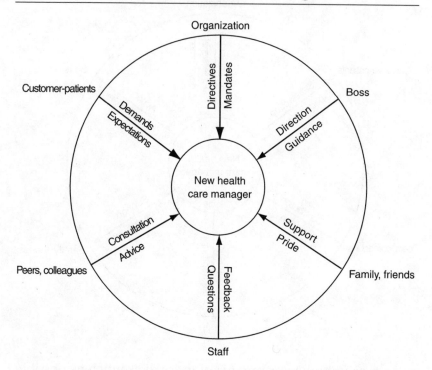

Organization

Customer-patients

Boss

Demands
Expectations

Directives
Mandates

Direction
Guidance

New health
care manager

Consultation
Advice

Support
Pride

Peers, colleagues

Family, friends

Feedback
Questions

Staff

implicit or explicit. For example, an implicit directive might be that you maintain the highest moral and ethical standards in the delivery of your particular segment of health care service. However, if this directive is written into the organization's code of conduct, its mission statement, or a set of organizational standards, it is explicit.

Therefore, it is vital during your management team orientation that you learn what organizational directives for management conduct are in place. Include them in learning the organization's history, the style of management encouraged by the organization, and what type of individuals seem to be role models in the organization. Determine which managers seem rewarded by the organizational system. It is likely that they embody the standards and characteristics that the organization values, and their professional conduct can serve as a model for your own.

Figure 2.2. Outgoing Communication Guidelines.

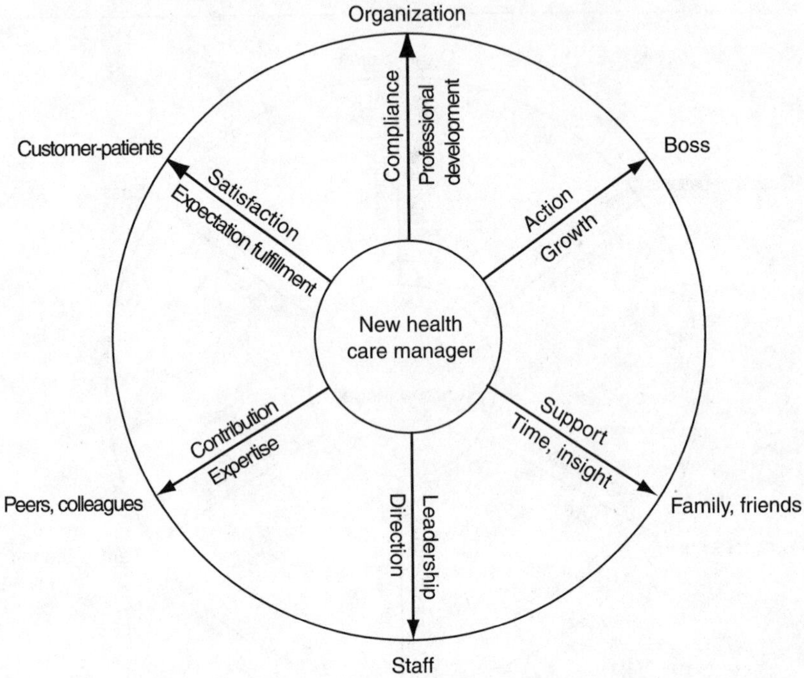

Organization

Customer-patients

Compliance

Professional development

Boss

Satisfaction

Expectation fulfillment

Action

Growth

New health care manager

Contribution

Expertise

Support

Time, insight

Peers, colleagues

Leadership

Direction

Family, friends

Staff

In researching your organization, read as much as possible about it, particularly newsletters, annual reports, and any newspaper articles or other sources of local information. Questioning staff, colleagues, and supervisors who have been with the organization for a long time can provide you with accurate and meaningful insight. The public relations office, human resource department, and development office are also good sources for this kind of information.

Your Supervisor

Your supervisor will provide you with a certain amount of direction in how to conduct your job. This can include a history of your departmental responsibilities, some background into the department's prior performance, and perhaps some insight into individual members. Your supervisor also should provide you with a set of expectations she holds for your department, and these should be detailed as explicitly as possible. Try to gain insight into suggestions your supervisor might have for attaining departmental goals and objectives by specifically asking questions such as

- What are the major objectives for this department, in your view?
- What would be the keys to success regarding my management performance?
- How often should the two of us meet to discuss departmental issues?
- How do you perceive your role as a potential mentor in the process of my transition into this new management job?

The mentoring guides in Appendix C of this book contain a complete series of guides that can assist your supervisor and other senior managers in your organization in their mentoring efforts. More specific direction on beginning a progressive relationship with your immediate supervisor is also forthcoming in this chapter.

Family and Friends

In your previous position, you probably had autonomy in your responsibilities and worked a fairly set schedule. However, as a health care manager, your time is not really your own. Now the demands of your job and the needs of your staff pretty much dictate your working hours. For example, if an emergency requires your presence at the hospital, most likely you will be there—even if it is your scheduled day off or hours past the end of your shift.

Being on call in your new capacity obviously can put a strain on personal relationships, and although most of your family and friends support your new role and share in your career progress, they might have difficulty adjusting to the shift in your working hours. It is imperative that you take a proactive, rather than reactive, approach to this potential problem. Do not wait until conflict surfaces in personal relationships before communicating to friends and family the demands of your new role.

Accordingly, take four basic steps during your management orientation:

1. *Orient your family to your new job.* If your organization runs an open house, bring as many family members as possible. Not only will they get the opportunity to see your facility, they will get to meet your coworkers, staff members, and supervisor. This will give them some insight into your coworkers and work environment and an understanding of the dedication required in health care in general and your new role in particular. They will see that your job is not a nine-to-five proposition but that the job demands are the primary determinants of your working hours.

2. *Bring work home.* There are two reasons for doing this. First, even if at home you are still involved with work, it is probably better than staying at the office and depriving your family of your physical presence. Second, at home you can take breaks to join in family activities. Remember to maintain some perspective, however, by not letting homework become a habit once you complete your management orientation.

3. *Do not bring work home pointlessly.* There is no point bringing work home that can be easily resolved the next day or on your next shift. Nothing is more unfair to family and friends than for you to be at home dwelling on a problem you cannot solve until you return to the office.

4. *Keep the communication constant and open.* Let your family and friends know whether an emergent situation might preoccupy your time. For example, if your hospital is undergoing a major construction project, bring home some information about the construction program to share with your family and friends. Let them know the reason for the construction project, share the plans and activities with them, and explain any involvement you might have in the project. Get their input on how best to deal with the prospect of spending more time at the hospital. If the construction project will require extra hours on Sunday afternoon, a member of your family might meet you at the hospital for lunch. If the construction project requires your putting in longer days, get a handle on your children's scheduled activities so that your work commitment does not conflict with some of these important activities.

After six months on the job, you will have oriented yourself to your new role, made the necessary steps toward making the transition, and now must establish some norms that will assist in your personal relations. Certainly, the challenge of balancing work, family, and friends can take an entire volume to explain, let alone resolve. However, by using these four suggestions for handling this area of incoming communication at the outset, you can make a smoother transition onto the management team.

Your Staff

As a manager, you will seek and receive feedback from your staff on a variety of issues. These can include technical issues involving your department, individual concerns relative to the job, and suggestions on improving performance across the department. While installing yourself on the management team, share information as appropriate with your staff and get their input and suggestions. This vital exchange can help you form a progressive frame of reference in dealing with key management issues.

For example, suppose your organization is about to implement a bonus-incentive compensation system. After attending several management meetings on this issue, you are curious about what the employee reaction might be to the proposal program. You might therefore discuss the issue in a department meeting, in a one-on-one setting with several of your key employees, or informally within the context of your ongoing discussions with your staff. These efforts will give you a frame of reference you can use in your management discussions and will help refine the bonus-incentive compensation system within your organization.

Peers and Colleagues

Peers and colleagues—that is, your fellow managers—will rely on you to provide technical expertise in key areas. In exchange, they will provide their technical expertise when appropriate. I'll discuss the keys to this segment of management communication in more detail later on in this chapter.

Customer-Patients

The most important player in this incoming information circuit is the customer-patient. In your former staff role, you probably had many occasions to deal directly with the demands of customer-patients. However, this communication was probably directed primarily to a specific technical issue or a particular request for assistance. As a manager, you will receive all communications from customer-patients, or at least be a party to all communication originating from that sector. Fundamentally, you will take the lead in answering customer-patients' requests, handling their complaints, and incorporating their input into the general management strategy of customer-patient service.

Pay particular attention to the concerns of customer-patients and integrate known customer-patient perceptions into your management communication and orientation processes. Significant information provided by the customer-patient that might help educate the organization on ways to deliver better service should be added to your intermanagement communication. For example, if you are the physical rehabilitation manager of a small hospital, you might receive specific complaints or compliments about the way physical therapy was provided for a particular customer-patient. However, the same customer-patient might also comment on the hospital's billing system, its parking facilities, or how cooperative the security and reception personnel were in helping the patient find your department. All of this should be incorporated into your data bank or one of your management journals or notebooks and relayed to the appropriate individuals in your organization.

As shown in Figure 2.2, outgoing communication-information flows from you to the six recipients along the circuit. The kinds of communication you send differ. As you read through this chapter, you will find many specific suggestions and strategies you can implement in maintaining a positive level of performance as a management team member.

Management Orientation

Initially, your participation in management meetings should center on absorbing as much information as possible about your colleagues, departmental interrelationships, and essential communication strategies needed to work cohesively within the organization. Basically, you try to learn as much as possible from your new peers.

Getting to Know Your Management Colleagues

The starting point for this orientation process is educating yourself about the talents, skills, and activities of other members of the management team. One approach is to arrange a series of individual meetings with your colleagues. Try to schedule extensive one-on-one meetings with all managers who are closely related to your function.

For example, if you are a personnel manager in a large metropolitan hospital, the departments closely related to your management efforts would have a large employee population—nursing, support services, and operations, for example. If you work in a rehabilitation setting, all other rehabilitation-related departments (such as physical therapy, occupational rehabilitation, and social work), of course, are closely related to your mission. If you work in the business office, certainly the financial and accounting departments are areas in which a close alliance of effort exists. To determine which departments are closely related to yours, answer the following four questions:

1. Which department(s) seem to have a natural similarity to the department I manage?
2. Which department(s) do I communicate with the most frequently?
3. Which department(s) have I found myself spending the most time in ever since becoming a manager?
4. Which areas have similar personnel and mission objectives and work with the same type of customer-patient as my department?

Learn as much as possible about the areas you define as closely related departments. This is an instance where communication and information definitely lead to greater action and better productivity because shared perspectives can lead to improved efficiency and effectiveness. Spend some time with the manager of these departments, asking questions about their basic mission and major objectives and how your department and theirs might work more closely and progressively toward achieving the common goal of providing stellar customer-patient service.

In a similar vein, try to orient yourself as much as possible with the responsibilities of your other management peers within your organization. This orientation process can be less formal and may not require as much time. For example, if you are director of personnel in a small rural hospital, you might want to have lunch one day with the pharmacy director. Even though the pharmacy director might manage only six people, he still might have some personnel needs to discuss with you, some suggestions you can use, or some potentially helpful insights into the organization as a whole. Once again, ask questions to seek as much information as possible. Establish a professional yet cordial relationship, and open a basic communication that will encourage your colleague to request information or assistance from you or provide you with insight or suggestions that might help make you a better manager.

Consulting and Collaborating

The next stage of your management team orientation is a two-fold process of

- Giving assistance to your colleagues who need your expertise
- Getting assistance from your colleagues when you need their assistance

The first part requires acting as a consultant; the second part requires seeking progressive collaboration.

In acting as a consultant within your organization, your first rule of thumb, as always, is to ask questions. The purpose of these questions is to clarify the basic problem at hand and to identify the area in which you might provide assistance. Some appropriate questions for problem solving include

1. What is the basic problem?
2. What effect has the problem had on your operation?
3. What have you done to try to remedy the problem?
4. What outcome do you desire?
5. What suggestions have you gotten relative to solving the problem?
6. Does your staff have any suggestions about the problem and how to solve it?

7. If either your staff or your supervisor have provided suggestions, which ones make sense to you?
8. What specific expertise do you need from me?
9. What do you want me to do immediately?
10. What are the specific areas in which I can assist you in making this a permanent solution?

These questions help isolate the cause of the problem, invite input, and seek to determine what your colleague's expectations are for your participation. You must then determine what information is needed to solve the problem and try to establish a list of options for your colleague to pursue.

Acting as a consultant to your peers is driven largely by a list of what to do and what not to do. There are several things you should try to do. Start by showing empathy for your peers who face the problem. Express your understanding of the problem once you have clarified it, as well as the problem's ramifications and negative effects, and determine how to obtain the outcome desired by your colleagues.

Your best approach to a solution is to consider what you would do if your were faced with the problem. How would you logically attack the problem? What technical expertise would you use? How would you attempt to solve the dilemma?

It is often prudent to try to establish a time frame for considering the problem once you have collected the needed information. Following the data collection process (asking your colleague the ten preceding questions), return to your own office and objectively consider the problem. Ask yourself five questions:

1. What is the major problem at hand?
2. Can the problem be solved?
3. What technical expertise is needed?
4. What four options can I provide to solve the problem?
5. What is the possible outcome of each option?

Strive to construct a list of four options for colleagues to consider. Even if you are only able to come up with two options, you are still allowing them a range of choices. If you do come up with four options, you will have applied your technical expertise in four ways. For your fellow team members, this will demonstrate your flexibility.

After making these determinations, respond to your colleagues in a timely manner. Restate the problem, and explain your four options and the rationale for each. After reviewing the options with colleagues, answer the inevitable question with candor, What do you think we should do? Advocate the best possible option but also emphasize that you respect your colleagues' decision and will give full support in any action chosen to solve the problem.

There are several things you should not do in acting as a consultant and resource to your peers. To begin with, do not be a know-it-all. Most individuals realize that health care management involves complex problem solving, and any individual who provides simple, ready-to-use answers probably will not enjoy long-term credibility. As a new health care manager, you have neither the experience nor scope of managerial knowledge to have the answers for every situation. So feel free to give your initial impressions and suggest ideas, but use nonautocratic language; for example: *One thing you might want to consider might be. . . . Something that might work would be. . . .* Be sure to reinforce these initial ideas with the pledge to consider fully all the options as quickly as possible.

Do not provide general information without specific details. An individual who asks you for the time does not want to know how a watch is constructed. In a similar vein, do not give a wealth of pedantic information or technical jargon that is not immediately useful. Try to be user-friendly in all your comments, provide solutions that can be easily understood by your colleagues, and express rationales that are logical and carefully considered.

Never assume anything when consulting with a colleague. Ask questions and give your colleague a full opportunity to provide as much information as possible. Do not "fill in the blanks" for someone who is presenting you with information. A lack of detailed information can lead to a lack of detailed analysis, which in turn might lead to an inaccurate decision, poor suggestions, or misguided information—none of which solves the problem.

Do not give information you are not certain of or information whose validity is questionable. If a colleague asks you a question to which you have no immediate answer, do not try to cover up the fact with a superficial or blatantly inaccurate answer; instead, offer to get back to the person as soon as possible with an accurate answer. Research information fully. Though recognizing that no solution can guarantee results, try to convey as much confidence as possible in the information you provide. Once again, rely on numerical data percentages, time, and money amounts—when discussing resources or possible outcomes.

Try to avoid advocating a solution you suspect is a major gamble. Anything you think might be too risky or questionable in terms of producing results is probably an option you do not want to present to a fellow manager. In the four options you present, try to identify risk factors, potential outcomes, potential downsides, or things that can go wrong.

In many consultation scenarios, your role is that of mediator and consultant, not advocate for one side over another. Nor is it useful to campaign for a position that is more favorable to you or your staff than another position that might benefit the entire organization. Mutuality of benefit defers to the interest of the customer-patient and the organization as primary concerns. Use tact in your communication delivery, as already discussed. Certain political players might attempt to draw you into conversations that demean upper management, another colleague, or a specific organizational position. Engaging in this type of activity will only harm your position in this endeavor and diminish your credibility and reputation in the organization.

Remember that the final decision rests with the individual who requested your assistance. Help the colleague make the decision; do not make the decision for her. Present as much information as possible, giving the benefit of your insight and expertise, and allow her to make the final call. This way, you are acting as a consultant, not an "insultant"; that is, you are not insulting a colleague's intelligence, experience level, or basic management responsibility but are helping facilitate a difficult decision and progressively develop her own management performance.

Finally, follow up with your colleague subsequent to your suggestion being implemented (if this is the case), and provide any additional support that might be needed. A good follow-up technique is to set up a file folder in your office for use by all your colleagues in the departments with which you interact. Establish a file each year for each of these related departments and keep your notes and correspondence in these files. This procedure will give you a natural follow-up system as well as maintain a chronology in establishing your own knowledge base of the organization and your technical expertise.

Getting Assistance

When you need assistance, a good starting point is to reverse the consulting process by preparing answers to the ten problem-solving questions listed earlier in this section. That is, begin by defining your specific need. Try to list the major problems you are facing and their effect, then garner some suggestions from your staff relative to how the problem is presenting itself and, more important, how it might be solved.

Try to collect as many examples as possible of how the problem has affected your department's workflow. Collect specific pieces of evidence that will help you illustrate to your colleague the extent of the problem, its scope, and its deleterious effect on your work role and those of your staff. The more illustrations you can provide and the more information you can convey, the more likely your chances become of achieving a specific solution.

In trying to define your problem, try to quantify as much information as possible; for example, drops in performance measured numerically, efficiency shortfalls that might be represented by percentages, and decreases in expediency of performance measurable in time gaps and monetary expenditure. Furthermore, try to present qualitative information that further defines the problem. This might include lowered staff morale, diminished customer-patient satisfaction, or your own gut instinct that you are pursuing a course of action that might lead to future problems.

Consider two other factors in preparing your presentation and request for assistance to your colleague. The first is a cause-and-effect relationship that might be apparent in the problem you are attempting to resolve. Make a list of causes that give rise to the problem and list the effect. For example, consider the personnel director of a small community hospital who is having difficulty recruiting nurses. The *cause* might be cited as a poorly placed newspaper ad, resulting in the *effect* that only a few nursing candidates applied for the open position. Or the *cause* might be explained as a poor job description, resulting in the *effect* that the applicants who apply for the open nursing position do not get a full impression of what is involved in the job.

The second factor in preparing to ask a colleague for assistance is the big picture. Be prepared to explain to your colleague how the problem affects the big picture of your activities. For example, in the preceding example of the open nursing position, the personnel director can simply cite that the open position has caused a shortage of nurses, current members of the nursing staff to put in an inordinate amount of overtime, poor morale in the department, and frustration among the director's personnel staff. Presenting a big-picture perspective makes *the* problem *our* problem, not just *my* problem. That is, the problem is defined in a manner that explains its negative effects on the whole organization, not just on you. This motivates your colleague to help you find a solution to the problem.

Now you are ready to get the assistance you require. To determine your source of assistance, simply make a list of four individuals in the organization who would be most likely to help you solve your problem. For the personnel manager at the small rural hospital, the list of four individuals includes the nursing director, the personnel manager's supervisor (the hospital's operations director), her recruiting assistant, and the chief medical officer. The first person on the list is usually the most logical person to turn to for assistance. (Your first impulse is usually your most appropriate choice.) In this case, the nursing director would probably present the most pertinent information toward solving the dilemma.

Toward this end, the personnel director (staying with the example) will now schedule a consultation meeting to request assistance from the nursing director. Five basic considerations should be reviewed in scheduling this meeting. First, the personnel manager should schedule the meeting in her own office so that she can have all the needed resources at hand to present her problem to the nursing director. In this case, resources would include newspaper ads, resumes, and other information that might help give the nursing director an idea of what the problem is. In other situations, such as the emergency room or the maternity ward, it is even more important to have the meeting on the turf of the requester. This way, your assisting colleague can literally see the problem at hand.

The second consideration about the meeting is to prepare a presentation that indicates the problem at hand. The presentation would include all the input, evidence, examples, cause-and-effect dynamics, and big-picture relevance of the problem. The presentation should draw on several of the communication C-factors, discussed later in Chapter Sixteen, which in this case are the *cause* of the problem, the *criteria* for solving the problem, the *clarity* of the presentation, and the *consequences* of the problem, and any other factors that would help define the problem.

The third consideration for the meeting is to seek input from the individual providing assistance. Five questions would help gather this input:

1. Have you ever seen a problem like this before?
2. What is your initial reaction to this problem?
3. Do you think I am overstating or understating the problem? (In what manner? Why?)
4. Do you have any initial solutions or suggestions at this time?
5. Is this specific area one in which I can rely on your expertise for help?

The answers to these questions should provide you with an overview of the type of assistance you can expect from your colleague. It will also help your colleague focus specifically on your objective and the problem at hand.

The fourth consideration about your consultation meeting is to ask your colleague what he would do in your situation. This can also be worded as, What do you think I should do in this situation? This is perhaps a more oblique way of getting at the same objective— to get your colleague to internalize the problem and present his insight into gaining a solution.

The fifth consideration is a follow-up strategy that will assist you in arriving at a solution. To do this, ask your colleague, once again, a series of questions:

1. What resources do you think I will need to solve this problem?
2. What recourse do I have in solving this problem?
3. When do you think you can give me some ideas on solving this problem?

4. When can we schedule a follow-up meeting?
5. What other resources should I consider?
6. What research should I do for solving this problem?
7. How can I get some relief from this problem?
8. How can I refocus my efforts?
9. Who else should be involved in this process?
10. Should I relegate this responsibility to another area of the organization or to another colleague?

The answers to these questions will provide you with a follow-up strategy. You hope that your colleague will subscribe to the same list of do's and don'ts that you enlist in providing consultation. In any event, by keeping with this strategy, you will be able to gain the assistance you need to solve complicated problems and to institute effective action in your management responsibilities.

Maintaining Your Relationship with Your Supervisor

Of critical importance to your success as a health care manager is the relationship you maintain with your supervisor. In the best of times, he can fulfill several positive roles: mentor, conscience, educator, and primary supporter. In the worst of times, your supervisor can fulfill negative roles: enemy, detractor, inhibitor, and destroyer. To make this relationship more positive than negative, there are several steps you can take initially in your management role—and especially at the six-month mark—to make the relationship a positive one.

Setting Goals

Establishing several initial goals with your supervisor is a very effective way of beginning a mentoring process and calibrating a sound course for your initial management efforts. A list of at least five goals that are achievable in the first year will provide you with the opportunity to learn and grow on the job. These goals should include tasks your supervisor sees as imperative to success on the job. To compile this list of goals in a chronological progression, consider the chart of twelve-month goals that appears in Figure 2.3.

The process begins with your supervisor assigning five goals he thinks are imperative to your work role. These can be from the job

Figure 2.3. Goal-Setting Progression.

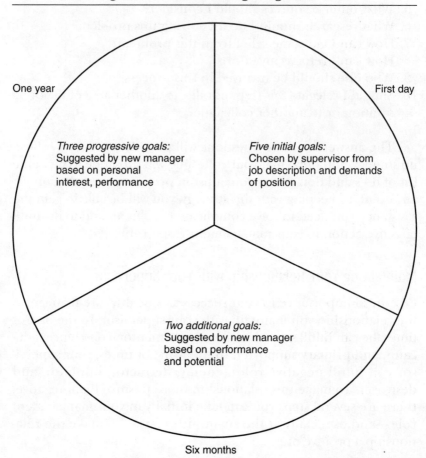

One year

First day

Three progressive goals:
Suggested by new manager
based on personal
interest, performance

Five initial goals:
Chosen by supervisor from
job description and demands
of position

Two additional goals:
Suggested by new manager
based on performance
and potential

Six months

description or the demands of the position as enhanced by your
supervisor's perception. These basic job-based goals should be
achievable in your first six months on the job.

At the six-month mark, you should add two goals to the roster. Suggest five goals to your supervisor for consideration, which
he will narrow down to two. These goals should be meaningful
and educational, and they should contribute to the success of your
department.

Finally, at the one-year mark, you should add three more goals
to the list, for a total of ten goals. This list of ten goals will become

your set of objectives for your second year as a manager. These final three goals should be submitted by you but should not be included unless you have achieved progress toward accomplishing your first seven goals. Incidentally, this goal progression is a good strategy to use with members of your staff who are achieving at a satisfactory or exceptional level of performance.

Maintaining Open Communication

In establishing a relationship with your supervisor, maintain open and ongoing communication. For example, hold regular meetings of fifteen to thirty minutes at least once a week. Regular meetings allow you to keep your supervisor informed of new developments in your work area, and they give you the opportunity to get his input on critical issues. If possible, these weekly meetings should be supplemented with monthly meetings, at least one hour in length, in which you comprehensively cover all issues vital to your management responsibilities and get your supervisor's full input and dedicated concentration on your management development.

Do not hesitate to schedule meetings with your supervisor, particularly in your first year. Crisis management meetings should occur as frequently as crises arise, especially crises that clearly are beyond the norm of your regular responsibilities. For these occasions, try to have in place at least one plan of action, if not two or three. Once you have established these plans, decide which one you think is potentially most effective. Then jointly review with your supervisor your suggested plan of action, as well as providing some detail about the crisis it is meant to handle. Doing so is in the interest of validating your plan, as well as gaining additional input. Prepare a draft of the plan before seeing your supervisor. Dumping an ill-conceived plan on your supervisor's desk is tantamount to dumping your management responsibility into his lap. It does nothing to encourage supervisory trust in you as a manager, and it certainly does nothing to assist in your development as a manager and professional.

Try to strike a comfortable balance between distance and closeness in your relationship. Depending on your supervisor's personality (and your own), the balance might lean more toward the distance of your regular meetings and scheduled activities. Another type of supervisor might want to meet with you at least once a day, even if it is informally over a cup of coffee. Try to achieve a comfortable balance that allows you the freedom you need to grow and develop as a manager. Discuss this openly with your new supervisor and simply ask him how often he thinks you should meet. This should lead, one hopes, to a happy compromise.

Other occasions you and your supervisor can share include attending meetings, seminars, and workshops together. This will give you an opportunity to add some dimension to your relationship while sharing your perceptions on the material presented. You might want to suggest sharing a reading list of journals and other information that you can make notes on and circulate to each other, thus increasing communication between the two of you while providing a common ground of professional interest.

Other joint activities include the selection and performance evaluation process you undertake as a manager. Any time you hire a new member of your staff you should ask your supervisor to conduct or sit in on an interview. Not only will this heighten the quality of your own selection efforts, it will give you and your supervisor the chance to design a structured system and mutually beneficial practice in hiring new members. By all means use the questions for candidate selection that are explained in the resource material in Appendix B.

All performance evaluations of your staff that you conduct should be reviewed by your supervisor. This allows him the opportunity to help you refine your performance evaluation techniques and to instruct you in the nuances of your organization's performance evaluation system. This should be a continuous practice throughout your management career, because it helps achieve the proverbial "one-over-one" performance evaluation sequence that is essential to the success of many health care organizations. This approach provides a logical review system in which a reviewing manager overlooks the performance evaluation efforts of all the managers who report to him or her in the interest of fairness, employee recourse, and equity within the system.

In planning work activities for your department and yourself, your supervisor's input might be valuable. Ask him to review the key objectives of your plan and give input about the best approach in achieving an objective. Also, try to get a sense of the style and substance your supervisor uses in executing a decision. Do not hesitate to ask what tactics, strategies, or approaches he would use in a given situation. This can be particularly instructive, as it will give you another viewpoint and alert you to possible pitfalls in your plan. It also might provide you with a more expedient way of reaching the same objective.

Remember, your supervisor's style does not necessarily have to be your style. But a supervisor who has a level of experience and expertise that is beyond your own can be a great help.

Ensuring Your Management Development

The final aspect to consider as you forge a relationship with your supervisor is your own management development. Be certain to discuss your career needs and desires whenever appropriate. This includes any training or education you might want to undertake relative to your own management development. Ask about the best ways to find the information you need, and express interest in your successful development. After all, your ambition reflects favorably on him for having selected you as a manager (if this is the case). Therefore, your supervisor usually will be amenable to most of your requests, provided they are within fiscal reach.

Maintaining Your Relationship with Your Peers

In your daily dealings with colleagues (other than when you need their assistance or are rendering assistance to them), keep in mind the following keys for management-team success. It is not surprising that all are centered on principles of good management communication.

Communication Through Daily Interaction

Open communication with your fellow managers and colleagues is essential. This openness should extend to providing forthright opinion, candid assessment of problems, and direct dialogue on key issues. To the extent possible, keep your communication with colleagues on an interpersonal, in-person basis. Unfortunately, many new health managers fall into the trap of sending memos on virtually everything. This behavior, especially to an experienced manager, can be interpreted as an affront or as being overly aggressive. Given the "hyperactivity" associated with health care management, it is more expedient to discuss things directly with your colleagues, and to do so in an open, honest fashion.

Strive to be receptive in all of your dealings with colleagues. Listen carefully to their new ideas and try to understand not only what they are saying but why they are saying it. That is, capture the rationale behind their thinking as well as the basic elements of their plans and ideas. Do not be too quick to dismiss any idea without full consideration of it, and maintain an open mind when your colleagues tell you of their new ideas or plans. Remember, it is quite a compliment for your colleagues to take you into their confidence and share their thoughts and ideas with you. Build on this confidence and trust by being receptive and not overcritical or aloof in management-team discussions.

Try to be supportive in all management team activities. Encourage colleagues to go ahead with their ideas when they make sense, but when appropriate caution them to potential problems. Volunteer your resources and time when they are needed—do not wait to be asked. Demonstrate a willingness to assist your colleagues, and hope that this courtesy will be reciprocated when you need support.

Approach challenges that confront your management team with a sense of creativity. Remember that creativity is the most important asset a health care manager can have in solving problems. Lend your creativity in group situations when required, and try to provide your colleagues with the benefit of a different slant on key issues. Contribute freely to the brainstorming process whenever possible and shed light on new circumstances and problems with your creativity and your technical expertise.

Never hesitate to be inquisitive when discussing work-related situations with your colleagues. Being a good health care manager is largely the function of asking the right questions at the right time. Never overestimate the value of asking questions of your colleagues. These questions can help them clarify their own thoughts and confirm the validity of their ideas, as well as provide you with information to support their efforts or give them the benefit of your technical assistance.

A good team member in any management setting acts as an inspiration and motivator to other members of the team. On many occasions your colleagues (and you) will become frustrated or disenchanted by the rigors of health care management. Try to make yourself available to give a needed pat on the back, pep talk, or demonstration of empathy. There will be many days when you will need a source of inspiration and some encouragement from your colleagues. Render this encouragement and motivation in the same manner that you would like to receive it. This encouragement is truly a valuable commodity, one that will be needed even more in the future as health care becomes increasingly complex and at times overwhelming.

Render assistance to members of the management team on a regular basis. If you see a circumstance in which your contribution could be valuable or provide a solution, offer it readily. Many times, health care managers feel as though they must take the burden of their problems on their own shoulders exclusively. Solving problems is a team effort, and the successful health care organization acts as a team.

So try to learn as much as possible from your colleagues. They are a tremendous source of information on the practice of health care management and on the provision of health care service. Their experiences have provided them with a great deal of anecdotal information that can provide numerous lessons for your own development. Benefit from your colleagues' experience not only by asking questions, but also by encouraging them to give you their insight as they deem appropriate. By being receptive and developing a reputation as someone who is willing to learn, you will receive the benefit of a valuable education.

Even though you may be new to health care management, you still have a certain amount of expertise from which your colleagues can benefit. Feel free to offer instruction in situations in which your technical expertise and insight might be constructive. If you see a need, do not hesitate to participate and provide guidance. You can certainly preface your remarks by saying, "I know you've been around here longer than I have, but here's an idea I think you might find helpful."

Volunteer any resources you have that colleagues might find helpful. These resources can range from a computer software program to a member of your staff with pertinent expertise. With the thought in mind that "nobody wins unless we all win," recognize that your human, physical, and fiscal resources do not belong to you alone but to the organization. You maintain control of these resources, but you should relinquish that control to individuals who are in need—that is, you are a team player. A true team player uses all of his or her resources for the good of the team, not the good of the individual.

Five Basic Communication Ideas

Consider five basic communication ideas when interacting with your colleagues.

1. Ask questions at all times, validate information, clarify ideas, and get as much information as possible.
2. Make suggestions as appropriate. These can be brought forth from your own experience, technical expertise, or simply from a creative surge you are experiencing. Your suggestions and input are valuable resources you provide to the team.
3. Provide new ideas regularly. Whenever you have an innovation or inspiration, particularly one that will benefit the entire organization, make it known to the powers that be. Bring your suggestions directly to the individual who is apt to use it most efficiently. In this way, you assist the individual and play for your teammate as opposed to playing to the grandstand. That is, you are using your idea to assist a colleague, not to glorify yourself.
4. Give colleagues second opinions without becoming a second-guesser. The distinction here is that in providing a second opinion you are genuinely concerned with giving your colleague another look at the issues, a view from another angle, or the benefit of a different "take" on a situation. A second-guesser subversively questions the actions of others with the intent of exposing the individual as incompetent or foolish. Make certain that if you give someone a second opinion you pose it directly and—what is most important—prior to the person's taking action. In this way, it becomes a true second opinion, not a second guess.
5. Remember that all your efforts should be gauged toward assisting the entire management team. They should not be merely for your own purposes or your own promotion within the orga-

nization. Show empathy for your team members, and you will find that your more experienced management colleagues will assist your development and take a genuine interest in your success as a health care manager.

Networking

As a new health care manager, it is vital that you build a network of individuals on whom you can rely occasionally for input and creative thought. (This is another topic that could take an entire volume.) The following nine suggestions can help you establish your network.

1. *Collect business cards.* Whenever you meet a management counterpart, either at your facility or elsewhere, exchange business cards. Counterparts, whom you may meet in the course of your personal or professional activities, include colleagues at other hospitals. These contacts might be potential sources of information. Keep these cards handy in a book or a Rolodex for easy reference, and classify them by state, business type, or title (for example, health care manager, radiology expert, or pharmaceutical supply).

2. *Join a professional organization.* Membership in a strong national or regional professional organization can help you develop in your area of expertise. The organization may be specifically related to your technical area of expertise, or it could be a health care management development organization. Professional associations offer tremendous educational and networking opportunities, as well as a range of publications that also might prove helpful in your management development. As is true with most such organizations, various standards of quality may be imposed on members. Therefore, if in perusing an association journal or newsletter you are impressed by the publication's high quality, it is reasonable to assume that you may benefit from attending one of the organization's meetings or seminars with a view toward membership.

3. *Become involved in community activities.* One of the unique qualities of health care is its standing within a community and its people orientation. Therefore, try to participate in a range of community activities that might build your base of contacts while

providing you with information about how your hospital is perceived throughout the community. Community-based contacts can include religious organizations, schools, social service agencies, or others that might be potential information sources beneficial to your career and your conduct within your health care organization.

4. *Use your calendar.* Invest in a week-by-week or month-by-month calendar with plenty of room to write notes in big boxes around each day of the week or month. Try to make at least one new contact daily, and record that contact's name, organization, address, and phone number in the calendar box. Furthermore, schedule some form of communication (phone call, note, letter) by placing the individual's name and number in a "contact" box for an upcoming week or month, as appropriate. This will ensure your keeping in touch with individuals by using your contacts and building a network.

5. *Questions, questions, questions.* When you meet a new contact, ask as many questions as you can without becoming impolite or intrusive. Ask about the person's background, areas of interest, and knowledge. Furthermore, ask about other individuals she may know who might help you gain specific knowledge in key areas. Most individuals are flattered by such questions. The attention enhances their feelings of self-worth and therefore they will be more than happy to provide you with critical information.

6. *Consider your internal resources.* Remember that your organization represents your biggest bank of internal contacts. Many within your hospital (or provider organizations) have expertise in an assortment of areas and already may have their own networks in place. Feel free to call on them and ask, "Do you know someone who . . . ?" This approach can yield important answers and information while enhancing your own network.

7. *Read critically.* Take full advantage of journals, newsletters, abstracts, and other professional literature. For example, authors receive correspondence on a regular basis from individuals who have read their books or journal articles and who desire additional information. (I have never failed to get back to someone who needs information, for instance.) The daily newspaper in your area, given health care's prominence on the public scene, is also a great source of useful information.

8. *Use mentors within your organization,* including *your supervisor or other senior members of the staff.* These individuals have extensive contact systems you can tap into and they can serve as resources. In turn, these individuals have their own mentors and contacts whom they have relied on throughout their careers and who might be helpful in providing you with necessary information.

9. *Join local health care groups.* Virtually every state in the United States and every province in Canada has its own health care group. The more populous areas in both countries have local health care groups at the regional and, in some cases, the municipal level. As a rule, membership in these groups is less expensive than in national groups; in many cases, these local groups are affiliated with larger national entities. The advantage of belonging to local groups is the opportunity to discuss specific issues that may be indigenous to your region. These groups can provide information on potential job applicants, pressing local issues, and future developments within your operational area.

Your contact network is a two-way street. That is, networking courtesies should be reciprocal. If you call someone when you need information you must also return their calls or answer correspondence when they need your assistance. Be a good citizen of your contact network, and you will find long-term benefits from your participation.

Conclusion

Being a player means being a strong team participant. During your orientation to the management team, the communication flow (incoming communication) will travel from six points of origin: the organization, your supervisor, your family and friends, your staff, your peers and colleagues, and customer-patients. The nature of the communication will range from organizational and supervisory directives to customer demands and expectations. Outgoing communication (from you to these six receivers) will range from your responsibilities for compliance and development to customer satisfaction and fulfillment of customer expectations.

Three key learning activities will dominate your management orientation. These are learning about your colleagues and how to work with them; learning how to be a consultant to and collaborator with your colleagues; and learning how to solicit your colleagues' help with your own problems and needs.

You will also spend this management orientation period (which begins around your sixth month on the job) forging two primary relationships. One is the working relationship you build with your supervisor; the other is the working relationship you build with your management peers.

Finally, during this period you will plant the seeds for growing a strong network base. You will cultivate your base of contacts by attending workshops, seminars, and other activities within your area of expertise; joining professional associations and reading their publications; becoming involved in community activities; structuring a mentor system; and asking questions at every point along the way. Have fun, enjoy the learning process, and give yourself enough credit to be an active management team leader and advocate as you develop your management style and strategy. After all, if your organization did not have faith in your promise and potential, you would not be in a management position.

Chapter Three

Establishing a Progressive Work Environment

As a new health care manager, your primary responsibility will be to manage and motivate your reporting staff, whose performance will define your success as a manager. Your primary objectives as a manager are to inspire top performance from each member of your staff, enable them to make a strong organizational contribution, and facilitate their positive growth and development. Your responsibilities begin on the first day, so you must already have a strategy for establishing a strong work environment that is conducive to your objectives of top performance, maximum contribution, and growth.

Your first challenge in assuming control of a work group is to establish some basic performance and policy parameters for achieving work goals. Next, implement a communication system that encourages all members of the staff to share information freely while enjoying a certain degree of comfort in their work roles. Once these tasks have been accomplished, seek to effect a leadership style that provides direction and guidance as well as support, thus increasing morale and individual motivation. Finally, despite any past history of acrimony or ill will within the department, encourage all members of the work unit to act as a cohesive team and a strong professional entity.

In undertaking all these initial management activities, be conscious that you are establishing precedent and building a foundation. Staff look to a new manager not only for work direction and inspiration, but also to ascertain the manager's style, approach, and strategies. Therefore, it is vitally important that you get off to a good start in establishing a progressive work environment, which can then be augmented and supplemented by the various management strategies detailed throughout this book.

In this chapter I offer more guidance on making the transition into health care management, beginning with the assumption of your supervisory responsibilities. I focus on how to gain staff support and encourage strong performance initially, and review the factors critical to establishing a progressive work environment. I begin by discussing how to construct a strong vision, garner active team support for that vision, and develop and communicate realistic policies and progressive work procedures with the intent of assisting you in creating a practical, innovative, strong, and ultimately successful work environment.

With all this in mind, I will focus in this chapter on the four factors critical to establishing a progressive work environment. As shown in Figure 3.1, these elements are visionary leadership, team orientation, open communication, and strong policies, procedures, and work conduct. These four factors are keys to progressive employee productivity and must be implemented in your initial efforts as a new manager.

In discussing these four critical factors, I will provide you with specific strategies to help you build a strong foundation for your ongoing management efforts. By recognizing the importance of these factors and then applying the strategies appropriate to your personal style and preferences, you can establish a strong environment that will empower your employees to perform at an optimum level.

Figure 3.1. Elements of a Progressive Work Environment.

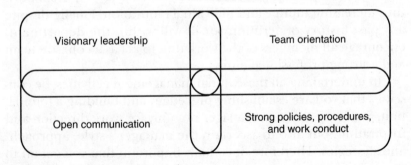

Visionary Leadership

Leadership is the catalyst of all action in any group. A military force cannot be deployed without the strong leadership of an admiral or a general; a country cannot realize its potential without stellar political leaders; an orchestra comes alive under a demanding conductor; and a talented athletic team shines under a great coach. The health care business is no different in this regard. A strong leader triggers positive action, provides the impetus for constructive and creative action, and leads his work group through difficult and challenging times with outstanding results.

Maintaining a Clear Vision

Visionary leadership, of course, begins with clarity of vision. A strong leader must maintain a clear vision of what she wants to accomplish with a work group. The adage *If you can dream it, if you can conceive it, then you can achieve it* captures the essence of visionary leadership.

Leaders who do not have a vision are not true leaders. People need to share a vision to get meaning from and excited about their daily responsibilities and individual work. A tremendous motivator for health care professionals—one that unfortunately is often overlooked—is the feeling that one is making a contribution to "the big picture." Health care professionals like to know that their efforts contribute to a greater, larger good. If a leader fails to provide a vision—a goal that provides customer-patients with solid health care, for example—the work group has nothing to get excited about and little inspiration during difficult professional times. To work through adversity—and we all experience adversity at some time in our work lives—one must have a sense of moving toward accomplishment of an important, even if difficult, goal.

To establish a vision, consider what you would like to see happen within your work group. To begin the process, list the five or six major goals you want your work group to accomplish in the first year. You can base these goals on your interaction and communication with peers and your immediate superior, as well as your entire frame of reference relative to your department. Write these goals on an index card, and keep it in your top drawer. Periodically—at least once a month—review this card. Make sure that you present the elements of your vision to members of your staff on a regular basis, beginning with the commencement of your management activities. Staff should feel that the vision is achievable, viable, and important to their professional aspirations.

A shared vision is a terrific motivator. Individuals who feel that the vision represents something that will provide them with a great deal of satisfaction and opportunity for career growth will be dedicated to helping make the vision a reality. The vision does not necessarily have to be measured quantitatively, so long as its content and achievement are positive and worthy of team effort. For example, a vision statement for a director of rehabilitation services at a small community hospital might include the following:

- Make every customer-patient feel as though he or she is the most important person in the building.
- Provide the opportunity for all of us to grow and develop every day.
- Provide the best rehabilitation services possible at all times.
- Support each other fully and give each other the benefit of our talents and personal attributes.
- Be totally uncompromising in pursuing the goal of making our customer-patients feel as though we did everything possible to assist them in enhancing their life and health.

This vision underscores the basic mission of the rehabilitation department and specifies five objectives that can be achieved, though they cannot be measured quantitatively. Subsequent to establishing this vision, the rehabilitation manager can involve her team in the vision process simply by asking them to list criteria that will ascertain whether the rehabilitation department has maintained focus on its vision. It is vital to involve the work group in creating the vision statement. The best time to do this, in the opinion of most health care managers, is after you have established the basic framework for the statement. The basic framework will give your group a foundation from which to work and will demonstrate your grasp of the department's goals as and your willingness to take the lead in this process. As you will see in a later chapter, this can become the catalyst for positive change, goal establishment, and performance evaluation. For now, understand that this helps define the leader's role, the department's aspirations, and the standards by which all performance will be judged.

Forging a Value-Driven Orientation

Another element of visionary leadership is the implementation of uncompromising ethics. Certain values and ethical principles should be incorporated into the work environment by the leader at the outset. Many health care work groups fail because they lack a proper ethical orientation. Volumes of books and a score of management development programs focus on medical ethics, but the concept of value-driven leadership is relatively new, though now widely accepted as a necessity by modern health care leadership. Many strong health care organizations have very sound value-driven leadership at all levels of the organization and enjoy a solid record of health care provisions and organizational growth.

The lack of value-driven leadership in a health care environment presents a number of problems. First, animosity can invade a work group in which ethical values are not an important or integral part of the everyday work process. Once again, the main catalyst in establishing a value-driven environment is the leader. If the leader fails to demonstrate value-driven action—actions that demonstrate decency and compassion, for instance—these qualities will not be valued and demonstrated by subordinates, and eventually this will have a detrimental effect on the department's performance.

As a new health care manager, try to determine which values are important for a health care department to maintain and enhance. A logical starting point is to examine the larger organization's values as they are expressed in the mission statement or in other organizational literature. The value-based elements of care, concern, compassion, and community should be part of your value-driven leadership strategy.

- *Care* mandates the provision of health services to customer-patients with the added "human touch" that all members of your staff should demonstrate when dealing with each consumer.

- *Concern* should be shown by the staff not only to customer-patients, but also to each other. Staff should be concerned about the welfare and development of fellow employees, helping each other through crises as well as sharing the joy of daily victories.
- *Compassion* is a cornerstone of successful health care organizations and should be present at all levels of a facility—including your department. Sensitivity and perceptiveness should be demonstrated by all team members toward the professional needs and desires of their fellow team members and certainly toward the customer-patient.
- A sense of *community (We are in this together)* should be promoted throughout the work group.

Initially, you might simply want to list these four value-based elements on a chalkboard or flip chart and encourage discussion among team members about the importance of each one. Discussion might center on the definition of each element, the importance that you as the leader place on each one, and how your team members perceive them to help contribute to success in the health care environment. This discussion can be enhanced by a short list of five or six additional value-based elements you think a health care team should have. These might include allegiance, dignity, optimization of resources, quality, societal awareness, and customer commitment (just to mention a few). The best strategy is for you to list another four values you think are important and have team members add to the list. This reciprocity makes the list more real, more pragmatic in terms of its relevance to your employees' activities; this approach also demonstrates clearly that you are a leader who encourages participation. Subsequent to compiling this second list, you might want to have it printed and distributed to all team members and incorporated into your management activities and group discussions. By doing so, you are making these ethics part of the everyday process, thus further underscoring their value in establishing a successful health care environment.

Demanding Top Performance

A stellar health care leader also insists on top performance from all team members. Individuals have different levels of talent and expertise, just as they have unique personalities. A health care leader is responsible for ensuring that each individual contributes at his or her own maximum level and strives to do so every day. As mentioned in Chapter One, effort is a key expectation. An individual who is allowed to get away with making only marginal effort within the work group is a threat to overall group morale.

An important team dynamic is the strength of each individual member. After all, a team is only as good as its individual members, just as a machine is only as good as the quality of its individual components. To carry the analogy one step further, all components must be completely functional, allowed to operate fully, and given every opportunity to succeed. It is possible that several individuals in your new work group may bot be performing up to speed. If this is the case, you must immediately correct the situation by making clear what your expectations are. For example, at your first staff meeting, you might announce the following six performance expectations:

1. Every member of this work group is equally important in attaining our group mission.
2. My primary purpose as your manager is to try to help each of you become as good as you can possibly be in your job position.
3. As long as you are collecting a paycheck I expect top effort, as does the organization.
4. Marginal performance puts all our reputations in jeopardy and will not be tolerated.
5. If you need assistance, support, additional resources, or guidance, ask for it; if you do not ask for it, I will assume that you have everything needed to get your job done.
6. Nobody wins unless we all win; therefore, recognize that your performance affects not only your future but the future of all of us.

By establishing these standards at the outset, you send a message to all your employees, regardless of individual performance level, that you expect maximum effort. The very good employees will take this as a sign that their efforts will be rewarded and that marginal performers are on notice. The steady performers, who maintain an average, acceptable performance level and output of effort, although encouraged to continue at that steady grade, may realize that you are open to assisting them reach an even higher performance level. You might underscore this message in your discussions with individual employees. And perhaps what is most important, the marginal employees—those not making a maximum effort and not performing at an acceptable level—will at least have been warned that you expect maximum effort and will closely monitor them. Of course, this in only the first step toward addressing negative performance. In-depth information on how to deal with marginal performers will be provided in Chapters Four and Twelve. At this point, however, you need only state your performance expectations and standards.

Using Power Wisely

Visionary leaders appreciate the ramifications of power and know how to use it effectively. In your new role as health care manager, you are the custodian of a trust between the organization and yourself. In effect, the organization has vested you with a significant scope of authority in formatting policy, executing decisions, and establishing plans for progressive performance. With this trust comes a certain amount of power.

There are two extremes at each end of the management power continuum. At one end is the new manager who is reluctant to use power; at the other is the autocrat. The reluctant manager does not want to exert authority over staff activities, holds back from making decisions, or perhaps tries to be one of the group. That is, this manager fundamentally does not want to accept the responsibilities of management and would rather maintain a low profile by being part of the work group. This stance causes problems because these managers cannot garner the respect necessary to have their plans and initiatives followed and carried through. Furthermore, they are in effect abandoning their responsibility to the organization and belying the organization's trust.

Your visionary leadership style should incorporate the proper use of power by exerting appropriate pressure when necessary to help realize the department's vision. Be firm but fair in the discharge of your responsibilities. By following four basic rules, you can get an initial sense of how to administer your management responsibilities in a way that properly uses your power base:

1. *Let people know you are in charge.* From your first day as manager, emphasize in appropriate words that you are indeed the manager and will make decisions. While expressing that you will make every effort to learn about the department, get to know each staff member, and basically undertake a learning curve in your initial few months, emphasize your intent to take appropriate action when necessary in the interest of achieving top performance.

2. *Let people know where you stand.* Again, at the outset, try to communicate some feedback to all members of your staff. Let them know when they are doing a good job in moving toward top performance and, conversely, when their performance is less than satisfactory. In this way you communicate to all of your charges that you are interested in their activities *and* are setting high standards for performance.

3. *Be forceful when necessary.* As mentioned in Chapter One, someone in the department—usually a poor performer—is sure to challenge your authority initially. When this happens, meet with the person privately in your office and tactfully provide specific evidence of their poor performance and contrast it to the high performance standards you have delineated. You must take an immediate stand with subversives or poor performers. (See Chapters Four, Five, and Twelve for more information about dealing with problem employees.) Not only are they testing you, they are forcing you to react in a manner that will demonstrate your management style to your entire staff. You must demonstrate clearly who *really* is in charge.

4. *Be action-oriented.* From your first day, never hesitate to make decisions (once you have gathered enough information) or to take appropriate action to enhance departmental performance. New health care managers often take too much time to make a decision or fail to empower their staff with the resources necessary to take action. Procrastination causes departmental stagnation and can cripple performance. (Decision-making strategies are provided in Chapter Seven.) Besides, your staff

will respect you more if you take thoughtful and timely action than if you take no action.

Finally, nowhere do I suggest that you become a maverick or autocrat but that you try to achieve balance between nonexercise of power and abuse of power. Keep this in mind not only in your initial management efforts, but also as you continue to develop your leadership style.

Establishment of Team Orientation

As a new health care manager, it is important to establish a team orientation to build a progressive work environment. This is a major topic of interest among health care managers because all departments, regardless of technical expertise, must function cohesively as a strong, coordinated team of professionals. It is difficult to select key members for a team, get individual talents to mesh into a unified whole, and achieve the synergy that drives a successful team. In later chapters (Chapters Five and Nine in particular) I give specific information on generating a strong team orientation among your staff. In your initial ninety days, establish a policy of team coordination by establishing standards for team achievement.

Principles of Building a Team Orientation

As a new health care manager, you will find it helpful to generate a sense of team orientation by first defining a policy—either implicitly or explicitly through your staff meetings—that defines the team orientation elements you wish to instill in your staff. This can be achieved by having your staff brainstorm a list of principles by which a team should be guided. Five basic principles for shaping team orientation might include

1. Clearly defined roles
2. A strong interest in shared objectives and goals
3. An open communication system
4. Resilience
5. Diversity of talent and perspective

Clearly Defined Roles

Team members should know their role on the team, and the team itself should have a defined role throughout the organization. Role definition is essential so that individuals can identify with their work role and with the overall mission of their work group. If roles have been previously defined in your department by virtue of pre-existing job descriptions and work group objectives, you have an advantage in this regard. If not, review primary work roles with staff members; compile, refine, or update a job description for each individual; and enlist the assistance of your human resource department to establish set job descriptions. Make certain that you have established an objective for your work group that specifies its relevance to the organization's big picture. In compiling this departmental mission statement invite input from your staff and team members by asking, *What is it that we contribute to our overall health care organization? What would happen to the hospital if our department was not here?*

Strong Interest in Shared Objectives and Goals

A winning team is goal-oriented. Accordingly, upon establishing (or reinforcing) team goals, ensure that all team members are committed to achieving these goals. If they are not, you might want to discuss why, either individually or in a group conference. Individuals may not be committed to department goals for a number of reasons. For example, a worker may not understand the goals, may be misplaced in his or her work role, or may simply be apathetic. You'll hope that your entire department is motivated by the goals and objectives. If not, check performance documentation. You may find that those who are not committed to the goals may not be contributing according to standards. If this is the case, consider placing them elsewhere in the organization or perhaps even terminating their position.

Open Communication System

Maintaining open communications with all members of your staff is essential. The easiest way to go about this is to hold regular staff meetings (biweekly or monthly) in which you discuss department objectives, recent events, and organizational information. A roundtable discussion in which all team members describe their current activities and other essential information can be helpful. Take time to discuss work dynamics with each member as frequently as possible; for example, by engaging in a one-on-one "coffee conference" once a week or simply by walking around the department and asking each person, How's it going today? Use the meeting format and other less formal methods to encourage cooperation and communication among all team members.

Resilience

Great teams are not defeated by adversity—they bounce back. Your department will not be perfect, nor will it operate under perfect conditions every day. As a result, adverse situations will arise that can have negative and demotivating effects. When these situations occur, call a staff meeting to ask these questions:

- What went wrong?
- How could it have been avoided?
- What have we learned from this?
- What will we do next time given the same circumstances?

By following this sequence, you give everyone an opportunity to learn from their mistakes, avoid reactive (as opposed to proactive) behavior in tough situations, and become more effective in their everyday work activities. As manager, take the lead in this discussion by admitting any mistake you might have made and acknowledging whatever might have caused a problem that was outside your department's power to remedy. This process provides a basis on which to generate progressive discussion, which can help turn negative situations into positive future action.

Diversity of Talent and Variety of Perspectives

The individuals in your department will have various types and levels of experience and, of course, different viewpoints and opinions on work activity. Celebrate this diversity by being open and perceptive to a variety of ideas, and encourage staff to share their ideas and perspectives. Many new managers make the mistake of trying to force "groupthink." Unfortunately, groupthink turns into "group stink." That is, by forcing individuals into one perspective or one common viewpoint, creativity is sabotaged and individual initiative is cut off before it has a chance to blossom. Ask people for their opinions, encourage them to share their opinions in staff meetings and other group communication forums, and reward creative behavior by giving individuals the opportunity to pursue ideas that might enhance effectiveness and efficiency within the department, thus contributing to the entire institution.

These five basic principles of team orientation should provide a foundation to assist you in formulating a policy of team action. By using these strategies, you will take the first step toward setting a policy of team action.

Other Considerations in Team Building

Several other ideas may also be incorporated into your philosophy, if not your policy, on establishing a progressive work team within your department. These ideas revolve around the needs for common values, clarity of purpose, and growth and development.

As stated earlier, a good team should have common values based on a sense of allegiance to the team and respect and dignity for all team members. Furthermore, the same value-based elements that go into your visionary leadership style should be reflected by individuals in your department. These elements include fortitude, commitment to customer-patients, societal awareness, and visibility in all work activities. (By now you should have ascertained which values are important to the organization and to yourself as the manager.) Try to reinforce these values among your team members by praising actions that demonstrate staff commitment to these values. For example, if one staff person puts in considerable voluntary overtime to help another whose work load is currently overwhelming, this clearly demonstrates allegiance. By giving public recognition to contributing individuals before their peers, you reinforce the standards you want to see the entire team embrace.

As already discussed, having a clear vision is vital, which you as visionary leader must provide. However, make sure your staff understands two aspects of the vision and its effect on all team members. First, they should understand the purpose of the vision; that is, they must know the answer to the question, Why are we here? The purpose should be clear and underscored by everyday activities and management decisions. Second, they should understand that for the good of the group they sometimes will be called on to sacrifice their individual goals. As a health care professional, certainly you can recall numerous times when your manager asked you to pitch in on a group project that took your attention away from your own objective. Expect nothing less than that from those who work for you if you desire strong team orientation among your staff.

Finally, as team leader, expect to act in a mentor capacity. Staff growth and development is part of your responsibility, so take time to act as a teacher as well as a leader. At the same time, remember that staff are experts at their particular jobs and that a confident leader is not afraid of or threatened by strong individual contribution. In essence, a confident leader never feels threatened by a strong and competent staff; in fact, strength derives from this dynamic. Let your team know that you trust them, and you will find that trust is a two-way street. When you exhibit trust in their professional expertise, they will place their trust in you as a leader and a primary action agent within the work group.

Open Communication Systems

Open communication is essential to establish a progressive work environment. Cultivate a wise policy of open communication, direct dialogue, and honest direction and feedback in all your work activities. This should start on day one of your management responsibilities and be nurtured throughout your tenure as a health care manager.

Communication as a topic can fill several volumes. It is a recognized academic discipline in and of itself. A great deal of information in this book is dedicated to your efforts to communicate as a health care manager. As noted earlier in this chapter, communication is a key to performance and therefore is vital to your success in this role.

Establishing a Communications Mechanism

At the start of your tenure, strive to facilitate communication among your staff and between you and your staff in several ways. First maintain an open communication mechanism so that individuals feel comfortable approaching you with problems and questions. An open-door policy allows you to be physically accessible to all staff members. It also mandates use of staff meetings, as discussed previously, and daily conversations with all members of your staff. Critical to your success in establishing an open communication system is asking the right questions. Ask people about their responsibilities, daily activities, new projects, and anything else you deem relevant. This kind of probing demonstrates your interest in their work and encourages them to share their insights, opinions, and other revealing information.

Seek to communicate directions clearly and cohesively. Let the individuals on your staff know what your goals and aspirations are for the department on a regular basis. Furthermore, provide specific direction to individual members of your staff whenever appropriate. At the risk of micromanaging, give people the benefit of your experience and insight as they pursue their own work objectives. Most important, let people know as soon as possible what your expectations are for their work performance, as well as your standards for work achievement.

Express your support for your team members' efforts. This is perhaps the best encouragement you can provide. Let individuals know when they are doing a good job and how you and the organization appreciate their efforts. Health care managers often fail to tell staff members how their good performance helped customer-patients receive better health care service. Always give people this type of feedback if you can. For example, if housekeepers do a particularly good job at cleaning patient rooms, let them know that this will help the patients' morale and outlook as they recover from an illness. Try to emphasize this linkage to customer-patients as much as possible.

Demonstrate your respect for the expertise and contribution of all your team members at every possible opportunity. Let people have autonomy in their jobs until they show you that they are either incapable or not trustworthy enough. This freedom demonstrates your respect for their professionalism, encourages their individual growth and development, and inspires them to greater performance. Your confidence in them can be communicated verbally through words of encouragement and motivation but can also be expressed nonverbally by simply staying out of the way when your individual members are busy or pursuing an important objective.

Clarifying Expectations

Once you have explained generally (at the outset) what work norms you intend to implement throughout the department, these norms can be distilled into finer protocols. For example, memos can communicate how much overtime you expect from each employee, the dress code and appearance mandated by the organization, specific protocols for communicating with customer-patients, or any other working condition you want to establish as a department standard. It is essential to do this within the first ninety days of your management tenure so that you can avoid confusion or contradiction later. This clarifying of expectations will also help you establish a group norm that everyone will be expected to abide by, so that no one will be able to violate the group norm indifferently or contentiously without fear of reprisal.

I already discussed the importance of demonstrating your respect for staff's expertise. Making certain that you express a trust in the members of your department to do their job in a professional manner and to make a maximum contribution to the organization is also important to clarify expectations. Emphasize the contributions to the greater good of the department and the health care organization as much as possible, thus reinforcing the concepts of quality, responsibility to the customer-patient, and allegiance to everyone in the team.

Finally, use communication to demonstrate the human side of management. Demonstrate your own enthusiasm for your responsibilities through words and action, showing empathy and compassion for individuals in your department who might be struggling but usually make a strong effort. Give them assistance and find additional resources to help them get back on track. Use your listening and perception skills as much as possible in your inter-actions with your staff.

Policy Formation and Implementation

In discussing this final category of considerations for establishing a productive and progressive work environment—formation of specific department policies and compliance with policies for the organization—I examine several policy compliance issues and strategies for formulating appropriate department policy. Policies are usually drawn from ten basic areas:

Policy Mandates

1. Long-range performance goals
2. Immediate needs
3. Perceived action needs
4. Daily requirements
5. Accomplishment standards
6. Industry norms
7. Positive past precedent
8. Negative past precedent
9. Organizational mandates
10. Technical mandates

Figure 3.2 highlights the five essential elements of effective policy implementation.

Fundamentally, policies should be implemented with three basic objectives in mind:

1. They should help establish standards that regulate particular types of performance within the department or govern daily action.
2. They should add to the fluidity of action within a work group; that is, having set policies and standards in place allows a work group to achieve action quickly because the expectation for performance is already known.
3. They should reflect an organization's governing principles, which in turn reflect its values and commitment to the customer-patient.

Figure 3.2. Elements of Effective Policy Implementation.

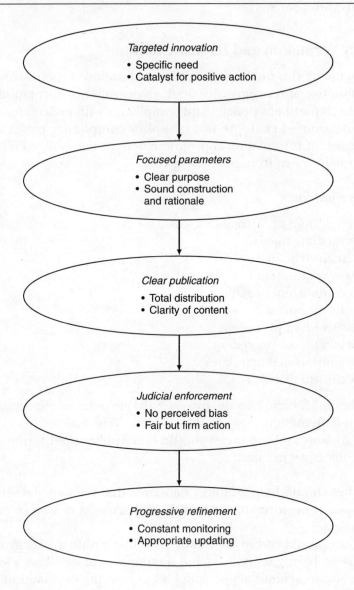

Targeted innovation
- Specific need
- Catalyst for positive action

Focused parameters
- Clear purpose
- Sound construction and rationale

Clear publication
- Total distribution
- Clarity of content

Judicial enforcement
- No perceived bias
- Fair but firm action

Progressive refinement
- Constant monitoring
- Appropriate updating

Several policies are of specific relevance to your initial tenure as a health care manager and are grouped under two broad categories. The first category encompasses fiscal policies. The second category includes all other policies (dress code, sexual harassment, personnel, and the like).

Fiscal Policies

As a starting point, try to establish with your supervising manager which fiscal policies you will be responsible for in your daily activities. These might include budgeting processes, expenditure reports, or any number of others.

Once this is done, make every effort to learn how to enforce these policies so as to ensure compliance with regulatory or legislative provisions. This might be accomplished by spending time with a financial analyst or other individuals from your organization's finance and accounting department. New health care managers often make the mistake of absorbing several volumes on hospital financial management, only to find that their particular facility's fiscal policies and procedures differ radically from those depicted in the textbook. By spending time with the appropriate expert in your organization, you are assured of learning information as it relates to your specific environment.

There are some general rules of fiscal policy, however, that apply in all cases, despite organizational differences. First, try to prepare your budget, if applicable, well ahead of time. Financial experts in the health care field suggest using a logbook in which you track typical expenditures throughout the course of the year. By doing so, you are completely prepared to compile a prospective end-of-the-year budget that will be realistic while allowing flexibility to request sufficient resources for the upcoming year. By keeping track of your department's expenditures and financial demands, you can simply adjust the total of these expenditures at the end of the year with respect to inflation and other factors, and have a good general perspective on what your budget request should be for the following year. To get an even sharper picture when compiling a prospective budget, use your research abilities by gathering departmental expenditure data for the preceding three years.

To ensure that you are fiscally responsible, periodically review daily expenditures to determine whether department resources were used for their intended purpose and whether that purpose was fully achieved. Fiscal resources are extremely tight in today's health care arena and will probably be so for the next ten years. Therefore, keep reasonable control over your department's financial outlays and remain current with compliance requirements.

To further ensure compliance with fiscal policy, seek the input of individual key players in your department. Consider who among them spends the most money. Discuss expenditures with them— not necessarily with a view to cut the budget but to arrive at a reasonable understanding of how the money is spent and what returns it provides to your department. Key players can also give you vital input on upcoming major projects and contingencies that might require additional financial resources.

In all these activities, be careful not to let budget or other financial constraints unnecessarily guide your action. Keep the department informed and involved in the decision-making process in these situations. Key players can also give you vital input on upcoming major projects and contingencies that might require additional financial resources.

Following are five other suggestions that might assist you in budget planning and implementation of initial financial policy:

1. *Make a rough comparison between your department's contributions to the organization and the department's expenditures.* Include all revenue your department generates for the organization and major cost savings that are a direct effect of the department's actions. For example, an education department in a large community hospital might compare the amount of money saved by more effective hiring practices resulting from a training course to the previous cost of employee turnover and other related negative costs.

2. *Try to get a handle on the operating costs in your department.* Rely on your professional expertise to review the work role performed by the department as a whole, as well as by individual employees. You might identify opportunities for cost-saving strategies that would require additional funds to implement.

3. *Keep the paperwork moving.* Quickly process all paperwork that is related to fiscal expenditure. For example, make sure that invoices are reviewed and processed as soon as possible. Nothing could be more detrimental to your reputation as a health care manager than the perception held by individuals in your organization (or by outside agents) that you are incompetent because your failure to process paperwork efficiently and in timely fashion led to loss or delay of income for the facility.

4. *Conduct a detailed cost-benefit analysis of your department as a whole.* Once again, unless you are specifically knowledgeable about health care finance, enlist the help of a professional. This will go a long way toward gaining the objective of fluidity of action alluded to earlier. Consultation also is another means of using available support resources.

5. *Conduct an analysis of employee contribution.* Once you have settled into your role as manager review the contribution made by each team member. A contribution analysis can have implications for the organization's compensation budget. For example, many health care managers discover that certain full-time or part-time positions can be altered or eliminated, thus saving costs for the institution and ultimately the customer-patient. Changes in job status have to do with the difference between downsizing and rightsizing. *Downsizing* refers to employee terminations caused by organizational inefficiency or poor performance. *Rightsizing* means using the appropriate number of human resources to accomplish a task. If you discover the possibility of making a rightsizing move, discuss it with your superiors and over the course of a three-month period closely examine the contribution made by the employee in question.

Other Policies

Other policies address issues including but not limited to dress code, sexual harassment, and the work environment (employee relations, for example). Although specific policies are addressed in the context of their respective chapters, the following list is an overview of the categories of policy you will be asked to enforce.

- *Action-mandated policy.* These policies are installed due to a specific action the organization is taking or because of a crisis situation that must be met. Examples include policies governing activity during new construction, compliance with a local health care emergency, or response to new legislation.
- *Personnel policy.* These policies consist of issues related to the general administration of personnel and human resource activity. Examples include compensation and wage policies, equal opportunity policies, and recruitment policies.
- *Work environment policy.* As you will see in Appendix A to this book, work environment policy is usually an implicit determination made on the part of the manager relative to activities within the work group. Examples include employee fairness, communication within the department, and other interpersonal relations on the job. Certain work environmental policies can act in concert with personnel policies.
- *Technical policy.* These policies regulate technology-specific activities. Examples include rehabilitation services, pharmacy services, and pharmaceutical (prescription) delivery, laboratory services, or any other activity related to a specific technical field.
- *Operational policy.* This body of policy refers to the conduct of activity (operations) in the health care facility. Examples include policies governing the dynamics of work flow, standard department operating procedures, or organizationwide protocols. Unlike work environment policies, which usually are established and enforced by the department manager, operational policy is established and enforced by the provider facility (for example, hazardous waste disposal).

As a manager, you are custodian and executor of your institution's policies and a proponent of a system that generates these policies. Therefore, you must be familiar with all policies and apply them intelligently in your area of responsibility.

Politics and the Work Environment

Unfortunately, exercising your talents as a health care manager will probably be tested by overtly political behavior. The word *politic,* whose Latin origin refers to "the group process," has degenerated into meaning "the negative interaction of individuals who seek power or self-gratification in an unjust manner." Although this definition might seem particularly harsh, it is nevertheless important that you stay on your toes and try to avoid political quagmires in your work environment.

As a health care professional, you probably experienced overtly political behavior. In formulating the plan of this book, I was advised by several CEOs to be sure to include a section on politics. Their comments all shared the sentiment that politics were indeed negative, unnecessary in an organization but unfortunately a fact of life. Their fondest hope for new health care managers is that they will artfully be able to avoid politics in the interest of providing stellar, progressive services to the customer-patient and to the health care organization.

Common Political Problems

With this goal in mind, let us review briefly some of the problems created by politics. First of all, *politics inhibits productivity.* Generally speaking, workers are not particularly motivated to perform well for individuals who are more politics-minded than performance-minded. A great deal of time is spent avoiding power plays and preparing for counteractions. Consequently, productivity suffers, and worst of all the customer-patient is deprived of receiving the full range of services the health care organization is capable of providing.

Politics stifles creativity. Because politics can promote paranoia, team members may be reluctant to share new ideas or work in a group process that encourages creativity or innovation. As a result, staff growth and development are compromised, or top performers relocate to a less political or, better yet, nonpolitical environment. Again, the customer-patient and the organization suffer.

Without question, *politics cripples teamwork.* Individuals who are suspicious of each other, have limited respect for each other, and are simply "trying to keep their heads above water and knives out of their backs" are unlikely to foster true integrated team action. If your goal as a manager is a value-driven environment, such resentment among team members, avoidance of open communication, and lack of shared values and objectives certainly do not contribute to that goal.

Overt negative politics alters communication. Examples of overt negative politics include altered messages, altered presentation of messages, or flat-out noncommunication in certain situations. Politics begins once a third party enters the picture, creating an unbalanced dynamic and opportunity for two people to discuss a third person—often in an uncomplimentary manner. In the health care workplace, politics is evidenced by cloistered communication and interpersonal conflicts that jeopardize goodwill and progressive movement toward goals.

Politics destroys value-based elements that are critical to a successful organization generally and to your department specifically. Three areas in particular are at risk.

1. Politics destroys allegiance and loyalty among team members and to the overall objective.
2. If politics is allowed to fester, team members begin to question the leadership of someone who allows the situation to impede the workflow.
3. Group morale begins to diminish until finally individual employee motivation begins to erode.

Signs of Overtly Political Behavior

Whenever a premium is placed on politics as opposed to performance in the health care environment, political behavior is highly inappropriate and potentially destructive. Five basic indicators can signal overtly political behavior:

1. *Double-talk.* Individuals who tell one story to one person and an entirely different story to another are double-talkers. Their motive is to cover the bases on a particular issue, deliberately create disharmony, or simply try to pit two people against each other.
2. *Backstabbing.* Backstabbers overtly pledge allegiance to you and your ideas but covertly downplay them and insult your intelligence. This has a funny way of getting back to the source and is something you should be aware of.
3. *Power mongering.* Power mongers try to control everything. These individuals are also called *turf protectors* or *empire builders*

because they often use resources and territory as the principal focus of their subversive efforts. As a new health care manager, you may fall prey to a power monger's claim of being in charge of something that in fact he or she has no control of. More frequently, such a person will falsely claim to know a specific facet of the health care business. Once again, time will help you identify such behavior.

4. *Victim role.* Some individuals claim that the organization is out to get them and that you had better watch yourself. People with this mind-set and demonstrating this overtly negative behavior are more interested in their own survival than in assisting their fellow workers through the health care mission.

5. *Game playing.* Game players use phony behavior in trying to engender support. They play games with fellow staff as well.

Methods of Dealing with Overtly Political Behavior

As a manager, how do you deal with politics? Whether the politician is a member of your staff or a colleague, five solutions can be useful.

1. *Avoidance* is easy. Try to stay out of the way of political behavior whenever possible. If avoidance is not feasible on a daily basis, keep all contact on a business level and discuss only business issues. If someone tries invariably to shift the focus to a politically oriented level, firmly return them to the issue at hand. Do not delude yourself into thinking you can change this person. Remember, your primary managerial responsibility is to bolster staff motivation and productivity while contributing to your facility's goal of high-quality patient care.

2. *Confront* the person and let her know that you are aware of her political intent. For example, if you are asked a loaded question, simply counter by asking another question such as, *Why are you asking me that?* or *Why is that of so much interest to you?* You risk incurring wrath, but you will at least discourage overtly political behavior.

3. *Disclosure and support* works if the troublesome individual is someone on the management team or someone who reports to your own manager. Simply present evidence of the political behavior

to your supervisor, without judgment or opinion. Use objective reporting. For instance: *You know, a funny thing happened the other day. I was talking to (name), who seemed persistent in wanting to discuss (topic).* This approach indicates your apprehension in dealing with this individual and signals your need for specific assistance.

4. With *direct input* from your own manager, you can actively enlist support. Simply tell your supervisor about the problem, review the evidence, and ask directly for assistance: *What would you do if you had this situation?* (Note: If you perceive your boss to exhibit excessively political behavior, you might want to request the help of another mentor within the organization in dealing with this behavior.)

5. Gather *documentation* as evidence of political behavior by colleagues or staff. The more examples you collect, the better case you can make for termination (if the person is staff) or for limited contact (if the source is a colleague). Record evidence or examples of notable political behavior, and be sure to handle reports tactfully.

Continuing the Transition

As you continue your transition into the management role, consider the following twenty-five suggestions to help you establish a progressive work environment:

1. *Temper dreams with reality.* Do not expect to be perfect in your initial efforts or assume that your new dream job will not have some nightmarish moments. Be optimistic but not naïve.
2. *Temper reality with dreams.* Recognize that you are trying to strike a balance between your aspirations and your daily activities but do not lose sight of your vision. Incorporate the goal of providing high-quality health care with the reality of daily challenges and objectives.
3. *Ideas are your greatest resource.* You were probably promoted into management because, in part, not only are you intelligent, you are also creatively resourceful. Try to come up with a new idea daily. Do not be afraid to try out innovations, particularly in the areas of problem solving, planning, and project management.

These are the greatest resources you can contribute to your organization.

4. *Tomorrow is your saving grace.* Despite how difficult today's problems might appear, there is always tomorrow. If your commitment to health care management is for the long haul, look forward to the next day. Try not to dwell too much on the problems of today.

5. *Learn from your mistakes.* You will find that the "bad" things that occur will be more instructive than the "good" things that occur in your initial tenure as a health care manager. Accordingly, try to learn from mistakes and then commit to avoiding the same mistake.

6. *Learn from your successes.* When things do go right, make a mental note of what you did to obtain a positive outcome and try to understand why it went right. This retrospective analysis will help you construct a progressive plan for a future action.

7. *Try to be understood, not accepted.* You will never be accepted by everyone. Personal or professional bias is part of the human factor and may always challenge your people skills (discussed in Chapter One). As long as the people on your staff understand objectives and the performance standards you hold them to, everything else is secondary.

8. *Play for the long term, not short term.* Do not burn yourself out in your first ninety days on the job. Usually, your first year as a health care manager establishes your foundation and gives you the opportunity to make mistakes, learn, and grow. Adhere to reasonable expectations. Prepare for the long term, keep some balance in your life, and enjoy the experience and opportunities offered by your new role.

9. *Some days are better than others.* Enjoy the highs of the good days, and learn from and then dismiss the bad days.

10. *It is all good work.* Whatever the current work activity might be, it serves the larger good of providing health care to someone who is ill. Remember that whenever you become frustrated or bored with an assignment.

11. *Some jobs are more fun than others.* You probably know this already from your previous experiences in health care. This fact remains true in management. Health care management is an

adventure every day, but like Alice's adventures in wonderland, it has its ups and downs. Try to find satisfaction, happiness, and some enjoyment in every task.

12. *People will fool you.* People are unpredictable. Do not expect to peg them, that is, assume that you understand a certain personality because you have worked with that type of person before. Always be perceptive, observant, and listen to *why* as well as the *what* of conversation.

13. *Steady players work with the system.* You will find that at least 60 percent of the people in your department will work within the system, provide you with satisfactory effort, and require only that their goals and directives be clearly defined.

14. *Dynamos will define the system.* About 10 to 20 percent of your staff will define the system by their own stellar effort and outstanding performance. Make sure that you encourage these individuals, use them appropriately (and tactfully) as role models, and review their goals and objectives often so that they stay challenged.

15. *Marginal performers will try to beat the system.* Unfortunately, 10 to 20 percent of your staff will try to dodge the rules or challenge your authority. From day one, keep a close watch on these individuals, document their performance, and be ready to use the performance documentation and termination procedures outlined in Chapter Twelve.

16. *There is no right answer for every situation.* Each situation requires logic, your gut intellect, and creativity to find a solution. There is no magic bullet.

17. *Build a point of view.* Use your own subjective insight and judgment to establish an opinion on organizational objectives. Try to develop this point of view over the first six months on the new job. Then form a perception on the activities not only in the department but throughout the organization.

18. *Feel free to offer your point of view.* One of the things you are paid for is your expertise and vital contribution as a department manager. Hence, offer any ideas and suggestions, when appropriate, that might increase the organization's effectiveness and foster its progress.

19. *Expect the unexpected.* Once again, there are no set solutions or guidelines for every situation you will encounter in health care

management. Be ready to deal with situations that are outside the norm and react in a positive and constructive fashion.

20. *Do not expect the expected.* Once you have completed a set plan and established a set of expectations, do not believe that anything is necessarily locked in. Be flexible in your thinking and creative in your reactions.

21. *Trust your instincts.* At the end of the day, these are the best resources that you have: your instincts, your intuition, your common sense, your logic, and your creativity. Trust your instincts to be the trigger for the rest of these valuable assets.

22. *Do not worry about being persuasive or convincing, concentrate on being honest.* If as a manager you present an honest case to your colleagues, supervisors, and staff in a forthright and direct manner, you will probably get the support or resources you require.

23. *Losers create problems for themselves.* Individuals who create problems out of thin air for themselves and others will prove to be negative performers. Workers who have fallen into the habit of creating negative, self-fulfilling prophecies will have to be completely documented and eliminated from your team.

24. *Steady players handle problems.* The majority of your staff (the 60 percent referred to in item 13) will react well to a problem once you have defined it for them and provided the direction and resources needed to handle the situation.

25. *Dynamos anticipate and circumvent problems.* Your best players constantly seek to improve the status quo. Using this learning curve as a basis for performance standards throughout your department goes a long way toward creating a progressive work environment.

Conclusion

Upon assuming your new role as a health care manager, build (or maintain) a progressive work environment that promotes optimal patient service delivery. This will be difficult without first having a departmental vision that complements the larger organizational vision. Furthermore, your vision must be based on clear-cut values (yours and your organization's); for example, conscientious use of your new authority.

A progressive environment also relies on a team approach. This involves at least five components: clear definition of roles, strong interest in shared goals and objectives, open communication, resilience, and diversity of talent and perspective.

You will also need to foster an environment that operates on sound policies and procedures that are applied consistently. Some policy areas have to do with principles of sound financial management and adherence to regulatory and legislative policy and compliance. Others have to do with the overall workplace environment (policies on dress code, sexual harassment, fair and equitable compensation, and the like).

Strive to keep your department's environment free of overtly political behavior. Signs include double-talk, backstabbing, power mongering, playing the victim role, and game playing. In this chapter I have suggested strategies for dealing with this kind of behavior and preventing politics from impeding your goals. The key goal, of course, is providing top-quality patient services.

Finally, I have offered a number of pointers to help you continue the transition into the management role. These range from being grounded in reality to foreseeing and circumventing problems.

Chapter Four

Managing the Nonplayers

Every organization, despite its best intentions at creating and maintaining a quality workforce, has a certain number of employees who can best be categorized as nonplayers. As demonstrated in Table 4.1, the nonplayer presents a unique set of challenges to any leader, especially a new health care manager. Many experienced managers do not have the essential skills to diminish the negative impact of the nonplayer or to remove the nonplayer from the organization toward a more suitable career path.

In this chapter I examine the characteristics of nonplayers and provide field-proven strategies to diminish their impact in a progressive work environment. This task may be one of the most important of your initial responsibilities, because nonplayers always seek to test a new manager. Remember these three maxims regarding nonplayers:

1. Nonplayers are comfortable in their resistance to change and positive challenge and rarely change their work approach.
2. Unlike a health care patient, who wants to get better, nonplayers have no desire to improve their performance or contribution to the organization. In essence, they thrive on negativity.
3. The steadies and superstars in your department will welcome positive management handling of nonplayers, and will provide support and appropriate peer pressure if the leader begins the process of eliminating nonplayers' negative impact.

Table 4.1. Superstars, Steadies, and Nonplayers.

Group Composition	Percentage of Total Group or Department
Superstars	15–20
• Stellar performance	
• Thrive on challenge	
• Define the system	
Steady or Strong Players	60–70
• Satisfactory performance	
• Strive to succeed	
• Support the system	
Nonplayers	10–15
• Questionable performance	
• Self-centered	
• Eradicate the system	

Communication, Psychology, and Roles of the Nonplayer

An important facet of communication is the interplay between psychology and roles in the communication process. Some individuals draw on psychology as part of their communication style and in playing a specific role. In this section I discuss the psychological roles some individuals assume in communicating and describe measures you can use to deal with these individuals and the effect their roles can have on your management efforts.

It is important to remember that some individuals communicate by assuming roles for a number of reasons. For example, they might be conditioned to playing these roles because of their upbringing and their relationships with families and friends; their perceived image within the organization and the way they have been conditioned to respond, react, and communicate with others in the organization; or the way your predecessor set communication standards and expected individuals to communicate in departmental activities. Whatever the motivating factor may be for assuming their role, it is important to understand the roles, how they affect the communication process, and how to manage them in the interest of departmental progress and performance.

In the following section I examine twenty of the most common communication roles in a health care workplace to assist you in identifying the roles played by certain members of your staff. With each role description I suggest a strategy for dealing effectively with that role type. These roles are usually played by team members and are described accordingly. However, managers have been known to play these roles as well.

The Ego Appeaser

Ego appeasers constantly appeal to someone's self-esteem to make a point or to elicit an action they desire. This approach is often seen in marketing; for example, in sales appeals to "the man who has everything," "the discriminating buyer," or "life's winners." The workplace is a natural setting for ego appeasers. For example, they might say, *You must do this because . . . you're the only one who can get the job done,* or *you're the only one I can trust with this assignment,* or *you're the best person for the job.* This ego-appeasing ruse becomes manipulative over time and, as people become wise to it, it becomes insulting.

A counterstrategy is to ask ego appeasers directly about their need to constantly compliment others. For example: *Do you realize that your compliments might be seen as being manipulative?* It is also essential to explain to them that this tactic is shortsighted and perceived as manipulative. Finally, it is incumbent on you as a manager to suggest a more productive way for ego appeasers to interact with people, perhaps by use of mutual benefit or another progressive tactic (such as appeal to authority).

The Conformist

Invoking the norm is a tactic used by conformists who have identified a particular norm within or outside the organization. For example, conformists might say, *We must do this because all the hospitals in our area are doing it.* A conformist manager might use this tactic on an individual by saying, *I want you to do this because everyone else will be doing this.*

A benefit of conformist communication is that it can make a point and encourage action by appealing to the need to be part of a group or (for some workers) to meet an unspecified standard. However, the negative side of this tactic is that it does not particularly inspire creativity, and in some cases it might ask for acceptance of a substandard level of performance. For example, if a hospital is unique to its state and has a mission different from other hospitals in its state, there is no need for it to do what every other hospital in the state is doing. Likewise, if an employee has a specific set of duties, it is not necessarily essential that he or she does what every other employee is doing.

Use of this tactic can be helpful when discussing a compliance issue or in trying to implement a group standard. But beyond that, conformist tactics in communication should be avoided because they appeal only to average performance, not stellar achievement.

The Authority Broker

Authority brokering is a popular approach used in marketing all the time. Whenever you see "Nine out of ten doctors recommend . . ." or "Many leading hairdressers say . . . ," authority brokering is at work. In the health care environment, authority brokers rely on the following kinds of statements: *We must do this because the Joint Commission says so. We must do this because Doctor So-and-So says so.* Use of the pronoun *they (They said we must do this)* is a prototypical example of the invoking of authority that identifies the authority broker.

In issues that require compliance, such as regulatory affairs and audits, this tactic might be useful. Beyond such situations, however, discourage its use because basically it is management by intimidation. Furthermore, if as a manager you cite an authority other than yourself to get something done you are abdicating your authority and position as a leader.

The Activist Without a Strategy

Appeal to action is a device in which a goal is stated and individuals are encouraged to contribute to its attainment. Politicians sometimes make emotional promises to achieve objectives without detailing a strategy. The politicians' constituents are excited and ready for change, but nothing ever really gets done. Herein lies the problem with appeal to action.

Whereas it is vital to state the desired outcome of an action, it is equally important to delineate the steps to be taken to achieve that action. Asking your staff for suggestions on how to achieve a goal is a great start. Appeal to action, therefore, is a good opening gambit, but a manager who does not follow through by asking individuals their perceptions on how a goal could be achieved and what action must be taken to reach that particular goal is an activist without a strategy.

The Agreement Junkie

Sometimes individuals, including managers, fall into the communication trap of seeking a consensus on everything they do. Appealing strictly to a team orientation or to the common good is not always enough to get a job done. Seeking consensus often encourages passive-aggressive behavior; that is, individuals will agree to aspire to a particular goal but will not take any action beyond that agreement.

Specific action steps to achieve the goal must be delineated. Once that is done, it is not necessary to have universal agreement before taking action so long as there is basic management support for the action. Therefore, if a majority of coworkers support an action, the manager must endorse the action, even if some individuals still might not be fully supportive. It is better to risk not having full support than to risk inaction by waiting for universal agreement.

The Nonplayer

Certain individuals in your department invariably will not participate in any communication whatsoever. They see themselves as superstars who are valuable to the organization purely on their own individual merits. In some cases, they might just politely listen and accommodate your viewpoints, as well as those of their colleagues, without any contribution or verbal interaction of their own.

It is tough to recondition nonplayers. For whatever reason, they might be very comfortable in being noncommunicative and nonparticipative in group activities. As manager, you can ask non-players two questions: *How will this affect your role? How will this affect your particular job?* If neither question engages nonplayers' partici-pation, you may have a three-pronged recourse: to inform them of actions and their job objectives, measure their performance accordingly, and simply accept the fact that they are neither strong communicators nor group enthusiasts.

Note, however, that if these nonplayers are also nonperform-ers, another communication exercise should take place. That would be the counseling and probation process that must occur prior to terminating a nonperforming employee. (See Chapters Twelve and Seventeen for specific guidelines.)

The Sympathy Player

Certain individuals may play off sympathy. They need a lot of atten-tion and tend to demand extra support. They might also feel in sympathy with, or compassionate toward, others in the organiza-tion but to a fault.

The problem with sympathy players is that they inject too much emotion into the work process. Accordingly, in communicating with sympathy players, stick to the issues by redirecting all conver-sations to specific outcomes and action plans. Any needless plays for sympathy must be countered with the questions, *Why do you feel you need extra attention? What kind of extra support do you need from me?* If this becomes a chronic problem, address it as a performance problem, not a communication problem. Once again, documen-tation of poor performance must take precedence over inter-personal interaction.

The Empathy Player

If many of your staff previously were your peers within the depart-ment, it might be quite natural for some to make statements such as, *I know how you feel; I know what it must be like to in your position.*

Both positive and negative motivations could be involved in such a play. From a positive perspective, a former peer (and possi-bly your friend) is simply expressing support for your position. In that case, ask for his or her ideas and input on whatever problem or issue you are discussing. From a negative perspective, if you suspect insincerity or a ploy, ask, *If you know how I'm feeling, then how would you solve the problem at hand?* Once again, depersonalize the issue and use the questions cited above as a strategy to refocus the conversation on action, not emotion.

The Exempt Player

Many individuals in health care organizations feel that their work roles are so unique that what applies to others in their department does not apply to them. When individuals confront a work discussion by saying, *That's great but it doesn't apply to me,* your natural follow-up question should be, *Why does this not apply to you?* If the answers are not satisfactory, you should then have the individuals delineate specifically why their position is so different that the issue at hand has no effect on their work roles. If they are unable to do this, take them aside in a private meeting and say that from this point on you expect them to look at things from a more universal perspective. In this instance, appeal to ego might be a useful tool. Tell exempt players that they might have a different perspective that is important to the conversation and might be useful in arriving at a solution. Otherwise, if a negative pattern persists, you probably have contrarians on your hands.

The Contrarian

Contrarians will argue or contend with anything you say. They use expressions such as, *I've got a problem with that,* or *I have a sense that this won't work.* Contrarians can be very detrimental to the group process, because they can refocus attention on why something cannot work, as opposed to what must be done to make it work.

To resolve the contrarian problem, use confrontation. Counter the I've-got-a-problem-with tactic with a challenge to define the solution rather than redefine the problem. In response to *I have a sense that this won't work,* ask contrarians what they sense will work. Force contrarians to get off of their negative viewpoint and onto a more positive one. If confrontation does not work, it may be time for a counseling session in which you ask contrarians why they feel a compelling need to be negative and to constantly question your judgment and the input of colleagues. Usually a persistent contrarian is a poor performer whose work should be documented and dealt with accordingly.

The Consensus Builder

Consensus builders like to get everyone's agreement prior to taking action. They often act as office politicians in trying to garner agreement for a particular issue (or complete disagreement on a positive issue). They can be an asset if they help support you in taking action, or they can be extremely detrimental if their actions are negative. In many cases, consensus builders are unproductive because they stress the process over the product or outcome of an action.

In dealing with consensus builders, allow the positive actions to follow their logical course. In essence, if consensus builders help you build a positive consensus and support for an action, they should be allowed to assist you. If they act negatively or spend an inordinate amount of time building a consensus, counsel them on the importance of taking action as opposed to trying to accommodate the nuances of every individual viewpoint. Remember that the worst liability about a consensus builder is the time wasted in building a consensus rather than getting a majority agreement and taking action in a timely manner.

The Passive Aggressor

A passive aggressor is a sneaky person who agrees with you in a face-to-face meeting but subsequently does an action that is counter to what he or she originally agreed on.

Passive aggressive individuals are among the most destructive in the health care workplace. Usually they are poor performers, insecure personalities, and antipathetic toward group achievement or group success. Accordingly, their subversive tactics should be documented and dealt with quickly and resolutely. A major problem in today's health care environment is that passive aggressors are overanalyzed by their managers rather than dealt with aggressively. Do not fall into this trap. Instead, document subversive behavior, counsel the individuals (use the techniques described in Chapter Twelve), and take appropriate action before their detrimental effect destroys not only the communication process within your work group but the very achievement of your group and its performance activity.

The Activator

The activator sparks discussion and tries to take a positive slant on many issues in a conversation. This individual can be a terrific ally in group discussion. Activators love positive results, are genuinely enthusiastic, and can help get your point across.

Recognize activators by their vital signs. In addition to their positive viewpoints and can-do approach to all situations, activators put the good of the organization at the forefront of their viewpoints. They are naturally energetic, and because their enthusiasm is contagious it is a valuable tool to help you mine the talents and abilities of all your staff. Activators are naturally supportive and selfless individuals; they are very secure with themselves and pursue the health care initiative as a passion, not a burden.

Enlist activators in all your efforts, provide them with as much support as possible, and guard against their one potential risk factor—overenthusiasm—by defining their role clearly and expressing your appreciation for their activity at every juncture.

The Take-Charge Artist

Take-charge artists volunteer for everything and anything. They can be overwhelmingly enthusiastic in conversations and want to participate in every activity. They can dominate communication, seem to know everything, and are often labeled power mongers or control freaks.

Take-charge individuals must be watched very closely. From communications standpoint, their "air time" must be limited, and directives must be given very clearly. Stress the *who, what, where, which, how, when,* and *why* of what they do by using the questions in Appendix A relative to providing work direction. If they develop positively, take-charge artists can become activators; if they develop negatively, they can become any one (or more) of the negative role players discussed in this section. Hence, take-charge artists also can be quick-change artists.

The Victim

In many of your communication activities as a health care manager, you will encounter victims, people who feel the whole world is out to get them. The victim role will emerge in meetings and in individual conversations. In group activities or in one-on-one interactions, these players will say, *We are always the ones who have to* (fill in the action).

When you hear these verbal cues, the problem once again might be a performance issue. Victims can be workaholics, or they can be chronic complainers who never contribute anything. Once you have seized on these verbal cues, document these individuals' performance. If they are positive, strong contributors to the organization, the source of the problem is probably workaholism. If so, enroll them in a stress management program. More often, unfortunately, victims are simply nonperformers and chronic complainers. Once again, documentation and insistence on performance-based communication (set goals, set objectives) and coaching or counseling become your main tactics.

The Martyr

The first cousin, if you will, of the victim is the martyr. The only difference between victims and martyrs is that martyrs complain only after they have completed a task, whereas victims complain throughout the task.

Martyrs need a lot of positive reinforcement. Encourage their performance, express your appreciation, and try to engage them in positive conversations. If their personality is such that they are simply chronic complainers anyway, make a determination about the pejorative effect that this trait might have on the overall organization and the morale of other team members. Ironically, martyrs often become the source of amusement for others in the department. Coworkers are often amazed at how much a martyr will complain about a particular situation, despite having been successful at and completing the task effectively. If this is the case, the effect of this role is benign. Only when the martyr's communication becomes a burden to others in the department should it become a source of concern. If this happens, ask the martyr why he or she feels the need to complain to everyone, explain the effect of this negative complaining, and demonstrate how it counteracts strong performance. This usually serves as a strong wake-up call to a martyr.

The Doubter

Doubters never believe anything will work out. Doubters can be found among staff, peers, or superiors. A simple tactic to use with doubters is to ask, *Why do you think this will not work out?* Strive to get doubters to tell you specifically why they think a planned action will be futile or have negative consequences. Then decide for yourself whether the argument has any validity.

Recognize that some individuals are doubters simply by nature; they question everything or speculate automatically about the downside of any venture. Doubters can act as touchstones when you make plans, for they are ever ready to tell you why something might not work out. The key here is the degree and effect of negativity that the doubter evokes. If the negativity reaches a critical point, counseling is in order. In counseling these individuals, however, recognize that you will not change their personalities. Simply explain the negative effects of constant doubting and encourage a more positive outlook and expression.

The Theoretician

The biggest complaint against negative individuals in the area of health care training and development is that they are too theoretical. This same lament can be applied to certain individuals within your department and sphere of influence. A theoretician speculates about the possible angles of situation or outcome without regard to its practical aspects.

A theoretician must be constantly challenged with the question, *How does this practically and realistically affect what we are talking about today?* You must compel the theoretician to face the reality of each situation and to present useful information that can be used immediately. Failing to do this not only will hurt departmental progress, it will compromise the theoretician's development.

The Screener

Screeners create a smokescreen in any given situation by using another issue, a false premise, or an outright fabrication to divert your attention from their poor performance. For example, if a screener who is a housekeeper failed to clean a particular patient's room, the screen, or the excuse for not doing his or her job, might be lack of mops, the patient's being in the room, or your failure to tell him or her directly to clean the room. Individuals who create these illusions do so for their own gains to prevent positive action.

The Grandstander

Some individuals who work in health care settings would probably be better off working in Hollywood or on Broadway. They are compelled to display a great deal of emotion and need a lot of attention. They could be negative or positive performers, or individuals who are steady players. In any case, grandstanders seem to enjoy the communication process to the extent that it becomes an outlet for their own emotional outbursts and thespian abilities.

You can capitalize on the grandstander for your own purposes. For example, if you need a strong emotional reaction to make a point, rely on the grandstander to do so by providing cues. Simply direct the question, *What do you think?* to this person. If the emotionalism acts as a detriment to your delivering a message, simply direct them to *Calm down, relax, and tell me what you really think.* Many grandstanders might have taken on this role because of family or cultural ties. Grandstanding might be the most difficult behavior to modify, so simply recognize it and manage it for the most progressive outcome possible in any given situation.

Managing Nonplayer Resistance to Change

The greatest threat to organizational renewal is the nonplayer's attempt to undermine the change effort. As we have discussed, a nonplayer is an individual whose performance might be barely adequate but whose behavior in the health care institution can be described as subversive, apathetic, or self-interested. Nonplayers become particularly fearful during all stages of organizational renewal, as they will now have more responsibility and must work harder, and smarter, than before.

In a failing health care organization, nonplayers are condoned because leadership lacks the fortitude to confront them. In a sense, managers who accept the nonplayers' detrimental behavior are not qualified for leadership in today's health care environment, where the nonplayers can cause poor morale, poor service, or in extreme situations, death.

In this section, I discuss the twenty excuses most often used by nonplayers to derail the renewal process. For each one, I define its basic psychology and provide a field-proven, effective strategy to counter it.

LINE 1: YOU DON'T LIKE ME!

Basic Psychology

A favorite nonplayer strategy is to make all work issues personal. When nonplayers are asked to work harder for the renewed organization, they will try to make it a personal issue between the manager and themselves, not a business imperative. Because most managers want to be liked, they fall prey to this particular tactic. It is more important to be understood and respected, however, than liked and accepted.

Recommended Response

It is not an issue of whether I like you personally or not; what I don't like is your performance, and here's two examples to discuss. At this point, the manager should present, honestly and accurately, two examples of how the nonplayer is ineffective, incompetent, or inadequate.

LINE 2: IF MY PERFORMANCE IS SO BAD, MAYBE I SHOULD QUIT.

Basic Psychology

The nonplayer recognizes that most managers want to help and assist their employees. Nonplayers therefore believe that in the opinion of a manager the greatest failure can be the resignation of an employee.

Recommended Response

If you've decided that you cannot meet the performance expectations that we now hold for all individuals in your position, I will accept your resignation immediately. This reply shifts the accountability for the nonplayer's future actions from the manager to the nonplayer. By using the pronoun *we*, the personal issue is removed and replaced by the business issue of whether the nonplayer wants to meet the new organization's requirements. In most cases, the nonplayer will not resign, but in some happy instances they may. Under no circumstances should a resigning nonplayer be rehired. In the majority of cases, this will be the last time that the nonplayer plays this particular game.

LINE 3: I'VE GOT A PROBLEM WITH THAT.

Basic Psychology

As discussed previously, this is a favorite trick of the nonplayer. The nonplayer's intent is to force the manager to wrestle with a problem that cannot solved, thus losing credibility with the nonplayer, as well as the rest of the staff.

Recommended Response

A solution to your problem would be more useful, and a better use of our time. Can you provide one? Again, this places accountability for the problem solving where it should be—with the individual employee. If this employee can recognize a problem, certainly she is intelligent enough to suggest a solution.

LINE 4: WE TRIED THAT BEFORE BUT IT DIDN'T WORK.

Basic Psychology

Here the nonplayer is focusing on the old organizational structure and attempting to dredge up unfortunate past history.

Recommended Response

Tell me what will work now. This forces the nonplayer to deal with the here and now of the renewed organization; it also sets a precedent that the past is only useful if it is positive.

LINE 5: IF IT AIN'T BROKE, DON'T FIX IT.

Basic Psychology

A nonplayer is threatened with anything that is new and more demanding, as well as unfamiliar. Accordingly, they resist *any* form of change.

Recommended Response

So-and-so just had to downsize because of that type of thinking. The manager should cite any well-known health care organization that was forced to dismiss any number of employees—and unfortunately there are many. This response demonstrates to nonplayers, as well as the other staff, that downsizing of the wrong kind occurs when individuals wait to be acted upon instead of being proactive.

LINE 6: I'M DIFFERENT.

Basic Psychology

Most nonplayers have usually been employed by the organization for a long time. Therefore, they believe that they should be treated specially because of their tenure and experience. Rather than trying to force the nonplayer into uniformity with the rest of their colleagues, the manager should exploit the "differences" of the nonplayer tactfully.

Recommended Response

I would expect more from someone of your experience and tenure. This again places the burden for positive action and progressive thought on the nonplayer. Because most nonplayers dwell in negativity, this effectively negates the complaint.

LINE 7: IT'S NOT IN MY JOB DESCRIPTION.

Basic Psychology

Most nonplayers can cite their job description completely and use it as an excuse for not assuming new duties. The manager can ask nonplayers to redefine their job description by using the position analysis technique described in Chapter Twelve.

Recommended Response

All of us recognize that our job descriptions are only 70 percent of our actual responsibilities. Let's talk about the duties all of us are now expected to perform. This response sends a strong message to nonplayers that a wider range of responsibilities will be expected of them and that they are part of a cohesive, interdependent unit, not simply individuals entitled to a paycheck for only doing 70 percent (or less) of their job position's scope. Strict adherence to that description is, in reality, dereliction of duty.

LINE 8: THAT WON'T WORK.

Basic Psychology

Most nonplayers enjoy creating doubt, suspicion, and apprehension in the workplace, which reflects their overall negativity and general dissension with positive work goals.

Recommended Response

What will work? Once again, the manager must shift the focus from redefining the problem to solving it.

LINE 9: WE'VE ALWAYS DONE IT THAT WAY.

Basic Psychology

The nonplayer loves to dwell in the past.

Recommended Response

There will be more change in health care in the next two years than ever before—that way won't get it done anymore. This recommended response can be followed by a reminder that the organization has just gone through an extensive renewal process to come up with a new, better way of doing business. Either the nonplayer will be part of the solution, or she will become an ineffective part of the problem—and be treated as such.

LINE 10: SEVERAL OF US THINK THAT . . .

Basic Psychology

The nonplayer is trying to enlist group support for negativity and contentiousness.

Recommended Response

That's probably just your opinion. And it probably is. Many managers make the mistake of asking, *Who else believes this?* which plays into the hand of the nonplayer, who then answers, *Well, that's confidential.* By stripping the nonplayer of perceived group support, he is isolated correctly.

LINE 11: I'M STRESSED!

Basic Psychology

The nonplayer is using stress—a valid feature in the health care workplace, especially during reorganization—as an excuse for nonperformance.

Recommended Response

Give me a specific example, or, *The patient is the only person owed a stressless existence.* Unless nonplayers can provide a specific example of how they are unduly affected by stress, this again is merely an excuse, not an honest work concern.

LINE 12: I'M NOT COMFORTABLE WITH THAT.

Basic Psychology

The nonplayer is using the issue of job comfort—which could be legitimate under different circumstances—in a nonvalid manner.

Recommended Response

What will make you more comfortable? Or, *The patient is the only individual owed comfort.* Once again, the manager must seek to make the complaint specific, work related, and legitimate, or handle it as it probably is—as a sneaky excuse for nonperformance.

LINE 13: THAT'S NOT PROFESSIONAL.

Basic Psychology

Most nonplayers confuse professionalism with their intention to do things the way they want to do them.

Recommended Response

Define professionalism for us. Nonplayers will have difficulty doing this and will merely revert to reciting how they have been victimized by the new system. Once again, by using *we* or *us* instead of *me* or *I,* the manager can negate this nonplayer tactic.

LINE 14: THIS ORGANIZATION DOES NOT PROVIDE QUALITY SERVICE.

Basic Psychology

With the emphasis over the past several years in the health care environment placed on an array of quality service initiatives, the nonplayer can suggest that the reason for their lackluster performance is found in a lack of commitment to health care quality on the part of the organization. In essence, the contention is that the organization, not the nonplayer, is the entity which is not performing at a high level.

Recommended Response

If what we're planning and undertaking currently takes care of the patient in a more effective manner, how it is not quality-driven in intent? The nonplayer must now innovate a better approach to performance, or simply desist in offering this excuse routinely when pressed for improved individual performance.

LINE 15: COMMUNICATION IS A BIG PROBLEM!

Basic Psychology

As discussed throughout this book, communication is a complex process and therefore can be cited by a nonplayer as a problem at almost every conceivable juncture.

Recommended Response

If I tell you what to do, when to do it, and how to do it, and I communicate to you in a style that is understandable, I have not failed you, you have failed us. The power of pronouns, action orientation, and the twenty-five suggestions to establish a progressive work environment discussed in Chapter Three are used in this response.

LINE 16: YOU WON'T LET ME TALK.

Basic Psychology

The nonplayer is suggesting that the manager is trying to prevent him from speaking, when really the manager is probably trying to curtail complaining.

Recommended Response

I'll let you talk. We just don't need to hear constant complaining and whining. The best solution, obviously, is to be honest and direct in calling the nonplayer's behavior exactly what it is—unnecessary complaining.

LINE 17: YOU'RE RACIST (SEXIST, ETC.).

Basic Psychology

The nonplayer is maliciously trying to interject illegalities into the work discussion.

Recommended Response

If you truly believe that I treat you differently from other individuals in your work position, we will postpone this discussion until I can get a third party to join us. Under no condition should managers try to handle this without the assistance of at least their manager, if not the CEO. At this point, the nonplayer should prove discrimination by concrete examples, or be properly documented for slandering the manager.

LINE 18: WE DON'T TAKE CARE OF
THE PATIENT ANYMORE.

Basic Psychology

The nonplayer is trying to use patient focus to further self-interest.

Recommended Response

The entire purpose of the renewed organization is to take better care of the customer-patient, as most of us understand. By citing the renewal process, and in the absence of specific examples by the nonplayer, the manager additionally enlists the unspoken support of all staff for the renewed organization.

LINE 19: ALL OF US ARE SCARED.

Basic Psychology

Once again, the nonplayer is trying to derail organizational renewal by suggesting that everyone is afraid of the process.

Recommended Response

On the contrary, I think you're wrong, because it is quite apparent to me that most of the staff are committed to the renewed organization, as evidenced by their recent actions and behavior. Once again, the manager is specifying that this complaint is centered on the nonplayer, not on the work group.

LINE 20: I LIKED IT BETTER IN THE PAST.

Basic Psychology

Apparently, the nonplayer, who now has more responsibilities, would love to return to the past. Doing so is inconceivable, unrealistic, and foolhardy.

Recommended Response

As we have discussed over the past several months, a new organization is necessary for the new demands that our patient and our community have for us. Notice that the emphasis is on patient, community, change, and renewed organizational strength, which is exactly where it should be.

Although the list is not all-inclusive, these twenty excuses are among the more obvious games that the nonplayer plays. By applying common sense and fortitude when using these responses, the nonplayer's effect can be diminished, if not nullified, during the entire organizational renewal process.

Working with Potentially Difficult Personalities

Many individuals in your department might be gun-shy. For example, they might never have been encouraged to be creative or, worse yet, might have been punished for trying out a new method that did not yield immediate positive results. Naturally, these persons are somewhat wary of offering new suggestions for fear of being shot down. Therefore, personality type is a factor in how you approach creativity in your management agenda.

In categorizing the personality types on your team as they relate to the creative process, consider the motivational factor of work interest. People who demonstrate work interest in all of their job role activities are motivated by several factors. First, they are genuinely interested in their work and are intellectually engaged by the content of their technical specialty and assigned duties. Second, they find a sense of intrigue in their work; they enjoy dealing with problems and finding solutions, meeting new challenges in their work area, and encountering technical innovations and applications. Third, people who are truly interested in their work role seek creative solutions and enjoy becoming knowledgeable about their jobs. This last factor is crucial to the success of establishing a creative environment, and you must reinforce it in your supervisory efforts.

Certain personality types are not compatible with the creative process, however. These personality profiles must be identified and factored into your decisions making when considering how to build a creative environment. Some of these noncompatible personality types are

- The contrarian
- The half-stepper

- The leaner
- The problem person
- The sixty-watt bulb
- The passive aggressor
- The superstar

The Contrarian

In examining personality types that might cause problems in creating an innovative environment, your purpose is not to stereotype individuals but to establish a list of culprits who might derail the creative process. One such category is the contrarian, an individual who will argue or contend anything and feels committed to act negatively on any work issue. Contrarians often do not even achieve a satisfactory level of performance, because they are constantly challenging the status quo from a negative viewpoint. Contrarians tend to be argumentative and are ever dissatisfied with the workplace, if not their own individual work role. Contrarians not only affect their own individual workflow in a negative manner, they also can have a contagious effect on others in the department. Because contrarians are overwhelmingly negative, and often are achieving at a less-than-satisfactory level, they are very difficult to bring into the creative process unless they are challenged outright.

To challenge contrarians, use a questioning process that puts the onus on them to come up with a solution. For example, if contrarians cite something that does not work, ask them what will work. If they answer *I don't know*, charge them with coming up with a plan (by a certain time) that will work. You cannot let contrarians off the hook; that is, you must constantly challenge them to come up with solutions and not simply to take counterpositions to everyone in the department, especially you, the manager.

The Half-Stepper

A half-stepper does not apply a full effort to any work activities. Often you will find that half-steppers were coddled by your predecessor and might possess one specific skill or have mastery over a particular body of knowledge that inclined your predecessor to excuse the entire range of the half-stepper's poor overall performance. For example, the individual might be a technician particularly skilled at one high-usage application but unfortunately does not make a similar effort, or possess the same technical proficiency, with other assigned responsibilities. Half-steppers do not like the creative process; they find it threatening because of its potential to identify areas in which superlative effort is required. They are very comfortable in their current role and have established a comfort zone from which they do not want to be jarred.

In establishing a creative environment, begin by approaching half-steppers in the area in which they are most proficient. Solicit creative ideas relative to the things this person does best. Furthermore, establish specific performance goals by using the material throughout this book that will increase the breadth of their performance contribution. This will set a new expectation for the half-steppers, whose comfort zone will be redefined to allow for creativity by using their area of strength as a center point from which to bolster proficiency.

The Leaner

Another potential negative influence in the creative scheme is the leaner. A leaner is someone who relies on the actions of others to get things done and often camouflages as a team player. A sure symptom of "leanership" is the *we* point of view that crops up in work discussions: *We did this.* There is very little *I* in these conversations. Once again, you are dealing with an individual who seeks to exploit a positive image by keeping a low profile and not fully embracing a leadership role in work activities.

Leaners are not openly against implementation of a creative plan. On the contrary, such workers usually will get on board with a new program, if for no other reason than simply to survive. Therefore, recognize that these individuals might lack sufficient self-esteem. Try to get them involved with the more positive members of your team by assigning them to work with your stronger players and by exerting your own personal influence to get them to play on the right team. Encourage leaners to give you creative input, and cite them personally when they do make a positive contribution.

The Problem Person

Problem people certainly can have a deleterious effect on the creative process. There are two kinds of problem person. The first always has a problem with anything going on in the workplace. They often use the phrase *I've got a problem with* . . . and, like the contrarian, usually accentuate the negative. Problem people are usually very technically proficient and extremely intelligent but use that intelligence to redefine problems and look to the negative rather than making a positive contribution. It is possible that such individuals feel they should be manager but recognize that it is more comfortable to be a second-guesser.

The second type of problem person is an individual who deliberately causes problems. These people might be openly uncooperative—for instance, with other individuals in the department—or they might exacerbate problems by not participating fully or not providing the full range of their resources and input in attacking a work situation. In short, they endeavor to throw a monkey wrench into work situations in a very subtle, sneaky manner to prove that they were right all the time. These troublemakers can be very dangerous not only to the creative effort but to your ongoing efforts to establish yourself as department leader.

A helpful strategy, one that can be used to manage both types of problem people, is to put the spotlight on them. Hold them accountable for every action and document performance and work activity closely. Furthermore, confront them tactfully and professionally when they make statements like *I've got a problem*. Each time you hear it, challenge the problem people directly to come up with a solution to the problem they just defined. Do not hesitate to do this, as timing is very important in dealing with these individuals. Also, never relinquish control of management discussions to problem people; give them an equal opportunity for input, but never allow them to lead a conversation or to belabor a negative point to a nonproductive end. In following these suggestions, you will define right away your relationship with problem individuals, which will send a strong signal to the problem people as well as to anyone who may be considering joining their ranks. Over time, the problem people will either be phased out or restructure their participation in a more positive manner.

The Sixty-Watt Bulb

Certain individuals who might raise barriers to the creative scheme are characterized as sixty-watt bulbs in a 120-watt world. These individuals do not have a lot of creative input to offer, either by virtue of poor work habits, adaptation of a noncreative thinking style, or any number of other factors. Individuals who might fall into this category also include those who like to do everything by the book. They are very comfortable in a structured environment, do not wish to adopt a more flexible stance, and are not particularly interested in generating creative solutions.

There is very little that you can do with a sixty-watt bulb. You can hope that by including them in group activities and other strategies discussed later (in Chapters Six and Ten) you at least foster enthusiasm about new activities and occasional participation in new, creative solutions and programs. However, recognize that many people are comfortable simply putting in a fair day's work, getting a decent wage, and going home at the end of their shift. Remember also to distinguish between the sixty-watt bulb and the half-stepper. The half-stepper more often is a performance problem; the sixty-watt bulb simply is not necessarily motivated toward creativity or toward doing anything different from the norm. Documentation is essential for dealing with the half-stepper, whose performance problems must be addressed. In the case of the sixty-watt bulb, encouragement and communication are the keys, and as long as no performance problem is evident, these individuals must be accepted as a fact of management life.

Some sixty-watt bulbs might be constitutionally inclined toward middle-ground performance or simply not interested in distinguishing themselves by performing at a higher level. Nevertheless, they still fulfill the basic requirement of the job position and maintain a fundamental loyalty to the organization. As a manager, it is vital for you to realize that not all workers are interested in excelling above and beyond the work of their peers or in participating in group activities in a leadership role, yet they are still capable and willing to make a solid work contribution.

The Passive Aggressor

You will hear the term *passive aggressor* repeatedly in management discussions. A passive aggressor is an individual who will agree with you in a face-to-face conversation but then either do nothing or do something contrary to the action contracted with the manager. A passive aggressor is a sneak. Passive aggressors are usually very intelligent and are more interested in playing games than in getting the job done. They are extremely detrimental to the health care environment, because their desire to play games and manipulate others can jeopardize a customer-patient's life. In terms of performance documentation, you must watch a passive aggressor very closely. In terms of the creative process, you must realize that passive aggressors might openly agree enthusiastically with any new programs and creative ideas, yet upon leaving a meeting they might exhibit any of the following behaviors:

- Talking negatively behind your back
- Discounting the importance or validity of the new program
- Enlisting the support of others in failing to carry out your plan
- Setting booby traps and other barriers to achievement of your goal
- Announcing to everyone in the organization that your ideas are invalid or unrealistic

The Superstar

Passive aggressors, like other personality types discussed here, might also exhibit behaviors that cut across category lines. In fact, they might very well embody the characteristics of the superstar. Superstars think they are above it all. Superstars are extremely proficient at one particular area of their job, but unfortunately they think they know it all. Many would be likely candidates for management but may not possess the interpersonal skills, attitude, and management savvy so vital for today's health care manager. Furthermore, this type of superstar might be an individual who is not in fact a superstar, whose achievement level might have fallen off due to failure to embrace new technology. Although he or she might have been a superstar in the past, this person is now no more than a steady performer.

In this instance, you have a prime opportunity to reverse the performance level of an individual. As you do your inventory interview upon taking command of your department, try to identify individuals who insist that they have a strong level of technical proficiency and truly have something to offer the entire staff. Immediately enlist them in your creativity efforts. Stress that you are counting on them for creative input and that you want to use their vast technical expertise and organizational knowledge as you pursue your objectives. In short, give them enough rope to hang themselves. However, you are allowing them an opportunity to provide creative input in a positive manner, and you will encourage this action so long as it does not become negative or self-defeating.

Conclusion

Dealing effectively with nonplayers is not an automatic process, and the strategies delineated in this chapter will increase in effectiveness in direct proportion to your ongoing experience. Remember four final guidelines as you undertake this often unpleasant—but ultimately necessary—set of responsibilities:

1. Always get an assist from peers or mentor managers if you need a second look at a nonplayer situation.
2. Keep in mind that nonplayers create problems for staff and patients; their self-absorption is always at the cost of poor health care service.
3. Nonplayers are adults and assumed to be professionals; if they have decided that they are unhappy in the present work environment, it is their responsibility to find work that is more compatible—perhaps with another employer.
4. Steadies and superstars will enthusiastically welcome the departure of nonplayers; ultimately, termination is the best solution to the nonplayer morass.

Chapter Five

Leading Through Conflict, Change, and Crisis

Invariably, health care managers must make the tough calls. This includes taking disciplinary action (including terminating employees and putting employees on probation), mediating conflict, dealing with internal customers, and an array of other potentially volatile situations. No matter what your technical background is or which departments you work in, inevitably you will have to manage tough situations—dissatisfied or even hostile customer-patients, for example. Because these situations can erupt immediately, you must be prepared with techniques to manage them.

In this chapter I deal directly and practically with an assortment of problems a newly appointed health care manager can encounter. Although no one solution meets all problems, the information in this chapter should prove to be a useful guide as you attempt to manage the gray areas inherent to tough situations. By adopting the strategies most suitable to your management style and work environment, you will take a proactive approach to problem solving and conflict management.

Next I discuss the symptoms of conflict within the workplace and pragmatic ways of resolving conflict among employees. Conflict resolution involves use of fact-finding processes, so I offer an adaptable approach to fact finding and a strategy for implementing conflict resolution systems into your responsibilities. I also provide some insight on counseling employees and resolving conflict in one-on-one counseling situations.

Because probation and termination are unpleasant realities of management responsibilities, I address these issues specifically, particularly when and how to fire someone. I conclude with a discussion on how to resolve customer-patient complaints successfully and efficiently, drawing source material from some of the most challenging complaints from physicians and union employees.

The Establishment of Trust

Regardless of the size of a health care work group, there are two elements that cannot be fully regained if lost. One is trust—the sense of integrity that exists between employees and their supervisor. If trust is lost or diminished through action and negative consequence, it is unlikely that it can be regained at its original level. The other element is pride—a sense of allegiance and high esteem that pervades the work group. Both trust and pride are valued commodities that link the supervisor and the individual employee. Trust, however, is the overriding motivator.

In this section I discuss how to establish trust in your work group. It is essential that you embrace these guidelines and try to apply them to your everyday activities. Unless employees have trust in your leadership ability, they may not be motivated to follow even the clearest direction. The consequence is that time will be wasted unnecessarily by challenges to your authority or misguided questioning of your decisions.

You begin to establish trust on day one of your tenure as a manager. Loss of trust usually results in the breakdown of group harmony and productivity; ultimately this loss of trust could lead to a manager's termination. Many new managers are filling vacancies created by predecessors who failed to elicit trust from staff and thus failed to elicit high-quality outputs. In the long run, the establishment of trust could be your most important asset as a health care manager.

Ensuring Clear Communication

Communication is the cornerstone for establishing trust. If you demonstrate a clear, open channel of communication, employees have the opportunity to explore the parameters of their relationship with you. Apprehensions can be addressed, questions can be answered, and directions can be ascertained through clear communication. Employees can gain a sense of their new leader's style through open communication. Without it, the perception can arise that game playing or selective communication is the new manager's modus operandi.

First, start building your communication strategy by remembering to ask questions frequently of all members of your staff. Use the questions provided in Appendix C, and focus specifically on asking them what can be done to make the organization better and what they need from you in order to become better workers. A second approach is to ensure that monthly department meetings are held so that employees can discuss work progress and so you can review your goals and objectives for the organization. A third strategy is to try to analyze which staff members need the most (or least) communication. Make an entry in your manager's logbook about how often you will meet with each individual on a one-to-one, interpersonal basis. This will give more reticent staff members opportunity to discuss issues they might not feel comfortable addressing openly in a meeting.

Many managers advocate an open-door policy. This is a good idea in theory, but in practice it requires some fine-tuning. Establish certain hours during which your door is indeed open and workers can have access to you. Ask your assistant or secretary (if you have one) to screen employee requests for meetings with you and to schedule them based on priority of need.

In addition to an open-door policy, apply the management-by-walking-around techniques. This strategy mandates setting aside a certain amount of time each day to simply stroll around your assigned area of responsibility, make sure that individuals have access to you, and ask questions in a nonthreatening manner. Again, this keeps the communication lines open while visibly reinforcing trust and making you accessible to your employees.

Holding Performance Reviews

Another way to establish trust is to pursue opportunities to review the past. Discuss with your staff areas in which their past performance was good or inferior. Ask for their suggestions on how improvement might be made. This can be done within the context of group performance or individual performance.

Reviewing Group Performance

Encourage staff to be direct and candid about their assessment of past performance as a group. Keep the conversation focused on performance, not on personality-based issues. For example, discourage reference to your predecessor's personality, that of individuals within the department, or other potentially explosive issues. In emphasizing performance, you discover areas for improvement and crystallize specific methods on how to improve performance throughout the department and within individual work roles.

Discussion about *what we are doing wrong* also helps establish trust. By acknowledging that the department is not perfect and that you as manager will not be perfect, you remind everyone involved that you share the human quality of imperfection. This listing of mistakes and opportunities for improvement is a good opener in establishing trust. Most health care workers are perfectionists who strive for ideal outcomes in all their assigned responsibilities. Accordingly, they are well versed not only on what goes wrong but why it went wrong. By reviewing mistakes and concentrating on where a problem may exist, your staff will appreciate your commitment to them and therefore feel free to share their thoughts on areas for improvement.

To use this strategy in a practical application, have all members in your department or work group brainstorm areas for improvement. Using an easel (as a group) or individual notepads, they can divide the page into three columns. In the first column staff should list the event or application that needs improvement. For the second column, ask your staff to focus in on things they can control or are doing right relative to the problems or challenges cited in column one. Also ask for suggestions for improvement as part of a commitment to the continuous quality improvement process to your work activities. In the third column, have them list situations and circumstances of which the department has either limited or no control.

Exhibit 5.1 shows an example of this charting system as used by one hospital's personnel department. The first column lists challenges, the second contains entries of things within the department's control, the third indicates problems with a project or process they feel are out of control.

In later sessions (or regular department meetings), you might want to discuss as a group how the team can become stronger. This could include another exercise on how the team can meet the needs of the customer-patient at an even higher level of quality and effectiveness. Five basic questions can be used in this regard and can be added easily to the agenda of your monthly meeting.

1. Where does communication seem to break down?
2. When do we operate as a team most efficiently?
3. When do we operate as a team least efficiently?
4. On a scale of one to ten, how would you rate the level of pride we have in our department (1 = very proud; 5 = no pride)?
5. What can we do better as a group?

Exhibit 5.1. Sample Identification Chart: Hospital Personnel Department.

Challenge	Under Our Control	Out of Our Control
Fill open receptionist position	a. Employee referrals b. Overtime contribution c. Alternate coverage in interim	a. Limited outside applicants b. No money in recruitment budget c. No local business school
Poor-quality training programs	a. Better preparation b. Use of audiovisual materials c. Improved scheduling	a. Limited training budget b. Time limitations of hospital management c. Prior administration's nonsupport
Implement new pay system	a. Good orientation b. Information pamphlets c. Continued question and answer sessions	a. Likely resistance b. Misperception (employees) c. Skepticism (managers)

As always, there is no magic answer to any one question. These questions serve to facilitate a group process for discussion of specific areas needing improvement and, more directly, address areas in which the unit can work more strongly as a team. Problems are defined and solutions are formed. (For example, patient parking might be a problem raised by the group, and rerouting of cars by members of the hospital security team might be the solution.) This, along with other strategies in this book, can be a logical (and immediate) starting point from which to establish trust. It also sets a precedent for discussing issues from a team perspective so staff view themselves as a group in which no one wins unless everyone wins.

Reviewing Individual Performance

People rowing a boat do not have time to rock the boat. That is, if you can immediately establish trust on an individual employee basis, each worker will be vested with advancing the group process. Sit down as soon as possible with each employee to discuss privately his or her job, perceived role in the organization, and needs. You should do most of the listening while the staff member does most of the talking. Prepare several questions to help frame this one-on-one meeting. The purpose of the questions is to elicit a specific response, guide the discussion, and initiate what should become a healthy manager-staff relationship.

Here are some suggested questions for these individual meetings:

- Tell me about your history here at (name of hospital).
- What do you need to become better at your job?
- How can I best support you in your everyday activities?
- What qualities do you look for in a supervisor?
- What short-term plans do you have in your job?
- What long-term plans do you have in your job?
- What are some of the major aspirations for your career?
- What advice do you have for me as I begin in my role as department manager?

These questions have been used by many health care managers in my consulting work and have reaped great benefits in beginning a strong manager-employee dialogue and providing a sound starting point in the manager–staff member relationship.

Setting Policies and Standards

In establishing trust, it is important to set standards immediately in your work role. As discussed throughout the text, it is important to communicate to all department members your policies and standards. These could be communicated via memo, or better yet, individually and in group meetings. These policies should include a simple overview of your management style, what your key expectations are for the department, and what you expect from each member in terms of job performance.

In the interest of clarity and simplicity, the best approach is usually to say generally that you expect four things from each department member:

1. Full effort
2. Clear communication relative to individual needs and desires on the job
3. Respect and dignity in the workplace
4. Compliance with all organization standards

Using this as a building block, you can present more detailed direction and standards in the near future regarding technical items, work projects, and interpersonal dealings. As always, by your own words and actions as a leader—which will be closely observed by all members of your work group—your departmental standards will become fuller, clearer, and more integrated into daily workplace activities. If people know where they stand and all individual members are "rowing the boat," trust flourishes.

Providing Clear Direction and Feedback

A system of clear direction and feedback is an imperative in the health care setting, where direction and timely feedback can spell the difference between good health and bad health and between life and death. Take every opportunity to instruct your employees, provide assistance, and give them the benefit of your technical acumen. This creates a sense of trust among employees, particularly when your input helps forward individual success. As always, asking intelligent questions is the hallmark of good leadership. Not only does it convey interest in the employee's activities, it demonstrates that you are in a learning mode.

Downplaying Minutiae

Another route to establishing trust is to downplay minutiae—trivialities that have little or no impact on overall departmental performance. However, use your judgment and exercise diplomacy. Something that might seem trivial or inconsequential to you might be very important to an employee.

For example, in one major metropolitan hospital, conflict and a lack of trust became a problem because of the way groups of workers took their breaks on shift. Basically, a personality conflict arose because a new supervisor mistakenly made a big deal of cliques going on break at the same time (which had been allowed by the previous supervisor). To remedy the situation and to underscore trust, the manager's new tactic was to state that he did not care who went on break with whom, just that everyone performed when it was time to perform. By stating this standard, as well as downplaying a small symptom that was really a sign of a bigger problem in the work situation, the manager refocused his staff's activities and performance emphasis to the point where the issue of break time became immaterial.

Reevaluating Operations Periodically

A final tip on establishing trust is to reevaluate your work group from time to time by using all the techniques cited in this section at various times throughout your initial year as a departmental manager. This includes having meetings, on an individual as well as a group basis from time to time, to reexamine the questions discussed in this section. By revisiting these areas, you will ensure that trust is part of the continuum of performance and departmental activity. In establishing trust, you now have a basis on which individuals will promulgate pride throughout the work group and leave most of the conflict of the past exactly where it belongs—in the past. Finally, the avenues of communication will be open and will become part of the everyday process to act proactively to avoid future conflict among department members.

Intradepartmental Conflict and Resolution

Despite your best efforts to establish trust throughout the work group and to avoid potential conflict, human nature will unfortunately create occasions for intradepartmental conflict throughout your tenure as a health care manager. Intradepartmental conflict is any conflict that takes place within your department or work group. In this section I will discuss the symptoms of intradepartmental conflict and present various solutions for resolving conflict so that progressive action and quality of performance become the department's top priority.

Symptoms of Intradepartmental Conflict

Initially, intradepartmental conflict takes place on an interpersonal basis. Interpersonal conflict, particularly within a work group, is potentially the most damaging type of problem a health care manager can deal with. If interpersonal conflict exists within a department and is not abated and healed, eventually it can have drastic negative consequences for the entire department—even implosion.

Numerous indicators signal intradepartmental conflict. Use your instincts and observations to examine the conflict in a cause-and-effect fashion. Following is a list of potential symptoms, their potential cause, and their effect on your department. The symptoms are examined within the parameters of a departmental relationship.

- *Anger.* Interpersonal adversity, loss of temper, lack of patience, or flat-out confrontational behavior can be exhibited in certain kinds of interpersonal conflict.
- *Avoidance.* Avoidance occurs when an individual declines to work with someone and simply avoids contact with that person. The effect is that work may not be done and establishment of the team process may be compromised. Avoidance is more subtle than anger, which is direct in nature.
- *Blame.* Individuals will often blame one another for mistakes, or cite another individual as a reason for their own inability or failure to perform. Blaming creates hostility among team members and betrays basic trust and pride in the organization.

- *Excuse making.* One individual will use another's behavior as an excuse for not performing a particular task. The individual may focus specifically on a personality nuance as being the problem that gets in the way of accomplishment. Another form of making excuses is to rationalize the negative behavior of others; for example, *Well you can't expect too much from so-and-so, you know how they are.* This form of excusing relies on a personality trait as the reason for nonperformance or inadequate performance.
- *Isolation and fragmentation.* Over time, certain team members may exclude one or more players because of personality conflict. The effect of isolation is that participation in the group process is jeopardized. Ultimately, there is a withdrawal of the resources needed to get the job done. Exclusion can occur to the point that workers may become isolated from the organization or organize their own faction. This fragmentation can become particularly deleterious in any group process, especially one that requires emergency response.
- *Confrontation.* Certain personality types are argumentative by nature, so that even routine operations are interrupted by confrontation and overall disruption of group harmony. This is a waste of time as well as a demoralizer.
- *Criticism.* Over the long term, an individual who is critical of everything and everyone in the department also creates a morale problem. Ironically, others respond to this behavior by becoming defensive and in turn critical of the chronic criticizer.
- *Erosion of performance levels.* Ill feeling, over time, leads to diminished performance among workers. Some staff begin to look for another workplace if the situation is not corrected by the manager.
- *Regression.* Continued erosion of performance leads to regression. In an era in which health care must be progressive, every employee's performance must contribute to its maximum potential.

Resolving Intradepartmental Conflict

To resolve intradepartmental conflict, an assortment of methods can be employed. These methods have in common a requirement to identify the symptoms, recognize the full effects of the conflict, and work through the issues with staff so that resolution can be achieved with confidence.

Identifying Symptoms

To begin with, identify the symptoms of conflict, using the preceding list as a basis. Look for the source of conflicts, specifically who is creating it and what the root cause may be. Note behavior or language that may provoke problems. This could include derogatory terms used to describe certain team members, the "silent treatment" directed toward particular team members, or outright verbal conflict or nonverbal hostility, such as glaring and gestures of disapproval.

Recognizing Effects of Conflict

Recognize what effect the situation may have on the entire group. First try to define whether the conflict is an individual versus a group problem, an individual versus individual problem, or a group versus a group (faction) problem. This will help you be more specific not only in identifying the symptoms, but also in finding a potential solution.

Try to quantify the person's (or group's) behavior as much as possible by recording in your logbook as many specific incidents as you can. Then use your notes to analyze whether the problem is related to poor attitude or to lack of interpersonal skills, team orientation, or technical ability. To educate the employee(s) and correct the problem later, you must be as specific as possible and collect as many examples as feasible. This evidence will help you illustrate the problem to the employee or group and provide the education needed to correct it.

Next, determine the full extent of an interpersonal problem—primarily whether it is limited to two or a few individuals or whether it is having a contagious effect on others in the department who were not initially involved. Try to ascertain whether a faction is being created by the problem, or whether one individual seems to be deliberately gathering support from others to form a faction. It is essential to stop the spread of harmful intradepartmental conflict as early as possible.

Working Through Issues

After collecting and analyzing your information, approach the responsible party (or parties) directly. In general, five steps should be taken to resolve intradepartmental conflict: separate and reach agreement on the issues, discuss harmful performance and its effects, explore the causes of conflict, state your expectations for resolution, and express confidence in arriving at a solution.

1. Separate the issues into two categories. First identify the business-related attributes of the problem—business outcomes, performance dimensions, and technical areas. Then list personal issues that might bear on the conflict. These include any of the ten symptoms set forth earlier—anger, avoidance, blame, and so forth—as well as your own observations from your logbook. Review this information completely with the involved party and reach consensus on the facts of the issues. If no one acknowledges the facts, you might have to state more directly your belief in their validity and supplement that statement with the pledge that you will not accept this behavior any longer.

2. Move the discussion to performance, focusing specifically on the business effects from the conflict. Cite work that is not being done; explain how the employee's (or group's) behavior affects other department members and how this behavior interferes with others' getting their jobs done. Discuss further how this behavior affects other departments and, most important, the customer-patients. By all means, use your own technical acumen to explain the specific negative consequence of the behavior and the danger if it continues.

3. Ask why this behavior has taken place and how it might be corrected. Try to get to the bottom of what the parties believe is contributing to the problem and how the cause might be alleviated. Following this discussion, present your own ideas on why the problem exists; however, spend most of your discussion on how the problem must be remedied.

4. State clearly, concisely, and resolutely your expectations, standards, and policies for future action. Explain what will be accepted by you as satisfactory behavior and what will be considered poor

performance or interpersonal conflict. Future actions might include probation or any other disciplinary action, including termination.

5. Finally, express your confidence that the situation will be corrected and ask whether particular assistance is needed to do so. Try to strike a delicate balance between expressing optimism that the situation can be corrected and underscoring the fact that continued poor performance and intradepartmental conflict will not be tolerated under any conditions.

As you deal with the difficult task of resolving intradepartmental conflict, incorporate two strategies into your efforts. The first is to do a good job of fact finding every step of the way. Fact finding is the process of collecting information from all involved parties before arriving at a decision. For example, when an intradepartmental conflict takes place between two individuals, you might want to investigate by discussing the situation with both parties separately and by asking them the same two questions: what they think the problem and root cause may be, and how the situation might be resolved. At that point, bring both parties together, present both ideas for resolution, and once again state your optimism for correction as well as your refusal to tolerate further interpersonal conflict.

The second strategy for resolving intradepartmental conflict is through policy compliance. Use as needed your facility's personnel policies and its expertise to resolve the problem. Also, rely on your own manager's input. In some cases, you might want someone from the human resource department or your manager to sit in with you as you seek resolution with the conflicted parties. This not only gives you some assistance and support, it also conveys to those involved in the conflict that this is a serious matter that will be dealt with resolutely. It does not demonstrate any weakness on your part. In fact, it shows strength because it indicates to the employee that you have the clout with which to resolve the problem. To further get this message across, take the lead in the conversation, state your expectations for the department, and promise further discipline if the problem is not corrected.

To gain the most benefit from your personnel policies, use both your documentation notebook to record counseling sessions and the performance evaluation. Clear documentation notes and subsequent notation on the performance evaluation will once again stress the importance to the employee or group that intradepartmental conflict is not an accepted mode of behavior on the job. Whichever approach you take, make sure that all involved parties understand clearly the consequences if performance and conflict are not remedied.

Interpersonal conflict, particularly within a department, is complex and can hinder progressive action. Again, it must be dealt with resolutely and in a timely fashion so that the majority of your department is not adversely affected. Remember, an array of individuals look to you for leadership. By not dealing ethically and promptly with interpersonal conflict, you not only encourage substandard performance, you also abdicate the trust and leadership your organization and staff expect from you. If the suggestions in this section are followed, this difficult area of management can become less burdensome and more productive.

Termination and Probation

Knowing *when* to fire someone is as difficult as knowing *how*. A health care manager at a client facility in the Southwest told me, "When I fire someone, I'm also firing their family." This statement underscores the difficulty attached to terminating an employee. Yet terminating employees is an unfortunate but necessary part of being a health care manager. When individual performance has deteriorated to the point of being counterproductive, it is clearly time for separation. In many cases, individuals are actually relieved when terminated, because they have become frustrated and ineffective in their work role.

Do not expect anyone to thank you for terminating them, however, or to admit that it was their fault for being terminated. Terminating an employee is a very difficult undertaking, and in this section I provide a ten-point checklist for signs that indicate that termination may need to be considered and discuss how to make the termination process as painless and productive as possible.

Disciplinary probation is generally a three-month process in which poor performers are given the opportunity, usually one last chance, to make good on their employment obligation. That is, the individuals have three months to turn performance around to an acceptable level. Most health care managers think that probation is a farce because if the individuals "behave" for three months, there is no guarantee that they will perform steadily for the rest of the year. In fact, they generally believe that performance will usually regress. Probation is generally acknowledged as a final step before termination, so I only touch on it in this section.

Discuss with your personnel department the probation policy at your organization; for example, when an individual should go on probation. In many cases, employees who are on probation will terminate themselves by securing other employment while on probation, thus saving you the headache of having to fire them. In this regard, probation is a worthwhile practice and should be used in conjunction with a performance evaluation for an employee who will be terminated eventually anyway. Beyond being used as a prelude to termination, probation has very little effect on performance enhancement. However, several guidelines can be used to help you decide whether to terminate an employee and if so, when and how.

When to Terminate

When should you fire someone? This question is asked at virtually every one of more than fifty seminars I conduct each year for health care managers and executives. The answer is not simple. Each case deals with a unique individual and specific circumstances. You should terminate an employee if more than seven of the following conditions are present.

1. *Chronic poor attitude.* An employee who regularly appears to be inflexible, overly aggressive or confrontational, irresolute, and tunnel-visioned and displays a poor work ethic and no sense of industry is a candidate for termination. Rarely are individuals who demonstrate these attitudes likely to change, because such outlooks are elemental to their personality and are life-conditioning. In an industry that requires high adaptability, appropriately assertive behavior, perseverance, and a strong work ethic, these problems, which probably cannot be corrected, are unacceptable.

2. *Poor interpersonal skills.* An individual who consistently demonstrates interpersonal behavior problems and creates conflicts, as discussed earlier in the chapter, might be a candidate for termination. In a people-oriented field such as health care, poor interpersonal skills do not make for long-term success.

3. *Negative effect on others.* When an employee's negative behavior creates intradepartmental conflict and the employee has been counseled several times about the effect caused by these conflicts, termination must be considered.

4. *Poor performance documentation.* If the employee's pattern of performance documentation over a one-year period has been largely negative, termination must be considered. Such individuals not only will fail to grow and develop on the job, they will actually regress to a level of performance that is less than what was expected for the current year. In short, individuals who have demonstrated a full year of poor performance have probably fallen into a pattern that will not be remedied by probation or another year on the job. In essence, they are absorbing a salary that can be better spent on a better performer.

5. *Gut instincts.* If you sense that it is time for the person to go, based on the first four factors cited in this section, termination probably is in order. Do not try to rationalize or overintellectualize your feelings.

6. *Counseling.* After a problem employee has been counseled by you, the human resource department, or other appropriate individuals in your organization and the individual still fails to perform acceptably, chances are the situation is unresolvable.

7. *Outside negative input.* If a customer-patient, peer, colleagues, or other department members have constructively criticized the individual's performance, most likely the performance is affecting the entire workflow of your department. To keep this problem from festering, termination must be enacted.

8. *Detrimental effect on the organization.* A poor performer who is in a critical work position can adversely affect the entire organization. If you have clear evidence that this is the case, termination must be enacted quickly to maintain exceptional organizational integrity and performance.

9. *Regressive patterns, trends, and habits.* A person who consistently demonstrates poor on-the-job behavior, inappropriate work

personality, and poor work habits—all substantiated by your own documentation—is a candidate for termination.

10. *Poor future outlook.* Ask, *Do you think the person will really turn it around?* If the answer is no, make your move.

Exhibit 5.2, an abbreviated checklist of the above indicators, can be used to help you evaluate whether you need to terminate an employee.

How to Terminate

Having determined that termination is necessary, you need to learn how to accomplish the task. Again, a ten-point checklist should help you through what is, at best, a difficult process.

1. *Explain documentation.* All prior appropriate documentation should be on hand for presentation at the time of termination. Explain in two to three minutes your overriding documentation and the reasons you considered termination as the only possible remedy. Documentation must be used as the basis for any discussion of termination.

Exhibit 5.2. Termination Consideration Checklist.

	Yes	No
1. Chronic poor attitide	——	——
2. Poor interpersonal relations	——	——
3. Negative effect on others	——	——
4. Poor performance documentation	——	——
5. Gut instincts say no improvements likely	——	——
6. Counseling attempts produce no positive results	——	——
7. Outside negative input	——	——
8. Detrimental effect on organization	——	——
9. Regressive patterns, trends, habits	——	——
10. Poor future outlook	——	——

Key: If more than seven items are checked it is time to terminate the employee.

2. *Recap performance counseling.* Quickly summarize all efforts made to resolve the performance problem.
3. *Get to the point.* Once steps 1 and 2 have been taken, get to the point. Tell the individual that you are terminating them for cause. If the employee already guessed that he or she is being terminated and says so, simply acknowledge it and move on to the next step.
4. *Have a witness on hand.* If you have never fired an employee, ask a third person (your boss or someone from the human resource department) to be present at the session. This allows you to have support on hand as well as someone to help guide you through the process.
5. *Allow a monologue.* If the person being fired feels like talking or wants to ventilate, allow them three to five minutes to do so. Then respond that although you respect his or her feelings, the decision has been made.
6. *Get closure.* Instruct the individual to leave the premises, but first explain the procedure for cleaning out his or her desk. If necessary, call security to escort them off the premises.
7. *Prepare the exit letter.* A letter of termination delineating cause and signed by the former employee should go in the personnel file, along with the person's comments, if any. Any other paperwork that completes the process should be included.
8. *Communicate with your staff.* Notify staff that you have terminated the individual and that you plan to fill the position quickly. You need not disclose the reasons for the termination. Tell them that it was your decision, but if they would like to discuss it further, they can come into your office on an individual basis and do so. If further discussion is desired, only the future of the department should be discussed, not the terminated employee (for example, *Now we will have to . . .*).
9. *Reject additional input.* Once an employee has been terminated, you need not accept further input from another employee. Your focus should be on the future, specifically on employee suggestions for filling the position. This keeps the termination on a professional basis.
10. *Fill the position quickly.* Quickly filling the position of a terminated employee is the best remedy for the situation. You have an opportunity to command trust and allegiance from your

staff by providing them with a productive, professional new colleague.

Termination is never easy, but by using these techniques and enlisting the support of your superiors and human resource staff, you can move through this difficult situation. Exhibit 5.3 is an abbreviated checklist to help you resolve the situation as effectively and efficiently as possible.

Dealing with Internal and External Customers

A final tough situation you will need to manage is dealing with the complaints of internal customers (such as physicians and unions) and external customers (such as patients and payers).

External Customers

In dealing with customer-patient complaints, again it is important to do fact finding first. Resources include the customer-patient and

---

Exhibit 5.3. Termination Procedure Checklist.

_____ 1. Explain to the employee the overriding documentation and reasons for his or her termination.

_____ 2. Summarize all previous efforts to resolve the performance problem.

_____ 3. Tell the employee you are terminating him or her for cause.

_____ 4. Ask your boss or a representative of your human resources department to witness the termination.

_____ 5. Allow the employee three to five minutes to talk if he or she wishes to do so.

_____ 6. Explain the procedure for exiting the premises.

_____ 7. Prepare a letter of termination for the employee's signature and complete any other paperwork required by your institution.

_____ 8. Notify staff about the termination and your plans to fill the position.

_____ 9. Reject further input from staff regarding the termination, except for suggestions on filling the position.

_____10. Fill the position as quickly as possible.

---

any staff members who might have dealt with the customer-patient. Ask questions and listen carefully to all information provided and take notes for accuracy and to show empathy for what is being said. These notes can also be used as a chronology in resolving the problem. Move proactively and try to head off future complaints by handling this one as quickly as possible. Use your perception to get a full picture of the situation and the basis for the complainant's anger or dissatisfaction. By all means, accept responsibility for any disservice and promise the customer-patient that definitive follow-up action will be taken and that feedback will be provided.

As part of the investigation stage, ask those who worked with the customer-patient their version of what happened. Use your facility's chain of command to get support whenever possible. Then resolve the situation by calling the customer-patient directly, explaining the problem, and writing a follow-up letter of empathy. Offer to provide any corrective action as appropriate, making certain to document the entire episode and refer requests for action to the appropriate parties. As always with interpersonal interaction, communication is key. By using the questions in Appendix C, you can more clearly identify customer-patient complaints. Remember, unlike a retail situation, where another product or a coupon can be given to a customer, customer-patients in the health care setting require empathy and the promise that a harmful action will not take place again. Very serious actions or requests from the customer-patient should be referred to the appropriate resource, usually your supervisor.

Internal Customers

In the case of internal customers—notably, physicians and union members—other strategies for handling complaints should be used. There are six keys to sound physician relations:

1. A strong organization orientation to meeting the legitimate needs of physicians in serving their patients
2. Inclusion of physicians in departmental activities and events
3. Consistent communication
4. Professional support

5. Shared views on meeting the needs of customer-patients
6. Cohesive efforts to ensure an effective and efficient flow of work

First and foremost, physicians should be made to feel part of the team. Hence, they should be included in as many activities and meetings as possible. Many health care organizations have physicians contribute to newsletters or involve them in strategic planning and hiring decisions.

Whenever possible, ask physicians for advice on how you can better support their responsibilities. Discuss every physician complaint with the medical director and physician in a three-way meeting. Again, use the questions appearing in Appendix C as part of your practicum, acting as quickly as possible and using all available communication channels. Many newly appointed health care managers create problems for themselves by starting off on the wrong foot with physicians. Get to know the medical staff, as well as all members of your organization, so that you will have access to all available resources when resolving internal customer complaints.

A final source of potential conflict within your organization's customer base is the union employee. With union drives being an ongoing presence in health care organizations, it is important to maintain your managerial equilibrium at all times and remain neutral during union elections and other labor relations activity. Answer all questions objectively; do not try to win over votes from individuals who are pro-union or those who are decidedly anti-union. Rather, try to provide support for individuals who are undecided and thus pressured by both sides. Reassure employees that life will go on despite the outcome of a union election, and stay close to your human resource department to keep up with developments and learn essential information you might need. Remember, union activity is no excuse for poor performance; therefore, continue to note poor performance in your logbook throughout union activity.

When dealing with all customer complaints, remember to show compassion, take command, and communicate with all responsible parties. The best way to enhance your credibility in conflict situations is to seek answers, decide on action, and execute that action resolutely.

Conclusion

In all conflict situations, do what is most compatible with your management style. Given that conflict is not a comfortable situation, and managing tough situations is not the most appealing part of your management agenda, trust your gut instincts and power of observation. By being concerned about the welfare of your entire staff as well as your customer-patients and colleagues throughout the organization, you will demonstrate a consistency that will help establish your credibility as a manager.

Keep in mind the following five factors of mediating conflict and managing tough situations: compassion, concern, communication, comfort, and command. These will help establish your managerial credibility, which is so vital to establishing trust and the personal power base you will need to manage tough situations effectively. Once you have used some of the techniques discussed in this chapter and established your own comfort zone with the strategies, these tough situations will be more manageable and your overall management systems more effective.

Chapter Six

Orchestrating Progressive Team Action and Individual Performance

Regardless of your team members' experience or rank within the organization, the task of creating synergy among individual talents to fuel a larger group effort is often problematic for new health care managers. Building a team can be a complex task. Trying to establish common goals, objectives, and shared dedication to a mission is one thing, managing and harnessing the abilities and talents of diverse individuals to move toward a mutual goal is quite another. If you examine the overall structure of your health care organization, you will probably find that it consists of many solid teams. Some departments may be stronger than others—perhaps their members have stronger talents, or maybe the group is more cohesive and works together more smoothly and efficiently. If the department is considered a stellar team, it probably has both these qualities. As a newly appointed health care manager, you can establish a team orientation reflecting these tenets.

In this chapter I discuss how to analyze a team and determine the potential contribution of each member to the team effort. I analyze work personality as it relates to health care, and conclude the chapter with a detailed discussion on establishing and then reinforcing a value-driven team orientation. Upon reviewing these concepts and considering their potential application to your situation, you should be closer to establishing a cooperative, progressive work group.

As you read through this chapter, think of individuals in your department and relate what you have observed about each one to the evaluation material presented in this chapter. Keep in mind your team's mission and objectives and what you perceive to be key potential obstacles to developing a strong team so that the presented material becomes realistic in your situation, effective, and more practical.

Conducting a Team Analysis

Great teams consist of great players. To build a team, first analyze the relative strengths and weaknesses of individual players, both current and prospective. In this section I discuss methods of analyzing strengths and weaknesses of individual team members and develop a system to assess the potential, performance, and contribution of each one. To begin with, you will need a notebook in which to enter your evaluations of each member (try to be as objective as possible). Use the seven basic resources described in the following subsections to make your analysis.

Performance Evaluations

Performance reviews and documentation include the evaluations completed by your management predecessor. Remember that under the best conditions performance evaluation is a subjective exercise. Personal bias on the part of your predecessor might have entered into the equation. While reviewing individual employee files, make copious notes about perceived strengths and weaknesses and the employees' development needs. Note in particular any comments on employees' ability to work with others and their contributions to the team effort. Try to gauge attitudes and interpersonal skills.

Firsthand Observations

Write down your firsthand observations of each employee's progress. If your "new" employees are former peers, you already may have opinions about their performance level and ability to work as part of a team. Remember that this logbook is a compilation of your own subjective notes; it is not a legal document or anything that can be used against you in any manner, so be forthright in your note taking.

Credible Secondhand Information

Upon assuming your responsibilities as department manager, interview each employee regarding their goals and objectives, aspirations, and opinions on how to improve performance on an individual and departmental basis. Only ask questions that relate specifically to your particular department's activity, current team orientation, and established group processes. These answers can be most telling in terms of individual attitude toward team cohesion and group contribution.

Selected Interviewing and Selection Data

Seek out any useful information uncovered during the actual hiring process for applicants screened by you or your predecessor. In most health care organizations, the human resource department has copies of interview score sheets or similar data that will give insight into the employees' attitudes, people skills, and team orientation. Most of these professionals are very skilled at extrapolating data obtained in the selection process that can be helpful in assessing potential team orientation. In addition, when conducting applicant interviews, always ask about teamwork experience and how highly group interaction is valued.

Probation Performance Records

Some health care institutions designate the initial three months of employment as a probation period. This means that a new employee's performance is closely monitored and assessed for a period of the first ninety days in a given job. More often than not, copious notes are taken by the reviewing manager and other individuals in the chain of command. Probation notes are a great means of determining the employees' team orientation, individual strengths and weaknesses, and a wealth of other information essential to determining potential value to the work group.

Job Description and Collective Department Behavior

Two other resources can help evaluate individual performance relative to team contribution. The job description, combined with your perception of the individual's ability to meet the performance standards delineated in the job description, is important. Vital considerations are how employees perform their jobs, conduct themselves in the workplace, and act as a source of information and supportive player, as well as their potential and promotability in terms of technical acumen. (Technical acumen, for example, would include how much a compensation specialist knows about the hospital's employee benefit program or how much a pharmacist knows about decongestants.) A simple standard to apply in this case is determining employees' present level of expertise and how vigorously they pursue new technical knowledge and business acumen.

Finally, perhaps the most telling resource of determining caliber of team orientation is simply to observe collective departmental behavior. The following five questions can go a long way toward determining employees' team potential:

1. Toward whom do people seem to gravitate in times of crisis?
2. Which individuals seem to be most willing to share technical knowledge?
3. Which individuals become actively involved in orienting new members?
4. Which individuals seem to work consistently in isolation?
5. Which individuals seem to provide leadership to the team by virtue of example, communication, and inspiration?

The answers to these questions, combined with the information from the above-mentioned resources, can go far in giving you a general perspective of your team leaders and followers. They can also give you an idea of who the more reluctant team players might be, and whom you might target for specific individual team involvement.

Qualities of a Strong Team Player

As you conduct your team analysis, several characteristics and work-related behaviors should be identified and quantified. In this section I review several of these qualities and provide guidelines for identifying them. I also present a profile to use in your efforts to select new staff members.

Figure 6.1 provides insight into what qualities a strong health care team member should possess. The model can serve as a building block in formulating a team blueprint.

Figure 6.1. Health Care Team Member Profile.

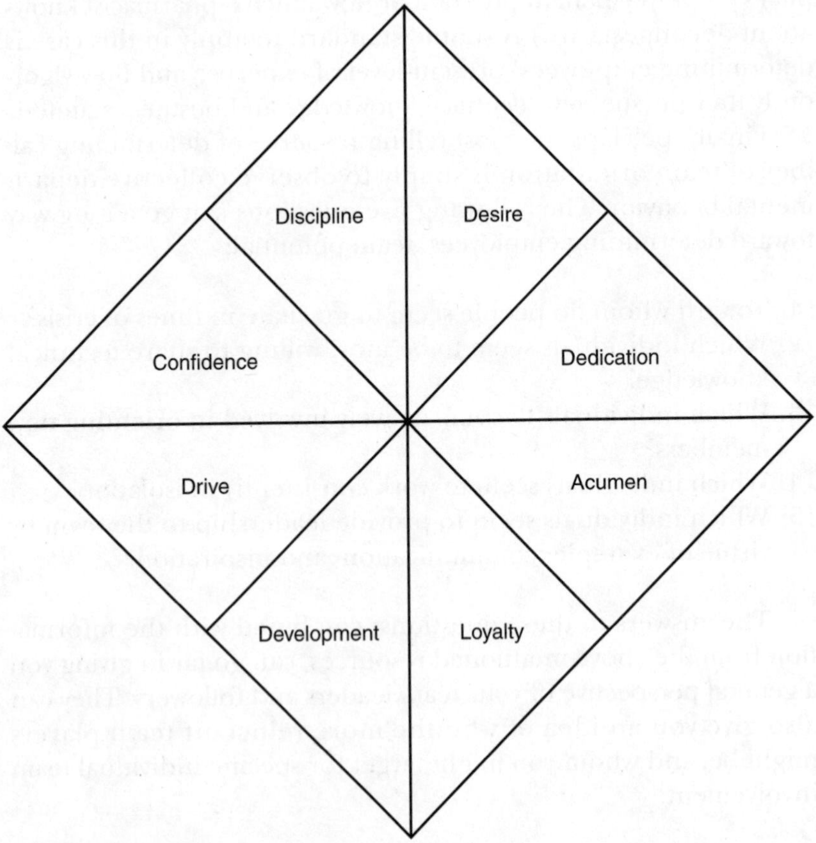

Drive

Each team member must have a certain amount of drive to attain individual and group goals. He does not need to be jump-started every morning or at the beginning of each shift. The drive toward performing strongly, learning and growing every day, being a motivator for others purely by example, expending energy and applying on-the-job initiative all characterize a stellar team player.

Confidence

All team members should feel self-assured about their technical ability and the resilience to perform under changing and critical circumstances. A strong player usually radiates confidence about departmental goals and everyday work activities. Customer-patients and fellow workers pick up on this attitude and therefore feel comforted by this individual's presence. They have the conviction that the job will get done and that when the going gets tough—an everyday occurrence in health care—the job will still get done.

Discipline

Good teams are disciplined. They steadily make exact determinations and seek all facts necessary to making a decision. They get the job done correctly the first time and do not cause little problems that can add up to big problems. Good teams know intrinsically what has to be done and how to do it; that is, they set their own objectives and determine a course of action for achieving those objectives with excellence. Their sense of discipline is self-perpetuating throughout the entire department.

Desire

Desire, best defined for our discussion as a hunger to get better all the time, is a constant motivator for the team player. An individual possessing this characteristic wants to help others and has a strong need to learn and grow on the job, which is a constantly available opportunity for anyone who works in health care. Team members who possess desire in this semblance do not need to be "hand-fed" with the promise of educational opportunities; rather, they seek out learning opportunities everyday and are perpetually fueled by this desire to become better at their jobs and stronger in their daily contributions to the organization, team, and patient's health.

Dedication

Strong team members emanate dedication to a common goal of providing stellar health care to all customer-patients. They are equally dedicated to all team goals, departmental objectives, and one another in providing help, guidance, and technical assistance. They are passionate in their allegiance to the health care profession and equally dedicated to providing whatever support is needed to meet the health care mandate of premium service delivery.

Acumen

The synergy of many technical talents working toward a greater goal makes the health care field so unique. Every employee on the payroll of a health care organization has a certain amount of technical acumen and expertise that they bring to the job every day. Whether that expertise lies in conducting a good lab assay, filling a prescription correctly, or cleaning a patient's room quickly and efficiently, strong team members bring their unique, essential ability to the workplace every day. Never taking a know-it-all attitude, a strong team player looks at every day as an opportunity to learn something new.

Loyalty

Team loyalty is critical in health care, and each player's loyalty cannot be selective or sporadic. The first loyalty, of course, is to the health care institution and its mission of providing care to its patient community. The second loyalty is to the department manager or team leader, and is demonstrated by following set objectives, providing feedback, and accomplishing team goals. The third loyalty is to the work group, to act as a positive participant who contributes to group goals. Fourth, the team members maintain a dedication to escalating their individual strong performance and progressive development on the job.

Development

Each team member should desire to grow and develop on the job. This development, however, expands beyond the parameters of basic technical growth. Strong health care team members seek to learn more about the health care business and understand the changing dimensions of the business. They know how to interpret the impact of change in the social environment and their communities, and they understand how these changes may affect their particular duties and the institution's mission.

An often-overlooked aspect of team member development is interpersonal skills. A strong team member seeks to learn more about individual personalities and the proclivities of fellow team members and what their professional preferences and personal likes and dislikes might be relative to performance. This focus on development of interpersonal skills contributes significantly to an ever-expanding knowledge base from which the employee can grow, prosper, and continuously improve the quantity and quality of their work contribution.

Analyzing Work Personality

In industrial psychology and management philosophy circles, much discussion surrounds a concept known as work personality. The work personality of a health care employee is basically defined as *how* a job is performed, as opposed to *what* is done. As public scrutiny and customer-patients' perception of health care delivery become more intense and keenly focused, the work personalities of health care employees become increasingly important.

In conducting a team analysis, you may find it useful to identify the attributes of work personality present in your team, as well as to study their effect on team performance. This effort can help you deal with employees who go to extremes in performing their jobs, thus creating performance problems for the team. For example, employees performing their job in an extreme manner are strong performers who become workaholics and pressure coworkers to work to their unrealistic standard. Several strategies and systems aid in analyzing the work personality of health care employees. One of the most widely used work personality profile systems, used by more than 150 hospitals, is the Quantitative-Communilogical Organizational Profile System (the Quan-Com System) that I designed in the late 1970s. The Quan-Com System has been endorsed by several major health care accreditation organizations, including the Joint Commission of Accreditation of Healthcare Organizations, the American College of Healthcare Executives, and several state and local regulatory agencies. (For further information, please refer to the *Handbook of Personnel Selection and Performance Evaluation in Health Care,* by Donald N. Lombardi [San Francisco: Jossey-Bass, 1988], pp. 27–57 and *passim.*) This system may be useful for studying your team orientation and work behavior by helping you more accurately determine the team development needs of your staff and the individual tendencies and liabilities of your team members.

The basic elements of this system are

- Attitude orientation
- People skills
- Managerial aptitude
- Team orientation

As they relate to the analysis of potential interactions and performance within your department, report in your notebook the behavior and actions that might indicate a prospective member's propensity for constructive or nonconstructive behavior in any of the four areas, which are described in the following subsections.

Attitude Orientation

Review each employee relative to a series of attitude orientation characteristics. These characteristics include adaptability, aggressiveness-assertiveness, perseverance, and work ethic.

Adaptability

Individuals lacking on-the-job adaptability are inflexible, reluctant to learn new methods or adapt to new ideas, and have difficulty relating to personalities unlike themselves. In contrast, people who are too adaptable are said to be wishy-washy, unwilling to take a stand, or chameleon-like, changing with any minor fluctuation in the work environment.

Individuals who demonstrate adaptability in good balance can adjust well to new methods and ideas with excellent practical results. They also are flexible in dealing with a variety of people, reacting proactively and positively to change, and developing not only a plan A, but also a plan B in accomplishing set objectives. In essence, these individuals are versatile and can accommodate change positively, function well in crisis, and set new goals readily as circumstances dictate. This behavior is illustrated on the adaptability bell curve shown in Figure 6.2. You can draw similar bell curves for other attitude orientation factors to chart pluses and minuses. Write the initials of team members who represent points along the curve relative to their behavior.

Aggressiveness-Assertiveness

Individuals who demonstrate aggressiveness-assertiveness are able to make a stand and stay with their objective without wavering in their position. These individuals take command appropriately in all business situations, and they are enterprising, direct, and persuasive in their business dealings.

Individuals whose behavior falls along the minus range of the curve (if you were to draw a bell curve similar to Figure 6.2) usually will not take a stand on major issues and are overlooked by

Figure 6.2. Adaptability Bell Curve.

Advantageously adaptable

Will adapt only if pushed

Can change course of direction readily

Totally inflexible

"All over the place"

-

+

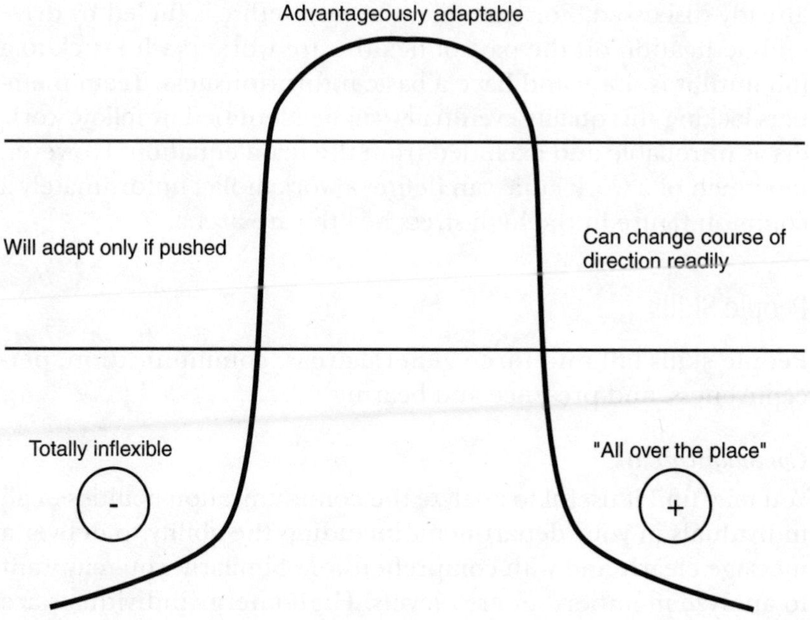

managers. At the plus extreme would be those who are too aggressive or pushy and who may be characterized as obnoxious, overbearing, or offensive. They alienate fellow team members and over time become isolated or, worse yet, they create unnecessarily difficult situations.

Perseverance

Perseverant workers are consistently persistent and tenacious in accomplishing a goal. They forge ahead tirelessly to a successful end despite situational obstacles. These players tenaciously assist fellow team members in the pursuit of group objectives.

Individuals who lack perseverance will quit at the first detour and usually bring someone down with them. That is to say, their malaise and resistance toward accomplishing a goal can act as a negative contagion and affect the morale and motivation of other team members.

Too much perseverance leads to tunnel vision; that is, these players are task-oriented at the expense of being mission-oriented.

Work Ethic

Work ethic is encompassed in some of the work personality factors already discussed. For example, the work ethic is fueled by drive and dedication on the part of health care workers who stick to a job until it is done and have a basic industriousness. Team members lacking this quality eventually will be identified by fellow workers as unreliable and excluded from the team equation. However, too much of a work ethic can define a workaholic, unfortunately a common figure in the high-stress health care arena.

People Skills

People skills fall into three general areas: communication, perceptiveness, and presence and bearing.

Communication

You may find it useful to analyze the communication abilities of all individuals in your department, including the ability to deliver a message clearly and with comprehension. Similarly, you may want to analyze members' energy levels. High-energy individuals are enthusiastic, enthralled by their work, convey a sense of electricity in their encouragement to others, and are eager to take on all new responsibilities and challenges.

Perceptiveness

Perceptiveness relates to the insight individuals possess in dealing with others. Perceptive workers understand the people equation in the health care team process. Those lacking in this quality focus on people only after a problem surfaces, as they tend to be oblivious to the people aspect. At the other extreme are "overly" perceptive individuals, who focus on personalities and interpersonal problems at the expense of programs, processes, products, and objectives.

Presence and Bearing

In weighing the concept of presence and bearing, simply ask yourself, *What would I think of this individual if he was the first person I came in contact with upon coming to the hospital?* The answer will tell you what customer-patients and fellow workers perceive about this particular team member. Presence and bearing—overall demeanor—denote the positive or negative impression created in a business situation.

Managerial Aptitude

Creativity is simply defined for our purposes as the ability to come up with new ideas and creative solutions to problems. Part of this aptitude is the ability to delegate responsibly to expedite service delivery and effectiveness of action. By exercising independent judgment, a worker makes decisions autonomously when necessary. Managerial aptitude relies on the ability to construct plans and make preparations for significant action.

Managerial aptitude might not be critically important in some areas. For example, if most members of your department are classified as nonexempt, nonskilled, or hourly employees, managerial aptitude might not be an essential quality. It is essential, however, to have team members who are relatively creative, can make plans, and use their own common sense in executing action. A preliminary analysis of each individual team member will disclose strategies for enhancing these abilities and managing individuals who demonstrate varying strengths and weaknesses in these work personality areas.

Team Orientation

This category of work personality analysis addresses the very issue of this chapter—team orientation. Strong teams cooperate, relate well to peers, are loyal to the organization, and have the requisite technical expertise.

Cooperation is the ability to work as part of a team and to interact cohesively with other team members. Truly cooperative individuals can coordinate activities with others, act as leaders within the team structure, and value team participation and group activity.

Individuals with no sense of cooperation act autonomously and in isolation from the team. They may become subversive and self-motivated to the point of destroying team morale and group interaction. At the other extreme are health care workers who are so team oriented that their individual contribution is suspect. These workers often use *we* instead of *I* when discussing their business situations and accomplishments.

Employee relations, an important component to team orientation, might also be described as peer relations, or the ability to work within a group when the term refers to individuals in a non-supervisory capacity. Individuals who relate well to peers enjoy a productive and progressive work relationship with other members of the team.

Loyalty and technical expertise have already been discussed, but remember that extremes in either characteristic should be avoided. For example, you would not want a subversive or disloyal team member, or one who lacked sufficient technical expertise. Nor would you want a player whose loyalty was misplaced or a pure technician who was unable to share information with a team spirit.

Performing a Work Personality Analysis

Using the four main elements of the Quan-Com System (attitude orientation, people skills, managerial aptitude, and team orientation), analyze the potential strengths and weaknesses of all team members relative to their potential to contribute to group goals. Like other areas of management, your preliminary judgment will be somewhat subjective and certainly not a quantitative exercise. Next do a preliminary inventory of each individual's preferences, tendencies, and liabilities (refer again to the adaptability bell curve in Figure 6.2). This can be done by dedicating a page in your notebook to each team member, and dividing each page into three columns that represent the individual:

1. Preferences for work assignments, and teammates with whom they enjoy working
2. Positive aspects of work personality
3. Negative aspects of work personality, and teammates with whom they dislike working

Having accomplished this, you are now ready to look at setting up a plan for team accomplishment, which includes determining what type of team you presently have and, more important, what type of team you want to have. By now, you already know that you have an assortment of talent and a variety of personalities and team orientations among current staff (the rule rather than the exception). In the next sections I explore what kind of teams you can construct and how to reinforce team orientation based on individual strengths and talents.

Establishing Team Orientation

As a new health care manager, chances are you are inheriting a ready-made team. No doubt your department has already been selected and has worked together under the leadership of your predecessor. To create your own team orientation and build (or rebuild) a team, first examine the current team. Even if you are the exception and are in the process of forming a new team, the following guidelines can help establish the standards you wish to incorporate into your team-building and team-orientation efforts. First look at what makes a strong, winning team. Eight qualities mark a winning team:

1. Motivation to excel
2. Credibility and respect
3. Progressiveness in taking action
4. Inspiration and the will to be successful
5. Talent and expertise
6. Allegiance to the group
7. Achievement orientation
8. Spirit and positive outlook

Motivation

A team that attains its stated mission successfully and effectively is well motivated. Motivation can come from a variety of sources, the first of which should be the department manager. Motivation can be positive, emphasizing encouragement and progressive action, or negative, emphasizing less-than-satisfactory consequences due to failure to meet team objectives.

Motivation also must come from the work group itself. Individuals must inspire one another to greater performance and support the efforts of all team members. Also, each team member must be self-motivated (as evidenced by drive, discussed earlier in this chapter).

Credibility and Respect

Because it is known for getting the job done, a strong team earns credibility and commands the respect of customer-patients and other departments. Strong teams have a wide base of technical knowledge and can readily provide whatever level of assistance is needed. Such teams are self-perpetuating, as they attract and retain other strong members.

Progressiveness

A progressive team grows continuously and develops expertise in an ongoing effort to enhance quality outcomes. Teams become progressive by valuing individual contribution, constantly attaining new technical knowledge, and experimenting with and implementing new methods of practices. Conversely, a regressive team loses ground and fails to participate positively in organizational activities, and its members are labeled as losers throughout the organization.

Inspiration

Great teams are inspired by their will to win. Their individual members are success driven, and their leaders reinforce the importance of succeeding. This combination is the basis for inspiration. So that teams remain inspired, clear goals must be established, outcomes must be defined, and methods of attaining success should be delineated by the leader with the participation of all members.

Talent and Expertise

Without the expert talent and ability needed to achieve desired ends, a team is doomed to failure. Talent encompasses technical knowledge, performance ability relative to current health care mandates, and awareness of business objectives within the context of those mandates.

Achievement Orientation

All teams want to achieve on an individual, group, and organizational level. In making their contribution, team members must be challenged to become the best they can be. Therefore, you must foster educational development, training opportunities, open communication, and goal attainment for each staff member.

Spirit

Team spirit can be described as supportive, positive, results-oriented, or winning. These adjectives relate not only to the perceptions others have of the team, but to something perhaps more important: the team's perception of itself. Losing teams are characterized as whiners, dysfunctional, or negative.

Conducting a Team-Type Analysis

Teams are formed for a number of reasons, and they either succeed or fail for a number of reasons. In this section I help you determine what kind of team you need and provide clues as to probability of success. I also guide you in taking an inventory of your current team so you can determine what type of team and team atmosphere you need to create.

Getting the Job Done

Some teams are formed simply to accomplish a particular task. Such teams can be described as matrix management groups and might exist only over the short term. In examining your department, determine whether certain individuals should be paired (or grouped) together for a specific function or completion of a specific task.

Recognizing Teamship

Poorly designated teams do not even realize that they are in fact work groups. Several individuals who work together on a constant basis may not see themselves as doing teamwork. A solution might be to designate a subgroup officially as a team; for example, if several individuals in your accounting department handle accounts receivable, you might call them the AR team. This method helps individuals form an identification, and it clearly delineates for the team the lines of support. It also increases their morale and sense of affiliation, while enhancing their communication flow—both within the new team and throughout the department.

Being Numerically Oriented

Every team should be numerically oriented. For example, an athletic team measures its successes by the team's won-lost record; a performance group quantifies its success by how much endowment money it receives and the number of performances it does in a given year. Teams must have a measurable goal (for example, repeating no more than a certain number of lab tests due to lost patient charts). Establish measurable numerical goals (significant numbers) using percentage, time, quantity, and fiscal indicators.

Some numerically oriented teams are "bottom liners," that is, oriented to success strictly as measured by numbers. For such groups (for example, an accounting department, which naturally is driven by numbers), set numerical goals to attain. You might prefer to use score sheets or some other device to chart progress over time. Use time-sequenced progress charts as comparison guides and, depending on your management style, share them at department meetings or post them in a prominent place in the department. This will serve as a constant reward and reminder for the group.

Defining Team Objectives

Some teams are thrown together basically because each member has a lot of talent. However, members' commitment is shaky because they have not been shown how to work together. Establishing a sense of cohesiveness through clarity of objectives is one intent of the continuous quality improvement (CQI) process. If faced with a cohesiveness problem, you might consider holding a group meeting for the purpose of defining objectives for the team, specifying how each talent can contribute to the group process, and allowing the group opportunity to answer the question, *How can we achieve collectively at the highest possible level?*

Another team may have medium talent but high commitment, perhaps a combination that is preferable to the first. Individuals with high commitment can sharpen their talent by working together and supporting each other's efforts to grow and develop. The cohesion demonstrated by this type of team can be used to increase interaction, define responsibilities, and identify ways to create synergy between talent and commitment effectively.

Using Star Players

Many teams have charismatic players who can have a positive or negative effect on the entire team. These individuals are usually very outspoken, typically have been on the team a long time, and have credibility with other team members. Seek out their allegiance at the beginning of your management tenure. If they affect the team negatively by virtue of their poor performance, document their performance, meet with them to put them on notice, and, if necessary, recommend termination. Provide positive performers with extra attention. Ask them how the team might get better and how members who might not be up to par can be supported. Enlist their support in developing the team and identifying areas in which the team can improve and grow.

In addition to star players, a team has steady players and low achievers. Use your superstars as role models and sources of positive motivation. Encourage their participation in group meetings. The steady players (probably most of the department) should be dealt with individually to learn their perceptions on how to increase performance, enhance goal attainment, and how they might contribute more strongly to the group. Underachievers are generally disinterested in their work and have no innate drive to improve on their activities. Document their work during performance evaluations, and, if necessary, recommend termination.

Establishing a Mentor System

Usually, a work group has a mixture of rookies, individuals new to the department (and perhaps the organization), and veterans, individuals who have been on board and working in the field a long time. This team mix can be used to great advantage if you implement a mentor system; that is, assign newer members to work with the more seasoned staff on a regular basis. Use your positively motivated veterans to help orient new employees, train rookies, and provide support for the entire department.

Using Veterans Effectively

Some work groups include individuals who have worked for the organization a long time and are experts in their technical field. These expert veterans can be a tremendous asset if most of them are motivated positively. Draw on this considerable resource by asking, *Given that you've been in this business for quite a while, what can we do to become even better?* However, teams whose veteran players appear burned out or complacent may need to have the fires rekindled. Try arriving at individual goals or discussing with the personnel department ways to boost the performance evaluation process so that tenure and experience can be rewarded in line with performance.

Recognizing Opportunity

Although it is a rare occasion, you might inherit a team of rookies. That is, the majority of players have not worked in the field for long, are new to the organization, or both. A visionary manager craves this opportunity to work with a clean slate. If this is the case, use the suggestions in Chapter Fifteen. Remember, however, that in this scenario, a disproportionate amount of time will be required for training and development.

Capitalizing on Familiarity

If your department players already know each other, have worked together for a while, and therefore know each other's strengths and weaknesses, use this familiarity as part of your orientation efforts. Begin your team-building efforts by asking individuals how they can improve, who they consider to be the stronger players, and what weaknesses the team may face as a group. Do not focus on individual weaknesses because employees may fear a witch hunt. Remember, take input from team members as subjective perceptions to supplement your own perceptions, not as an exclusive or definitive source of information.

However, teams that have never worked together and thus are unfamiliar with individual dynamics again provide the opportunity for you to work with a clean slate. Your main strategy should be to establish policies and operational procedures. Additionally, much effort should be directed toward educating your staff concerning your own objectives and desired expectations and toward developing individual goals for all members.

Capitalizing on Past Successes

If the majority of individuals on your staff worked in departments that have been successful, you have a great advantage. Primarily, these individuals will contribute to the motivation, spirit, and inspiration necessary for a winning team. Usually these individuals are steady performers who know how to win. Use them as role models, sources for suggestions, and proponents of positive contribution.

On the flip side, individuals who have worked in groups that have not been successful, or that have been depicted as losers, may have difficulty responding to positive motivation. If this is the case, you must impart three messages to the team. First, encourage them to focus primarily on the present and the future. Second, ask their opinion why past contributions were so unsuccessful and what their perceptions are on improvement. Third, use performance assessment and observation to determine whether the cause for poor achievement lies with the individual (or certain individuals) or with some other dynamic (for example, outdated policy, budget cutback, or suspension of the training program).

Benefiting from a Family Orientation

Family-oriented team members are socially cohesive and genuinely enjoy interaction with one another on a personal level. This type of team has both advantages and disadvantages. An advantage is that people will naturally support each other and work cohesively. A disadvantage is that certain individuals may be considered "closet skeletons" of the family. Try to determine whether family dissension is due to performance or personality issues. Maintain objectivity—do not play the matriarch or patriarch role. Neither should you arbitrate disputes. Attempt conflict resolution by keeping the emphasis on performance, and apply the strategies in the next subsection to underscore your role as a leader, not parent.

Allowing Independence

Some teams are predominated by experts with outstanding technical acumen in their specialty area. These teams often operate on the principle of autonomy: They are self-motivated, self-directed, and function more or less independently. Do not try enforcing a group perspective onto such a team; rather, take advantage of each member's expertise and meet with the team occasionally (not regularly) to share ideas. Keep the conversation tied closely to technical issues and ways in which technical data can be shared. Do not worry about socializing within this group or enforcing strict interpersonal standards. Doing so can have a counter-reaction—it can further distance these key contributors.

Maintaining Status Quo

Certain teams are very happy with the status quo; that is, they do not crave opportunities to improve their performance. Like the jaded veterans described earlier, these team members may need a new dose of motivation. Try to ascertain what might remotivate these individuals. Following are five suggestions for re-instilling motivation for the status quo team:

1. Explore new areas for creative activity.
2. Identify the performance dynamics of each individual member (what makes him or her tick).
3. Establish new goals for each individual.
4. Establish new goals for the entire department.
5. Implement a reward system; for example, employee-of-the-month status that incorporates time off as department needs dictate.

Work closely with both your supervisor and the human resource department to find positive ways to shake up the status quo team. Usually there is an inordinate amount of dormant talent that simply needs a wake-up call.

Identifying the "Collective We" Team

Certain teams are so group oriented that they see themselves as a "collective we" rather than a collection of individuals united in a common goal. These teams are considered to be "galvanized," meaning that they function as a unit and often will move only as fast as the slowest member or work only as hard as the laziest member. Sit down with each member to discuss individual goals and objectives, keeping the conversation focused on *individual* contribution. Discourage discussion of group activity, but without denigrating the importance of working cohesively. Clarify your position that the standard for excellence will be the expectations set by the best worker in the group.

Identifying the Leader-Oriented Team

A leader-oriented team, the easiest type for a new manager to inherit, will closely monitor the behavior and actions of the new leader and apply those standards and outcome observations to their own work. Therefore, strong, effective leadership (as described in

Chapter Eight) is the best strategy for generating progress on a leader-oriented team. Remember that in this case, as in all types of teams, your actions, words, and plans will be closely scrutinized and evaluated by all members of the team. So if you are fair and forthright in your actions and exhibit behavior that helps group progress, you are off to a good start.

Reinforcing Team Orientation

Remember, establishing team orientation is not an exact science; numerous strategies are available to help you constantly reinforce a team concept within your department. These strategies are drawn from the checklist of team qualities in Exhibit 6.1.

• The first strategy is to *establish common objectives* for the team. Let all team members know the objectives of the department and the main mission of the department in your estimation as well as

---

Exhibit 6.1. Checklist of Team Qualities.

Fundamental Attributes
- Common objectives
- Shared perceptions and perspectives
- Diversity of talent
- Open communication
- Appropriate knowledge base

Essential Abilities
- Ability to handle change
- Ability to motivate and inspire others
- Ability to bounce back from adversity
- Ability to grow, learn, and develop
- Ability to establish new goals for continuous improvement

Foundation Factors
- Strong leadership
- Clear direction
- Reinforcement of perspective and spirit
- Adequate resources and facilities
- Sound balance between control and freedom

---

that of the organization. Remember that management involves asking the right questions. Question your staff about their perceptions as to the main objectives of the department and the common goals toward which individuals should be striving as members of the team.

• Feel free to *share your perceptions* with all members of the team. Let them know what your opinion is on various organizational issues without appearing disloyal or lacking in allegiance to organizational objectives. This will encourage individuals on your team to share their perceptions and their perspectives on organizational initiatives, as well as their insight on how to achieve departmental objectives that will contribute to the good of the organization. Achievement is centered around the individual and enhanced by group action. Therefore, sharing of perspectives and perceptions is necessary to establish team orientation and vital lines of communication.

• Remember that diversity of talent characterizes a successful team. Recognize *individual talents* and ask for suggestions on how each individual's talent might be applied to the team. In the attitude surveys conducted by my firm, a number of employees have indicated that they have many suggestions but have not been asked by their manager to share them. The best source for learning how to create synergism between individual talent and group contribution is the individual department member.

• *Keep feedback lines open.* Encourage two-way feedback between members and yourself. Ask their opinions on your management style and on the way that the department is progressing toward stated goals. Listening skills and perception skills are important elements of decision making, as well as contributing to the group process. Again, use the questions in Appendix C as a model for asking the right questions on team achievement. Primarily, you're asking for how team members can better contribute to the group and who they can support to create a greater team effort.

• Good teams *have the ability to handle change.* Try to identify any changing dynamics or particular factors affecting your department as proactively as possible. Once again, elicit ideas from your staff about what is changing relative to their jobs and, more important, how they can best prepare to handle that change successfully.

- *Encourage all members to motivate one another* and support one another through transitions.
- The team's ability to *bounce back from adversity* is a hallmark of success. As a health care manager, you may have to reassign individuals occasionally to help team members who require extra assistance. Rely on veterans and stronger players to provide this assistance not only to help achieve objectives but also to increase team allegiance and individual motivation.
- Provide as many opportunities as possible for your team to *grow, learn, and develop*. Present as many in-service exercises as possible, and use the expertise within your department to present new ideas to the group. One strategy in this area is to have show-and-tell sessions in which team members explain to each other new principles, strategies, and methods of accomplishing technology-based ends.
- Hold meetings at least once a quarter to *establish new goals* for the department for continuous improvement. Review past goals and accomplishments, seek explanations for why goals were either achieved or not achieved, and seek input from the group concerning their perceptions as to why goals and objectives were (or were not) achieved. Make this a group process to ensure credibility as well as maximum input and opportunities for shared knowledge.
- Never discount the degree of scrutiny or underestimate the power of perception on the part of a team observing its leader. You must consistently provide *strong leadership,* using the guidelines offered in this chapter. As discussed in Chapter Four, exemplary leadership is fortified by executing decisions and actions that put the best interest of the team and the organization at the forefront.
- *Provide clear direction* on a daily basis, both to the individuals within the group and to the group itself.
- Take the time to *renew your perspective and replenish staff spirit* by conducting quarterly progress review, inviting suggestions, and encouraging participation.
- Always *make sure that your team has the resources needed* to get the job done. The key word in this sentence is *need,* and the vital necessities for performance should be provided by the organization with your assistance as the health care manager. Remember

that as circumstances change, the need for additional resources might change. Therefore, keep up to date on the needs and desires of your team and your subgroup.

• Keep in mind that *team orientation is a balancing act.* The balance between freedom and control, individual and group performance, and personal motivation and organizational spirit can be maintained mostly by clear vision, open communication, and progressive action. As a health care manager, recognize the importance of progressively analyzing individual strengths, team orientation, and using commonsense strategies to encourage team achievement and garner group performance.

Any attempt at introducing the practical precepts of ethics and value-driven action (VDA) programs into a health care setting must be anchored in realistic expectations, practical packaging, and a direct intent to produce meaningful outcomes and results. A specific needs-analysis must be conducted at the outset of the program to ascertain not only what will work, but perhaps more important, what will not work, or even be considered tenable, by members of the health care organization. This latter point is extremely important because the health care professional has been deluged with a variety of organizational development programs whose banality is insulting, irrelevant, and faddish. The outcome of such programs is usually one of two reactions:

So what? We still have problems, the hospital is still empty, and I'm gonna get laid off!

Leadership spent good money that could have been better spent on our salaries and needed supplies or saving jobs and taking care of patients.

These reactions destroy the trust that is required between leadership and staff in any successful health care organization.

Your organization's VDA development effort must not have a trendy name or any features that can be construed as phony, inauthentic, or faddish. The recent CQI craze among health care organizations has left a multitude of health care professionals with a justifiable antipathy for any trendy, insincere attempts at organizational renewal. Leadership must take a realistic outlook by accepting a commitment by a majority of organizational members to at least give the program a chance, as opposed to the unrealistic expectation for total consensus. There will always be dissension, notably on the part of the nonplayers who are self-absorbed, self-professed "victims" of anything and everything that the organization undertakes in a positive, honest attempt to better the workplace. If the VDA program is to be successful, it will stress

- Outcomes over opinions
- Product not process
- Results over remorse or retribution over past events
- Individual accountability and performance contributions to the organization
- Meaningful intents and objectives
- An approach different from total quality management and other failures of the process-oriented, "psycho-babble" era

To accomplish a real-world, practical organizational development process, four words—pride, accountability, commitment, and trust (PACT)—have worked successfully for us in health care organizations from Hawaii to Oklahoma to Maryland to Saudi Arabia.

Pride

A major motivational factor in any organization, health care or otherwise, is the sentiment of genuine investment in the organization through action and performance that is inspired by pride in the organization. A seemingly eclectic roster of organizations such as the United States Marine Corps, the Xerox Corporation, and the Girl Scouts all have withstood various travails and organizational strife and have developed and advanced through time and change due to the feeling by their members that each was, simply, part of the best.

Popular phrases such as "send for the Marines," "make a Xerox copy," and "Girl Scout Cookies" did not enter the lexicon accidentally.

Accountability

The worst statements that can be uttered in a health care workplace within hearing distance of a customer-patient are, *That's not my job. We don't do that here. I don't know.* All these excuses convey clearly to the listener that the speaker does not care about patient health or customer service and, moreover, confirms the worst suspicions harbored by the customer-patient. The VDA program must stress individual accountability and positive action that is a credit to the organization and a clear responsibility to upholding organizational mission and objectives.

Commitment

The commitment to the principal four constituent groups of a health care organization is mandatory to the continued success of the organization and the individual. In the proper order, these four constituencies must be the everyday targets of optimum performance by all members of the organization:

1. Customer-patients, who ultimately drive the organization and control its destiny, and who display their commitment to the health care organization by virtue of its patronage as demonstrated by emergency room visits, physician support, and participation in fundraising
2. The organization, which demonstrates commitment to the employee by providing employment that represents the opportunity of using all of one's talents in the pursuit of providing health care services to those in need of healing
3. The team-department, which coordinates and synthesizes individual talents into an expert, competent, able group who can fluidly provide service in an efficient and effective manner
4. The individual, whose commitment to maximum professional and personal development is facilitated by daily delivering top effort in all endeavors

Trust

Perhaps one of the few absolute certainties in industrial psychology is the importance of trust and the inability to regain trust after it has been breached. Employees, physicians, specialized staff, and volunteers may have the same reaction to a real or even perceived abridgement of trust: *If you burned me once, you'll likely do it again!* The manner in which new leadership initiatives are introduced must be authentic, straight-shooting, and clear if any hope of building or regaining trust is to be realized.

Operationalizing a Value-Driven Action Program

Once a commitment has been made to developing and implementing a value-driven organizational development effort, the innovation and installation of several strategies should be initiated. Eight fundamental programs can be customized, introduced, and incorporated into the fabric of the health care organization at a relatively low cost and with minimal consultant or other outside effort. This latter point is vital, as the perception that any organizational development program has been developed by a consultant for the benefit of the consultant's wallet rather than the progress of the organization's four main constituents is the precursor of failure for the entire program implementation.

The following eight programs fit into the organizational development efforts at most health care organizations:

1. *House rules.* A list of strategies for customer-patient relations that can be printed on a laminated card can be a good reminder for standards and can serve as valid performance criteria. At Pascack Valley Hospital in New Jersey, these standards, linked to their "Whatever It Takes" customer service program, were listed on the flip-side of each employee's name badge. Outstanding performance was rewarded with a merit bonus—a needed incentive for any people-development program in health care.

2. *Time lines.* The future plans of the organization, as well as a general review of its organizational performance over a yearly period, can be easily published as a time line depiction of organizational performance and shared with all employees, physicians, and volunteers. The Veterans Administration (VA) Medical System in Hawaii, consisting of four separate facilities on four islands, found that the publication of time line reviews and time line strategic plans in an annual report for the coming year was a terrific conveyance of getting commitment and understanding from all members of the four facilities.

3. *Targeted selection system.* Organizational standards, such as the CARE factors (community, accountability, respect, and excellence) at the Shore Health System in Maryland, can quantify performance standards at the essential how-we-do-it level. The Shore System and

other organizations we've worked with have also used a structured selection system replete with a set of seventy-five open-ended questions and interpretive guides to help in making sound decisions about the recruitment and selection of top job candidates. The interview questions and cues in Appendix B of this book provide a great start to implementing a structured selection system.

4. *Criterion-based, values-driven performance evaluation systems.* A major motivational tool for both the marginal performer and the superstar employee is the annual performance evaluation. However, when the performance evaluation is merely a checklist review of the existing job description, it becomes virtually impossible to distinguish the great performer from the "goldbricker." At Jane Phillips Medical Center in Bartlesville, Oklahoma, a performance evaluation that measures how the individual performed relative to job specifications, *and* assesses the CARE or PACT factors of attitude orientation, people skills, and team orientation, *and* recognizes contributions made beyond the set job description has been a key element in the renewal of this important, urban, nonprofit facility.

5. *Volunteer education.* Consider for a minute how many volunteers are present every day in your health care facility. Whether you measure by numbers or percentages, the likelihood that they become instrumental in the perception formation of your customer-patients is very high. Holy Cross Medical Center in Los Angeles found that inclusion of the volunteers in every educational forum ensured that the volunteers were on "the same page" as the paid staff members and moreover that a clear understanding was established regarding essential house rules and performance standards.

6. *CRI surveys.* Attitude surveys have been used to the point of tedium and inefficacy over the past ten years. It is a fair assumption that their impact has become negligible due to overuse and the confluence of media and organizational input, which leads the survey respondent to guess the right answer. The Change Readiness Index (CRI) is a scorecard system in which the respondent rates the organization in the categories of customer-patient service, organizational reaction and readiness to change, and overall organizational dynamics such as communication and morale. The VA Medical Center in Phoenix, Arizona, used the CRI to assess the

right strategy and approach for not only the commencement of a new leadership team, but also for strategy formulation in every new venture undertaken in their immense growth over the past eight years.

7. *Execugrams.* There is no such thing as overcommunication in a health care organizational setting. The use of periodic *execugrams,* which are correspondence from the CEO of a facility to all working staff members and volunteers, is an easily implemented management tool. At the Mercy Health System in Oklahoma, these messages were coded in green and contained information ranging from a favorable bond rating to news about the opening of a new clinic. The use of a color other than white for the execugram ensures that the document stands out from the missives usually delivered on white paper stock.

8. *Executive commitment.* The chief executive of every health care facility and their second tier of leadership—that is, all of the executives who report directly to the CEO—should undertake various new tasks with a renewed commitment to their own accountability. Many failing health care organizations like to expound on their commitment to employees, quality care, and all the other platitudes. Three questions can usually be asked to determine whether commitment exists at the executive level or whether the stated commitment to value-driven leadership is simply polemic drivel:

- When was the last time the executive walked completely through, around, and down all corridors and crannies of the facility?
- When was the last time the executive asked a random employee for any ideas on how to improve the facility at large or even about the quality of staff work life?
- When was the last time the executive asked introspectively, *Was I honest, direct, and hard-working in all I did on this day?*

If the answer to any of these questions is anything other than *today,* the outlook for the success of the value-driven action program is nil. In the final analysis, a commitment to decency, a sense of pride regarding the organization's mission, a deep-seated sense of leadership accountability, and a demonstrable ability to trust all those involved in the caring process constitute the ultimate value-driven action program. With such a program, the health care facility meets the charter of caring for those in need in the best traditions of American health care; without it, it's just another place where sick people go because they have no choice.

The most important choice is the decision made by the health care leader at every level to make value-driven action a daily, constant requisite of selfless service—not a fad or a "sometime" thing. The good news is that most of us in health care have a desire to lead a life worthy of our professional calling; the bad news is that we often get bogged down in nuances that cause disorientation from our precious mission. Renewal is easy if it is truly desired. I hope some of these ideas will give you a place to start.

Conclusion

Just as individuals are unique, each team is unique. Therefore, no one solution serves to establish team orientation. The worst mistake a new health care manager can make is to assume that a group of individuals with diverse talents and different perspectives will work cohesively and consistently. The team process takes time, so communication must be ongoing. Common goals must be stated and adjusted with changing circumstances, and positive motivation must be provided in healthy and abundant doses. The saving grace of establishing a team is that most health care workers are well motivated to provide stellar service to customer-patients.

Chapter Seven

Strategic Analysis and Decision Making

The ability to make timely decisions, exercise independent judgment, and gain positive results is the criterion by which a manager's ability is evaluated. Although there is no magic formula for analyzing data, considering options, and making a winning determination, there are several approaches a manager should take in arriving at decisions and taking action.

In making the transition from staff professional to manager, decision making will figure prominently among your new responsibilities. Until now, your decisions affected your technical performance as it related to your own individual work role. Now you will make managerial decisions that have direct impact on the work lives and overall performance of other individuals, namely your staff. In a climate where health care resources are limited, you must also make decisions that concern a number of areas: human resources, operational equipment, and financial expenditures, to name a few. Every decision you make will have consequence not only on the work life of others, but also on the long-term progress of your department. Although at first this responsibility might seem overwhelming, it is something you must confront on a daily basis. Your staff look to your decisions to direct their work activity, the organization depends on your decisions to help effect positive action, and customer-patients rely on your decisions for positive outcome with the health care they receive.

In this chapter I present several methods for coping with the pressures that are inherent in decision making and, more important, for adopting a decision-making process that is both realistic and progressive for daily use. I also look at fundamental aspects of the decision-making process, explore the ten phases of that process, and provide several strategies to help with what may appear a daunting responsibility.

Values Essential to Decision Making

Five essential values drive the decision-making process: accountability, adaptability, dependability, responsibility, and visibility.

1. As discussed in Chapters One and Two, managers must use all the tools available to them in accomplishing their set goals. In addition, they must be *accountable* for how those resources are used. In analyzing quantitative data and taking into account the potential ramifications of their decisions, managers assume accountability on several levels. They must be accountable not only for the decision made, but also for how the decision was determined, what data were analyzed, and which course of action was pursued in arriving at the final decision.

2. To demonstrate the flexibility needed for managing health care delivery in a turbulent business climate, a manager must embrace a certain degree of *adaptability*. This means being flexible in considering options, being able to deal with a wide range of people, and having a versatile business approach. Care must be taken, however, to avoid being too adaptable; that is, becoming wishy-washy or irresolute by constantly straying from an established course of action, or spending so much time considering options that the manager ultimately fails to arrive at a set course of action. Therefore, managers must reach a balance between rigid thinking and ineffectual leadership.

3. A health care manager must demonstrate *dependability*. As stated, staff depend on leaders to make timely decisions that, for the most part, are correct and specify a proper course of action. Constant reluctance to take stands or making decisions without benefit of communication or staff input will not promote the perception among staff and the organization that the manager is dependable, or worse, that the manager values enlightened input.

4. It should come as no surprise that *responsibility* is a key value element in the decision-making process. A strong manager

embraces responsibility for making decisions, takes ownership for them, and views the management role as a commitment to organizational excellence. This attitude mandates selfless participation in the decision-making process so as to consider at all times what is good for the organization and to consider both the positive and negative ramifications of a decision on staff and the entire organization. All of this must be done keeping in mind the organization's objective of providing stellar health care service to all its customer-patients. Managers who shirk responsibility may be seen as being overly political, figureheads, or worse. Even when managers delegate a particular task, they ultimately must take responsibility for the outcome.

5. As already discussed (in Chapters Two and Five), a manager must endure *visibility* in all decision-making activities. Visible leaders are present and on the scene, and in conducting their activities they are around to hear the cheers and the boos. Furthermore, a manager's visibility does not diminish in critical times or in situations that are out of the norm. At no time should a visible manager hear the question, *Who's in charge?*

A Ten-Part Process for Decision Making

Having committed to the five value elements that drive decision making, you are now ready to adopt a strong, objective process for making decisions. The plan I suggest consists of ten sequential segments that are appropriate for most situations that arise in a health care environment. It includes not only the critical long-term decisions, but the daily short-term decisions you must make that require quick action. Exhibit 7.1 illustrates this process, which is separated into three phases: conceptual, analytical, and performance.

The *conceptual phase* encompasses four parts of the decision-making process. The first part is *identifying* the elements of the decision to be made. This includes knowing the final outcome you desire, the action that must be taken, and the goal of that action. This step also includes identifying areas from which you will draw data and develop an action plan. These areas include data sources, those individuals who will help execute the decision, and decision outcome indicators. Identification also includes reviewing the impact of your decision, pinpointing which parties in the organi-

Exhibit 7.1. Ten-Part Decision-Making Process.

Conceptual phase	Identification (identifying the elements of the decision to be made) Collection (gathering as much information as possible relative to the decision to be made) Validation (ensuring that you have the information, defined courses of action, and objectives you desire and need) Organization (examining staff roles, qualitative goals, resources, and vision)
Analytical phase	Scripting (fine-tuning the plans, using specific date, and considering specific circumstances and situations) Presentation (communicating with stakeholders) Clarification (ensuring clarity of roles, needs, objectives, and plans) Listening (looking for indicators, progress, or new challenges to be faced) Perception (monitoring nonverbal communication, collecting subjective opinions, and assessing moods)
Performance phase	Action and reaction (persevering and making adjustments as needed)

zation will be most affected by it, and determining the most positive outcome that could be generated by virtue of your decision.

In the second part of the conceptual phase, you are *collecting* as much information as possible regarding your decision. This means reviewing all sources of information, receiving the perceptions and input of your staff and colleagues, and gathering as much information as possible relative to the decision at hand. Collection also incorporates investigation, meaning that you research the best possible way of achieving your goal and consider how others might have come to similar decisions and pursued their objectives. A certain amount of legwork is inevitable as you develop an initial course of action.

Validation, the third part of the conceptual phase, prescribes that you review all information collected, the course of action under consideration, and the objectives desired so as to ensure that these are indeed appropriate given the situation. In understanding this review, ask yourself three key questions:

1. *Have I collected as much information as possible?* Looking at your data sources, consider all of the input provided by them and make a determination as to how applicable the information is to your situation.
2. *Are my data accurate and up to date?* Consider whether the data are realistic relative to your particular situation, have current and timely consequences, and have direct relevance to the course of action you are considering. Furthermore, are the data truthful and reliable for providing an accurate picture and a credible source of comparison?
3. *How will I set an agenda?* Basically, this question has to do with establishing protocols and priorities. This means giving thought to who should be involved, what course of action to pursue, which data segments make the most sense and have the most applicability to your situation, and how you can best apply the information gathered.

Once you have explored these questions, the validation process is complete. You have determined that your information is clear, applicable to your situation, and helpful in designing a course of action.

The fourth part of the conceptual phase, *organization,* comes into play as you look at various formulas for decision making. You will see that this step can be the most important segment of the decision-making process as you examine the role to be played by each staff member, the numerical goals for achievement, the optimum use of each available resource, and (stated in military terms) the "conduct of the march."

The second phase of the ten-part decision-making process, the *analytical phase* (see Exhibit 7.1), has to do with fine-tuning the plan. In *scripting*, more specific plans are drawn out, specific data are used, and particular circumstances and situations are considered. As a manager, you will now consider all potential problems your decision might create, the positive gains that will be realized, and, perhaps most important, how you will communicate your rationale and action plans to your staff and other involved parties.

Hence, *presentation* allows opportunity for all parties to participate early in the decision-making process. However, they must also be clued in as to what action is being taken, why it is being taken, and how it will affect their work life. Participants must also know the expectations demanded by the decision and have the opportunity to communicate their perceptions of the problem, the specific impact of the decision on their work life, and, of course, any further suggestions toward making the decision and the prescribed action a successful endeavor.

Once the decision has been made and the action to achieve the objective undertaken, it is important to employ a *clarification* process. Therefore, ask yourself, as well as other significant players in the operation, the following ten questions:

1. Does everyone know his or her role?
2. Are all of the resources needed for this operation available?
3. If the necessary resources are not available, what contingency plans are in place?
4. Do all staff understand the overall objective?
5. Do all staff understand the rationale for the decision?
6. Do all individuals know the action agenda for the entire department?
7. Have all potential positive gains been enumerated?
8. Have all potential negative outcomes been identified?
9. Have all major concerns been discussed and resolved appropriately and efficiently?
10. Are most of your staff and other involved individuals (such as members of other departments, peers, and other significant members of the organization) reasonably confident of a positive result?

If the answer to question 10 is yes, the decision-making process up to this point probably has been a success. If the answer is no, however, you have two options. One is to re-analyze all information and review all preceding steps of the process to see whether others' apprehension and negativity are valid. The second option—the one that requires more managerial courage—is to review all your options, review your data, and if you still feel convinced you have chosen the proper course of action, proceed with it. *Remember: not all of your decisions will be popular.* Certain individuals on your staff will be contrary and negative regardless of what decisions you make. Individuals in other departments, as well as well-meaning peers, might also question your decision simply in the interest of ensuring that you have considered all possible options. The key for success in this case is to trust your gut. If your instincts and intelligence indicate that you are making the right choice, stay the course and pursue your objectives by reassuring the well-wishers and ignoring the doomsayers.

Be certain to keep *listening* throughout the action phase of the process. Once individuals have begun to implement your plan and move toward the objective, it is vital to listen for any indicators of positive performance, possible problems, and new information that might affect the action.

Perception involves screening intangible information; for example, monitoring nonverbal communication, collecting subjective opinions, and assessing the overall departmental mood. Do not try to read too deeply into moods or into the negativity of poor performers. Rather, try to gauge the morale of your entire department and remember that your positive outlook on the decision is a major contributing factor to the essential management dynamic of visibility. If you emphasize the positive and take supporting action accordingly, a visible example of appropriate action will be provided. Likewise, the management strength of being able to make minor alterations to a plan in the interest of improving action is part of adaptability, which is another management essential.

The final phase of the decision-making process is *performance,* which is defined by taking strong action or reaction through adverse circumstances, making minor changes to a plan when the need is evident, and communicating your rationale effectively throughout the process. Reaction entails monitoring the results of your action, responding to the concerns of individuals involved in the action, and adjusting the course of action as needed.

Practical Strategies to Support Decision Making

By adhering to the basic elements of this ten-part process, you at least have a framework for decision making and action planning. Specific strategies and tools for each phase help optimize the overall effect of the decision-making process. In the following sections I provide some strategies and tools for data collection and then review strategies and tools for data analysis and action planning.

Collecting Data

As already discussed, data collection and analysis is an important activity that takes place early in the ten-step process for decision making. Collect as much information as possible, and then make a timely decision based on the information at hand. Often, new health care managers have problems with this phase because of the misguided belief that a magical answer will solve all the problems of a particular nature. For example, if your organization has cut your department's budget, a new manager might believe that some magical solution will help deal with limited financial resources while somehow making the department staff feel good about the cut. Obviously this is a false hope, and although this is a universal problem in health care, unfortunately there is no right answer toward addressing the dilemma imposed by a limited budget.

New managers also make the mistake of believing that the more time that they spend collecting data, the more accurate their decision will be. Given the high visibility of a manager's position, too much time can be spent pedantically collecting information and becoming involved in a research process that instead of signaling a leader may demonstrate a manager who is afraid to make a decision. Not only is this perception extremely harmful to the manager's reputation, but the manager who spends more time on research than action does not inspire confidence or generate positive results on a consistent basis.

Therefore, two guidelines for data collection are as follows. First, try to obtain valid, realistic information; that is, do not expect a one-size-fits-all solution from colleagues or other sources. By recognizing that each situation is unique, you bring your individual style and approach to problem resolution. Second, recognize that the time frame for making a decision is as important as the decision itself. Once you have the information you need, rely on an intelligent gut feeling to arrive at an informed decision. Then initiate the action and begin implementation of your plan.

Studying Established Past Action

Several data sources should be part of your "homework" reserve. The first source is established past action; this includes what action predecessors or peer managers might have used in a given situation. Assuming their decision at the time was a correct one, you might gain some insight into the problem and a potential solution. Keep in mind, however, that what worked in the past may not necessarily suit current or future circumstances. Nonetheless, the overall dynamics of the situation might be similar and give you some clue for constructing your own plan of action.

Using the budget-cut example again, by exploring what your predecessor did, you might learn about the potential reaction your staff may have toward working with reduced resources. Furthermore, you might learn what your predecessor did "right," as well as what he or she did "wrong" in terms of staff reaction. By learning from others' mistakes as well as their positive contributions, you gain insight into what did not work and what did work. In a similar vein, you might ask colleagues for their ideas on what they would do or, better yet, what they did in the past to help staff deal with departmental budget cuts. In both cases, you will find valuable information that will provide you with a strong general frame of reference.

Researching Formal Reference

Another source of data is the body of formal references. Formal references are anything that might be construed as "book knowledge," including journals relevant to your technical area, management texts that offer pragmatic solutions, or your facility's manual of standard operating procedures. This last category includes specific protocols and policies your organization has adopted or specific bylaws applicable to the situation that you are currently confronting. Formal references can provide an important policy mandate and in some cases give clues for tackling your particular problem. For example, in addressing a budget cut that directly affects your department, you can consult your organization's standard operating procedures manual for fiscal management. Or you can review specific texts that suggest methods of achieving results with limited resources. Some books deal with presenting change in a positive light, and articles from financial journals might discuss ways of reconstructing budgets and making budget cuts creatively, without diminishing overall effectiveness.

Gathering Informal Information

The category of informal references might encompass your own insights, gained perhaps from a friend or relative who works in a management capacity in another industry (banking or school administration, for example). This person might be able to provide input by sharing how he makes decisions and effects action. Another source of informal information is reading material not directly related to the health care field. This body of work can include general management books or perhaps articles in journals and popular magazines.

Another informal data source on budget cuts might be an article in a business magazine about cuts that affect state government.

Analyzing Hard Data

In the data collection process, hard data should not be overlooked. Hard data can include any information that might have been generated by a questionnaire or survey, which gathers measurable facts. Measurable data, or quantitative information, can give you some outlook on the possible impact of your decision. Hard data on budget cuts can be gathered by reviewing organizational history relative to adverse reaction to budget cuts and employee perceptions toward dealing with them. For example, these five questions might be asked:

1. How can we best deal with the budget cuts?
2. What specific effect will the budget cuts have on our department?

3. What overall effect will the budget cuts have on our department?
4. How can we prevent the budget cuts from affecting the overall
quality of our patient care?
5. If you had to make the cuts, what areas would they affect?

Whether a preprinted questionnaire is used or questions are
asked informally in a meeting, the survey will generate data to assist
you in making your decision. It also will provide the benefit of
strengthening the communication link with your department colleagues and staff.

Weighing historical precedent in the data-gathering process
basically entails reviewing what worked in the past. This can also
be considered hard data. This review can be specific to your department or to circumstances in other departments whose dynamics are similar. One approach is to question individuals who were
involved in creating the precedent (to the extent this is feasible).
In most cases, newly appointed health care managers were previously staff professionals in the same organization. If this applies to
you, you have a natural frame of reference and point of comparison for looking at historical precedent that might have affected
you in the past.

If you were affected by a budget cut as a staff member, write
down what your feelings were at the time, how you perceived the
situation, and how you might have answered the five questions
above. Also review what your manager did at the time, what was
effective or ineffective, and what you learned from the decision.
Again, ask management colleagues how they might handle the
budget cuts, what plans they have, and what approaches they used
in the past in dealing with this ever-present dynamic of the health
care business.

Gathering Perceptions

In "gathering" perceptions, factor in the views and opinions of others who have had similar experience along with your own views and
opinions to arrive at a decision. The subjective nature of opinions
about budget cuts, for example, encompasses how others view the
cuts, what opinions they have toward coming to terms with them,

and what their overriding feeling is about how fiscal constraints affect their performance.

A word of caution: because perceptions are subjective, they must be kept in perspective; that is, taken with the proverbial grain of salt. Their validity is not absolute; nor are they necessarily 100 percent indicative of future action. Their purpose is to serve as a barometer of current mood and expectations. Therefore, they are only one component of the decision-making process.

Suppositions, also part of the perception collection process, include your educated guesses as to what will work. Visualize the impact of your decision and review all your options to ascertain what would work best in a given scenario. Ask yourself four "suppose" questions:

1. Suppose I follow plan 1—what will happen?
2. Suppose the worst that can happen, happens—how will I handle the situation?
3. Suppose the best of circumstances occurs—what course of action should I take?
4. Suppose I implement the decision I am now considering—what results will be gained?

While taking a subjective point of view during the decision-making process, discuss potential solutions with other members of your organization, particularly your supervisor. As your mentor, she is responsible for helping you in the data collection process, which will be furthered by gaining her suppositions and educated guesses relative to a particular situation.

Predicting the Advantages and Potential Disadvantages

An important element of data collection is consideration of advantages and disadvantages of your decision options. Who will benefit from your action? How might positive interpersonal effect best be achieved? Also consider when positive results might be realized, and set a time frame of realization of positive output.

Again using our budget-cut example, consider who would be involved with making the budget cuts, when some positive effects could be seen despite the cuts, and what the overall impact of the cuts might be. Set a projected implementation schedule and list the overall benefits, if any, that might emerge from the cuts.

At the same time, identify potential negative fallout. This includes adverse reaction, unfavorable perceptions that might arise from your action, and consequently the best way of addressing any negative reaction. By anticipating negative fallout, you have taken the first step toward addressing these problems and effecting positive action.

Following Your Instincts

The final element of data collection is trust in your instincts. Instinctual reaction gives credence to your insight into the problem at hand, the decision you have arrived at, and the action plan you will implement. It also mandates a certain amount of introspection, that is, considering the impact your decision will have not only on your staff but also on your own activities. Instinctual reaction also means trusting your intelligence and your ability to consider the facts objectively, subjectively analyze your data, and use your common sense to arrive at a course of action.

By using all the elements of data collection, you will achieve a comprehensive framework from which to make your decision. Remember to balance all these sources appropriately, given the nature of the action at hand. For example, in some cases hard data might carry more weight than supposition. What should be constant in all your decision-making efforts is the consistent application of all these sources creatively and realistically as you develop a conditioned habit of fully considering the range of your decisions, their possible impact, and their overall effectiveness.

Action Analysis

After collecting all significant data, you now must move to the action phase of the decision-making process. This entails reviewing all the information collected and setting a course of action and a specific plan for achieving the action. Action analysis allows you to examine the viability of your plan and try to predict whether your decision is sound and the course of action will be effective.

Reviewing the Data

Action analysis begins with a data review within the context of four essential factors. These factors are the environment, the various functions involved in the action plan, the business consequences of the action taken, and the historical precedent of the action. These four types of analysis—environmental, functional, business, and historical—allow you to examine every conceivable angle of a decision before taking action.

Environment Analysis

Environment analysis takes into account the theoretic and the physical environment in which you operate and the action plan will be undertaken. By using a charting system that is based on a concentric sphere of influence such as the one demonstrated in Figure 7.1, you can identify department objectives in undertaking the action and the action segments (as represented by arrows).

An environment analysis allows you to look specifically at the workplace dynamics while making your decision. The model shown in Figure 7.1 is based on the rehabilitation unit of a metropolitan hospital. This model will assist in determining areas that will be most affected by the budget cuts, identifying potential areas of concern, and arriving at some suggestions for undertaking the action.

Such analysis can also include other environmental concerns that cannot be charted clearly on a graph. One such concern is a major organizational change that will affect your decision; for example, drastic changes to operational revenue, human resources, or any other factors that affect everyday work activity. One factor is growth, which in the health care environment is occurring at a rapid pace. Growth gives rise to new opportunities that come with an expanding base of customer-patients and the resultant increase in revenue. Health care environments that are stagnant and demonstrate very little growth continue to suffer shrinking revenue and demographic contraction. These environmental factors must be taken into consideration as you formulate your action plan.

Certain indicators that are helpful in conducting an environment analysis can include your department's size, its daily volume of patient services, and the revenue the department generates. In

Figure 7.1. Sample Sphere of Influence Chart.

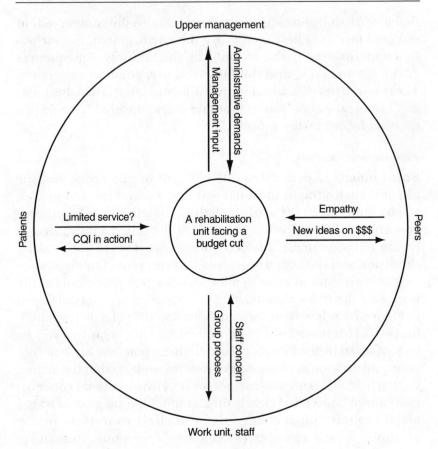

some cases, it might be helpful to sell your plan to organizational leaders based on the projected benefit (or benefits) of undertaking your action and following your decision. Less tangible environmental factors include the prevailing mood of the organization, employee morale in your department, and the administration's attitude toward your department. For example, a department that has direct patient contact traditionally has greater visibility within the organization and consequently gets quicker action and support for carrying out its actions. Hence, your department's status should be factored into your decision-making process.

Finally, environment analysis must take place over a time continuum. Seek to determine what the past status of the department has been, what its present conditions and objectives are, and what its future objectives might be. This viewpoint should be expanded to include the entire organization. Past, present, and future objectives that might bear on the decision at hand should be factored into the decision-making equation.

Function (Role) Analysis

A function analysis basically asks, *Who can do what to make this happen?* Try to draw an accurate picture of how you will use the various resources available to you, given their roles and functions. Begin with human resources. Do you have enough staff to carry out the action? Is the range of staff talent sufficient (for example, in technical ability) and balanced in terms of individual contribution? Consider the performance levels of the various individuals in your department. If your action plan is to be a group process, be certain to include the stronger players on your action team. If significant individual action is required, once again consider various individuals' roles, as well as their strengths and weaknesses, and then set your plan accordingly.

A secretary who works in a psychiatric ward provides an example of functional analysis. This individual would have a set of administrative abilities and would also have to fill the role of master communicator and, in a sense, liaison and internal consultant within the department. Accordingly, all these job tenets should be considered by the manager in reviewing the position and the player in the position.

The second phase of functional analysis concerns related departments and colleagues within the organization. For example, the action you have settled on and the decision you are about to implement might require the support and participation of other departments. You also might need the participation of specialists and other peers within the organization. Try to specify what roles or functions need be assumed by these individuals and what is required from all participants in installing your plan.

Next, consider what participation is needed by your supervisor. As your primary mentor, he will be invaluable in guiding you as you undertake the action phase of the decision-making process.

Furthermore, you might require specific action from your supervisor; for example, influencing another individual within or outside your organization who can further empower your efforts. If political clout is needed that only your supervisor can deliver, identify that role in your category of needs and enlist his participation as appropriate.

Finally, your functional analysis should cover benefits to the organization. Detail any specific advantages your organization might enjoy, and brainstorm any contributions or roles the organization can assume in supporting your decision. Analyze any negative or adverse impact specifically as it might affect the organization. With this approach to functional analysis, you evaluate every role affected by your action plan in arriving at a comprehensive strategy that will facilitate positive results from your decision and action.

Business Analysis

Action analysis is incomplete without analysis of business-related dynamics. To begin, consider the impact of your decision and its subsequent effect on the customer-patient. This means looking at what benefits the customer-patient will enjoy as well as anticipating potential short-term adverse outcomes the customer-patient might suffer as a result of your decision. The qualifier *short-term* is key here: If any adverse impact falls to the customer-patient, you have made a wrong decision.

To help bring your business analysis into sharper focus, construct a matrix consisting of two vertical columns. In the left-hand column, list the cost of your new program or action plan in terms of fiscal costs, operational resources expended, and its toll on your human resources. In the right-hand column, list all benefits to the customer-patient and the organization.

Underlying all aspects of your business analysis should be two key quality-related business themes. The first, CQI, should drive all your department's activities. Continuous quality improvement dictates ongoing quality enhancement as the incentive that fuels everyday activities associated with optimum health care delivery. The second theme, continuous business development (CBD), connotes a building-block approach to all departmental activities in management efforts. CBD is an important objective for new health care managers to achieve. Every effort undertaken by the department should be done to make the department a stronger, more progressive entity than it was prior to the effort. As a regular goal, the department should seek constantly to develop itself into a greater health care business component. The dynamics of CQI and CBD can be reinforced by asking yourself the following questions:

- Will my decision mandate action that is quality conscious?
- Will my decision result in action that will improve the quality of our services in particular and health care provision in general?
- Will this decision initiate action that will facilitate our departmental mission of progressive development?
- What future departmental or organizational goals might evolve from this decision?
- What will be the ultimate benefit of this action to the customer-patient and the organization?

Finally, in developing a business perspective through analysis, identify any potential negative impact and its possible business consequence. Specifically, what adverse effect could compromise appropriate use of resources (human, fiscal, plant, and equipment, for example)? How might visibility factors be negatively affected? Could customer-patients perceive that their welfare is not a top organizational priority? For example, might a construction project severely inconvenience customer-patients? These questions all speak to business dynamics that must be analyzed throughout your decision-making process.

Historical Analysis

Historical analysis takes into account past historical precedents established in your organization. As a starting point, consider precedents set by past action. What courses of action were taken that were similar in scope to the one you are contemplating?

Review from a political and psychological viewpoint where your historical backers and detractors might be. For example, the health care environment is not unlike other corporate cultures in that some individuals look with disdain on certain parts of their organizations. Specifically, in certain metropolitan hospitals, the human resource department is discredited because, according to detractors, it never seems to fill open positions quickly enough. Hence, whenever the human resource department tries to enact a new program, the department experiences a certain resistance from individuals whose positions may be on the line. However, line personnel (such as medical support services) hold human resources in high regard because the department facilitates the training and education that are so vital to the workers' roles. Therefore, enlist the support of potential backers in your decision-making process; they can help sell your new plan.

As discussed in Chapter One, the forces for change are exerting a tremendous impact in many health care organizations. The statement *We've never done it that way before"* is heard all too often. In light of changing dynamics such as ever-escalating competition and a variable fiscal climate, however, this statement fosters stagnation and can undercut a commitment to presenting new ideas openly and making decisions that explore new frontiers of organizational progress. A commitment to making history is a necessity in modern-day health care, where innovation and imagination in problem resolution spell the difference between success and failure.

Considering Relevance and Contribution to the Organization

Finally, consider all ramifications of your decision on the organization from the perspective of what it will contribute to the organization's goals. Again, by stressing the benefits of your action and gathering the appropriate operational and moral support, you can transform your decision from idea to action. To crystallize these ramifications, ask yourself the following ten questions:

1. How do my decision and action enhance the organization's commitment to the customer-patient?
2. How do my decision and action reflect the organization's stated values?
3. How do my decision and action contribute to attainment of the organization's stated mission?
4. Who should support this decision?

5. Who in the organization will automatically support this decision?
6. How can I convince nonsupporters of my decision's merits and positive contribution to the organization?
7. What are the overall benefits of the action to the organization?
8. How does my decision make the organization better in terms of effectiveness and efficiency?
9. How does my decision make my department a larger contributor to the organizational good?
10. What are two major benefits of this action that everyone in the organization will quickly recognize?

Action Planning

In this section I describe four strategies for formulating a comprehensive plan for action: the SWOT (strengths, weaknesses, opportunities, and threats) analysis, the military model, the parliamentary model, and the QUICK model (the acronym is explained later). Supplemented by two specific applications in Appendix A, I also offer suggestions for ways to apply these methods to your own decision making and action.

Each of these approaches can be used independently. Tried and true, they have been used successfully by health care managers and presented in textbooks on management for some time. Remember, take from these models and applications only what is compatible with your personal management style and appropriate for your institution's and department's needs.

I conclude the chapter with a closer look at communication—particularly as it bears on the four methods discussed. I also give some suggestions for monitoring your plan once it has been implemented.

Performing a SWOT Analysis

Performing a SWOT analysis requires you to take into account the strengths of your department—your own and those of your staff—in analyzing your action plan's effectiveness. Identify the strong players in your department, their areas of professional and technical expertise, and any supporters who can move your action plan forward. Then identify the positive benefits or contributing factors that affect positive outcomes.

Next, define the weaknesses, particularly those areas in which technical deficiencies are apparent. For example, poor performers might be resistant to change or to undertaking new responsibilities. Other weaknesses include resource shortages (notably operational, equipment, or financial resources). A major weakness could be any negative change that might arise from your decision, such as functional inconvenience or short-term inefficiency of operation.

Opportunities are to be found in your analysis of areas where you see a possibility to increase action (broaden patient services), gain support (win over detractors), or apply CQI to further justify your decision.

Conversely, threats include potential problems and long-term negative outcomes that loom on the horizon as you undertake your action. A threat is any element that compromises the generation of a positive outcome.

To understand application of the SWOT analysis, let's assume a training manager wants to implement a new program on interviewing and hiring job candidates. Use the SWOT sequence to analyze the action plan as follows.

Strengths

- The training manager's past experience in teaching interviewing skills
- A strong videotape education series the hospital owns but has not yet used
- Scheduled dates for management training already approved by the senior management staff

Weaknesses

- Interviewing is not a particularly popular topic among line managers in technically based departments
- The training manager is new and unproven, so some selling will be required
- No interview training has ever been presented, so skepticism is a likely obstacle

Opportunities

- The organization's plan to hire a number of employees over the next two years (already-established need) for the program
- Eagerness on the part of many managers to enhance their interviewing skills (they have never had to interview candidates before)
- CEO's "management mandate" or high regard for individual decision making by management (the manager has made a major, independent decision)

Threats

- The unlikely possibility of another type of training taking precedence in organizational importance (The fact that no interview training has ever been tried before, previously identified as a weakness, is not a threat but an opportunity to conduct training that is new and different.)

Having conducted this SWOT analysis, the training manager realizes that the balance is definitely in favor of implementing the new program. The decision is thus made positively, comprehensively, and progressively.

In performing a SWOT analysis (as well as the other techniques described in this section), divide a sheet of paper into four columns and create a list by using brainstorming techniques in each of these areas. If your lists are particularly long in the weaknesses and threats categories relative to the strengths and opportunities categories, you might want to reconsider your decision. Identifying these factors will lead you to the next step: finalizing your plan in such a way that strengths and opportunities can be enhanced and threats and weaknesses minimized. You can find a step-by-step application of SWOT analysis in Appendix A.

Employing the Military Model

The military model involves a five-part sequence.

1. *Define the objective.* Define a need or identify a desired outcome. In defining the objective, identify the optimum outcome you desire and the maximum result you feel can be achieved.

2. *Identify resources.* Identify all available resources, list their potential contribution to your action, and consider all related resources from other departments within the organization.

3. *Establish the plan.* Write down the specific action you require and establish a time sequence within which the action is needed. (I will explain this process further in this chapter, as well as in succeeding chapters.)

4. *Lay out the course of action.* Set up an incremental plan and establish time checkpoints in which certain objectives should be achieved. For example, if you delegate a particular task to an individual as part of your decision-making and action-execution process, you not only establish a final objective but also interim checkpoints for that individual.

5. *Provide closure.* Closure is made up of those final benchmarks of success that indicate that the plan was successful and the objective reached (such as an accomplished objective or attained goal).

Employing the Parliamentary Model

The parliamentary model is similar to the military model in terms of outcome but it provides you with another way of looking at plan establishment and action execution. This model is used in many legislative bodies and includes the following eight steps:

1. *Establish need.* Define the needed action and ultimate problem being addressed by the decision and the action taken.

2. *Define the optimum outcome.* What are the best possible results? How can maximum results be achieved by your decision?

3. *Conduct a stakeholder review.* Who is involved? Who has a stake in this action? Who needs to be in on the communication loop?

4. *List pros and cons.* Delineate the positives and negatives of the action taken.

5. *Make an option review.* Review all possible actions and alternative actions.

6. *Review potential consequences.* Consider all adverse reactions to your plan, as well as positive support that might be garnered.

7. *Formulate a step-by-step plan.* Establish a plan and allow for a general preparation and time sequence as evidenced by the infor-

mation collected in the data-gathering phase and confirmed by continuous contribution and communication with all parties involved.

8. *Analyze achievement.* Once you have reached the objective, analyze its results, considering the needed action and initial objective. This will give you the true measure of success and provide an educational and developmental opportunity for future decisions.

Employing the QUICK Decision Model

I devised the QUICK decision model as a five-part formula for executing action. Each letter of the acronym QUICK stands for a particular dynamic that should be followed in the action execution process:

Q = Question appropriate parties

U = Understand your objective(s)

I = Investigate all options

C = Communicate clearly to all concerned parties

K = Keep on top of things (knowledge, kinetic energy)

Communication with Stakeholders

Regardless of which tool you employ, remember that communication is a key element of management. It is especially so with decision making and action execution. Your effort to strive for maximum appropriate input from all parties involved in your decision-making process extends beyond the initial data-collection process to make the decision: You must also determine how effective your decisions and actions ultimately were by asking the parties involved.

Communication must be comprehensive, open, and (when necessary) repetitive. There is really no risk in being redundant when you repeat the importance of the task and underscore the basic objective you are trying to achieve with your action. Furthermore, make sure that you detail each aspect of the plan appropriately to key members of your staff and significant other players in your action plan. Individuals should be appraised not only of their part in the planning and execution phase, but also of the roles of others with whom they might interact.

In addition to simply reviewing the goals and mission objective, review and present your expectations as well. Your expectations make clear what specific level of achievement you want to accomplish toward your goal; that is, the margin of excellence needed to fully satisfy the initial need prompted by your decision. Again, staff, peer, and supervisory input are important. Be certain to set your goals realistically, without expectation of a perfect model of excellence in all your endeavors. By setting unrealistic and unattainable expectations, you create false hope and ultimately suffer the consequences of a disappointed staff and a disenchanted administration.

As you move closer to your goal, review progress periodically. Hold regular meetings with all significant players to discuss your progress and address any problems. Elicit the participation and suggestions of all players in resolving problems. For example, many senior health care managers are in charge of construction projects. However, they often fail to take the time necessary to brief their staff on progress or discuss particular problems that may be created by in-progress construction.

To summarize, four communication keys are important to the action execution process:

1. *Clarity.* Be clear and comprehensive in all communication with your team.

2. *Closure.* Bring all meetings and discussions to a positive end and leave no loose ends hanging (that is, all decisions and intermediate objectives are reached and the loop of communication is always closed successfully).

3. *Cohesion.* Make sure that your team works together as a focused unit by discussing their problems with each other in dedicated meetings. The key question to ask yourself in eliciting this type of communication participation is, *What have we learned up to this point in the project?*

4. *Command.* Once you have made a decision, take timely action. As emphasized throughout this book, the speed with which you undertake a decision is vital, and although haste makes waste,

you still must move quickly and positively toward your goal. Closely monitor progress throughout the project, and get continuous feedback. Doing so gives a clear indication about who is in charge and allows you to command the freedom to give direction and provide advice as needed. As you take command of the action-execution phase, avoid guesswork and unfounded assumptions on your part. Remember, data collection is a continuous process, and it becomes even more important once you have undertaken action. Remember also that being in command mandates a certain amount of participative management. Therefore, allow all members of your staff to become involved in the process, but without relinquishing your own authority.

This last concept calls for a kind of balancing act. As you assume command of action execution and watch your decision turn into the reality of performance, you must delegate a certain amount of control to your staff and other participating parties. While delegating control, do not delegate command. Ultimately, you alone are accountable and responsible for the action taken.

Quantification of Outcomes

Once you have reached your goal and desired outcome, clearly and objectively quantify the gains achieved by the action. Then compare these measurements to your initial decision-making criteria. Announce the benefits gained, both from a short-term and long-term perspective. Again, staff participation is the means to this end.

Review with staff what was learned—individually and as a group—as a result of your action. In doing so, your development as a manager will be enhanced by their feedback.

Recognize that no matter how effective your action was or how accurate your decision might have been, any action-oriented process is, in a sense, a trial-and-error education even under the best of circumstances. The more decisions you make, the better your judgment will become and, ultimately, the better your management style and performance effectiveness will be.

Try to list at least three or four lessons learned in the process. If your goals were reached, a need was fulfilled, or action was taken that led to improved service to the customer-patient, then you have made a significant contribution to the health care delivery process, which after all is your mission as a health care manager. Do not lose sight of this essential reward system as you go about your daily activities.

Conclusion

Decision making and action execution mark the scope of a health care manager's responsibilities. By having the courage, foresight, and intelligence to make a decision, you are applying the basic building blocks used by effective health care leaders at the top levels of premier organizations. The key concepts offered in this chapter in conjunction with the two strategic guides for decision making in Appendix A give you a starting point for executing your decisions and actions.

Making the tough call is one of the hardest jobs of management. By gaining the support of staff and other members of your organization who want to help you succeed, you can make progressive decision making and action execution an ongoing part of your health care management strategy.

Chapter Eight

Exemplifying Leadership Presence and Guidance

Leadership is a nebulous characteristic defined differently by industry type, situation, and individual preference. Countless studies and numerous books on the topic of leadership acknowledge various styles and approaches to cultivating leadership presence. In carrying out your new responsibilities, you will be expected to demonstrate leadership qualities. Not only must you set direction and policy, but you must also exemplify a style and strategy that will inspire performance and motivate individuals to attain their highest level of accomplishment.

In the health care field, leadership takes on a particular level of importance. Because crisis is an ever-present factor in health care management, leadership is essential to meeting critical objectives. Furthermore, because most health care workers are people oriented and value interpersonal skills, leadership presence is closely judged and monitored by staff. In addition, working with limited resources and close deadlines mandates that leadership be both effective and inspirational. Therefore, it is critically important that early on in your tenure as a health care manager you adopt a leadership style that is effective and that can serve as a building block for continuous successful performance.

In this chapter I explore leadership styles fully. What is more important, I analyze leadership impact from the perspective of cause and effect. Of primary importance to new health care managers, I suggest how to adopt a comfortable, effective leadership style that will provide optimum positive impact on your work group with maximum long-term effect. I also discuss various leadership influences from which you can construct your own leadership style and the process of developing progressive innovations in leadership. In looking at the great historical leaders cited in this chapter, you can gain some insight on successful leadership. I discuss various leadership criteria in light of employee and management expectations and basic leadership objectives. My intent is to provide you with a basic frame of reference from which you can establish a leadership style that will work for you.

Foundations of Leadership

There is no magic formula for great leadership; often it is defined more by circumstances and by type of fellowship with which a leader is charged by imperative. That is to say, the circumstances and types of individuals in your department have much to do with the type of leadership style you will find to be optimally effective.

However, a second part of the equation—your own preferences, personality, and predilections—is equally important. Your personal characteristics dictate the type of leadership style you will use, as they define what you feel comfortable with and find to be of maximum effectiveness in your daily activities. Accordingly, first examine the influences that played most prominently in developing your own leadership style. Then ascertain which ones were most influential in the development of your innate leadership identity.

Identifying Influential Leadership Styles

Figure 8.1 depicts the various leadership influences that might affect your thinking as you assume a management role. Role models from your youth are the primary sources of your leadership style. These include your family—parents and others who, charged with your upbringing, were the first leaders you observed firsthand. Primarily through their actions, they demonstrated a leadership style and management strategy that you naturally accepted (or perhaps rejected) as effective and incorporated into your basic value system. The combination of all the influences represented in Figure 8.1 serves as guidepost for the success you have enjoyed up to now in your health care career. In essence, they had a great deal to do with your now reaching a point in your career where you are enjoying the opportunity of becoming a manager and a leader.

Other role models from your youth might include favorite primary and high school teachers who demonstrated a style of leadership in classroom discussion, management of group activities, and efforts to inspire you in one of the most intricate processes of human endeavor—learning. You probably considered them subconsciously as role models based on their style of dealing with and motivating people, a style you admired, took subconscious note of, and have probably adopted throughout your career. Other role models might include youth group leaders—scout leaders, dance group leaders, or team coaches. All of these role models were expert communicators with vision and motivation—all essential elements of leadership.

No doubt you also were influenced by "bad" leaders, individuals you considered to be ineffective or individuals who have had a negative impact on you. Certainly you noted what these individuals did wrong, stored that information in your memory, and have since assiduously avoided mirroring their mistakes. Industrial psychologists maintain that we learn more from others' mistakes than

Figure 8.1. Leadership Influences.

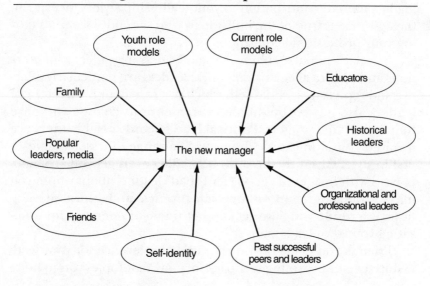

we do from their positive attributes. With this in mind, it is evident that much positive and negative learning was distilled through your early role models.

Current role models might include individuals within your organization whom you deem successful and effective leaders—former supervisors or administrators, for example. Perhaps leaders outside your health care environment—religious, community, or civic leaders—provide you with "action lessons." How these figures approach their responsibilities and conduct their activities educates you as to how you might lead and what choices you might make in the leadership process.

In a similar vein, consider the leadership styles among your professional educators, including college professors and training instructors under whom you studied. For example, it is likely that you had an inspirational teacher in college or nursing school. Perhaps even more than your primary school teachers, these individuals had a major impact on your perception. They were well versed in the technical aspects of your profession, provided constructive insight, and really knew their stuff. Furthermore, they may have gained the respect of everyone in your class or learning group, no easy feat. Naturally, you admire these individuals and emulate them as part of your communication and instructional process. Being a leader also entails being a great educator, so these individuals made a natural contribution to your leadership style. Once again, the converse is true of the individuals who set poor examples during your professional education.

In today's popular culture, certain leaders may affect your emotions and inspire allegiance. Political leaders are particularly effective and represent agendas with which you can identify. Great social leaders also have brought about tremendous change and have helped advance society. Political leaders and social leaders are inspired communicators who provide a range of lessons on leadership style. Given the breadth of media coverage, you are bombarded with images of "good" and "bad" leaders about whom you make value judgments on their effectiveness and ethical orientation. As a result, you have yet another frame of reference for innovating your own leadership style.

Friends and peers provide a frame of reference for your leadership style by providing feedback in a way that forces you to hone your people skills as you fine-tune your leadership approach. Also, there is a reflective value in our relationships with friends and peers. This means that the values we treasure in them are the same ones to which we aspire (like draws like). Along the same line, if friends or peers are successful in a particular pursuit, you observe closely how they became successful and then draw a comparison between their approach and your own.

Consider the following example: Assume that a peer within your organization is also a personal friend who was promoted into management a couple of years ago. You probably noted why she deserved the promotion, which you felt was earned without question. You then analyzed subconsciously what made your friend successful, and empathized with the trials and tribulations of her first year in management. You learned a great deal from this shared experience, which serves as a source of information and frame of reference as you undertake a management role. Both positive and negative experiences will remain in your memory and guide you as you now assume your own tenure.

Developing Your Leadership Identity

Along with the impact of friends and peers is your own self-identity. Self-identity might be thought of as a combined outcome of the influences in Figure 8.1. You have created you own self-identity with the following seven components:

1. *Observation.* Upon observing all the pros and cons represented by all of these influences, you made value judgments as to their efficiency and effectiveness. Furthermore, you detailed any particular nuance that you felt caused success or failure (cause and effect).
2. *Admiration.* You mentally recorded aspects of positive action by these influences that you admired and felt were worthy of your respect. These aspects then became basic sources of emulation, things you would aspire to once you assumed a position of authority.
3. *Identification.* Any positive result with which you identified from any of these influences will be something you use naturally now that you are in a leadership position. From a negative aspect,

anything these influences might have tried that did not work, that was not successful, or that you did not identify with strongly will not be part of your arsenal, or you will try the reverse. For example, if you saw a leader fail to attain success because he was too stern, heavy-handed, or tyrannical in his approach, you will naturally try to be softer, more compassionate, and more participative in your own approach.

4. *Trial and error.* Once you have observed, identified with, and admired a particular aspect of leadership, experiment with it on your own. If the experiment is successful, it will provide positive reinforcement and you will adapt this particular facet to your own style. If it was unsuccessful, you will dismiss it and probably not try the approach again. This is part of the natural progression of leadership adaptation and formation of style.

5. *Practicality.* As mentioned at the beginning of this chapter, your leadership style will depend a great deal on the circumstances and situations in which you find yourself and on the staff you inherit. Some aspects of leadership that you have observed and are willing to try might not be appropriate to your particular situation.

6. *Comfort.* Everything you observe is not necessarily something with which you will be comfortable. Comfort will determine whether you are perceived as being genuine or phony. Admiring something does not mean that you would be comfortable trying it out yourself.

7. *Development.* After you have considered these influences, you will put your own spin on your leadership application. This means fundamentally that you will customize the approach to your own means and desires. This is essential, as it gives you ownership of the leadership application, makes it uniquely your own, and embellishes and enhances it from a quality standpoint. In essence, you build upon the style characteristic, and make it even more effective.

Leadership influences are omnipresent and naturally at the forefront of your thinking when you assume a management role. They will set the foundation on which you will build your own leadership style. As you progress through your first year of management, you will find that your own actions become as important as your leadership influences and will result in a productive initial approach to leadership formation.

Leadership Dynamics

In this section I explore characteristics of historical leaders (another category shown in Figure 8.1), including Abraham Lincoln, Mother Teresa, Eleanor and Franklin Roosevelt, John F. Kennedy, Dr. Martin Luther King, Jr., Juliette Low (founder of the Girl Scouts), and others. I then discuss the universal characteristics of leadership. Finally, I offer some suggestions for strategies to ensure continuous leadership development.

Citing Historical Prototypes and Building a Leadership Matrix

In addition to mentors, predecessors, and early role models, you can call on your history classes to help define some characteristics of great leadership. Figures from American and world history most likely impressed you with their heroic actions and monumental achievements. Use Table 8.1 as a model for constructing your own leadership matrix, which you can use to help formulate leadership dynamics that suit your unique circumstances. The leaders listed in Table 8.1 meet many of the criteria specified in the preceding section. In the left-hand column, list your choices by name. Then in the right-hand column, list ten criteria by using a one-word, free association–type response. (Of course, each criterion will be subjective and, therefore, will probably apply to more than one leader.)

Look at Table 8.1 to see how this exercise can have practical application for your own efforts. The one thing most people remember about Lincoln is his nickname, "Honest Abe." Honesty is an obvious building block for effective leadership. It builds credibility and inspires "followership."

Franklin D. Roosevelt's imagination guided essential depression-era and wartime decisions that required creativity and ingenuity (relief and public works and "fireside chats," for example). He also enacted twenty-one pieces of legislation in his first hundred days in office, including the Lend-lease Act (support for war-ravaged Europe) and an assortment of strong social policies (creation of four million jobs, for example). A leader who is imaginative

Table 8.1. Sample Leadership Matrix.

Leader	Criteria
Abraham Lincoln	Honesty, integrity
Franklin D. Roosevelt	Implementation of innovative programs
Mother Theresa	Compassion, human spirit
Benjamin Franklin	Imagination, innovation
John F. Kennedy	Charisma, positive image
Dr. Martin Luther King, Jr.	Recognized that little things launch big things
Juliette Low	Value-based vision
Winston Churchill	Ability to get the job done
Mohandas Gandhi	Top priority was followers' best interests
Eleanor Roosevelt	Got her message across progressively, consistently, clearly, and with compassion

inspires performance and encourages others' creativity. In health care management, where shrinking budgets and tighter operational revenues are facts of life, there can't be too much insightful creativity.

A paradigm of compassion, Mother Teresa's mission was service to those in dire need. A great leader's compassion demonstrates his or her own humanity and assures followers that their best interests are taken to heart.

Benjamin Franklin's innovation, as differentiated from imagination, allowed him to use available resources to create new processes and products that had positive results. What could be a better example than his discovery of electricity by using a kite? He also founded the University of Pennsylvania and the United States Post Office. Certainly, universities and mail service existed prior to Franklin's intervention, but the fact that these two institutions have survived for more than two hundred years is a testament to his innovative spirit. Innovation is essential in a health care leader, who despite limited resources must arrive at imaginative solutions daily.

Few would argue that John F. Kennedy is as well known for his charisma as for his accomplishments as U.S. president. Charisma is embodied in many shapes and sizes, for the same quality that drew voters to JFK also draws basketball fans to Michael Jordan or followers to Billy Graham. Although all three have distinctly different personalities, their net effect is to garner attention and evoke positive action. This is an important quality in health care, where crisis management allows little room to question authority or wonder, *Who's in charge?*

Dr. Martin Luther King, Jr., made sure the little things added up to big things. Dr. King was never arrested legitimately for unlawful assembly because he made sure that all papers were properly filed with the appropriate municipal offices prior to each march or demonstration. In fact, he warned his staff that their failure to address any of these "little things" would result in discharge from the civil rights movement. Great leaders ensure that so-called "little things" are always taken care of; furthermore, they ensure that little things having adverse consequences do not come back to sabotage the positive "bigger things."

Juliette Low founded the Girl Scouts of America. Her values-based vision positively permeates our society today. The basic intent of the Girl Scouts, founded on allegiance to the country, commitment to others, and a positive spirit, developed from Low's initial vision of a multimillion-member organization. Given the people-oriented nature of health care service and the need for health care workers to share a vision and mission in their everyday activities, health care leaders need a vision that is based on values.

Regardless of circumstances—world war, economic depression, or social upheaval—Winston Churchill got the job done, and his successes bred tremendous loyalty among constituents. As emphasized throughout this book, your staff members want you to succeed; they also want success in their own efforts. Accordingly, you will find that success can be self-perpetuating; that is, once you start to get positive results, you will maintain the necessary "followership" and allegiance vital to long-term success.

Mohandas Gandhi always put the desires of his followers first. An ardent listener who never relied on aggression or force to make his point, he intuitively knew what people wanted and led them toward that objective. Great health care leaders know how to listen, understand the needs and desires of their staff, and attempt to help them reach their aims within the context of customer-patient needs and organizational goals.

Eleanor Roosevelt is known for her ability to get her point across. She was able to make cogent arguments in the public forum that produced worldwide progressive action. Her major accomplishments—triggered by her relentless advocacy and formidable presence—included the expansion of the International Red Cross, the reform of mental health facilities in the northeastern United States, and the creation of a world organization for promoting children's health and welfare, which many experts believe inspired the creation of the United Nations International Children's Emergency Fund (UNICEF). In a similar vein, a health care manager should always strive to get the point across clearly, compassionately, and comprehensively.

Identifying Universal Characteristics of Leadership

As you construct your own matrix and use it as a guide for your particular leadership innovation, there are other criteria you might consider upon completing the left-hand column. To begin with, a leader should be both short-term smart and long-term smart; that is, you must make good decisions for the short-term, but they should coincide with the organization's long-term mission. Doing so will create overall positive net effect of your activities and those of your staff.

Good leaders should also be visible. They make their presence known in any given situation, thus producing favorable results. Additionally, they are hands-on in their approach to leadership. Individuals know where to find visible leaders in times of crisis and when they need support. Such leaders are also ubiquitous; their presence is felt even when they are not physically on the scene.

Good leaders have a steady hand in all departmental circumstances and situations. They seek to manage the department responsibly and do not back away from making judgments. That is, they consider all the criteria necessary in executing actions, communicate the course of action clearly, and obtain positive results.

Consider the matrix in Table 8.1. There is no question that each leader embraced all the criteria. Furthermore, none of them openly used emotion inappropriately or became too negative in situations that required strength and a positive vision. Nor did they act as robots or automatons. Instead, they struck a balance by being inspirational in their view, showing anger only when appropriate, and never being dissuaded from reacting with the resoluteness demanded by the situation.

An example concerning the use of emotion in health care leadership might be helpful. A nursing director once remarked that she tries to avoid using profanity except on rare occasions. When she does use profanity, she says it is to inspire the performance of a negative staff member and to "really get someone's attention." Profanity aside, you should only use emotional outbursts when appropriate and when you seek to make a point. Remember that you do not have to be on an even keel all the time, but also keep in mind that you should stay true to your own style and personality during emotional moments.

All this is to say that leaders are human beings, subject to human emotions. Emotional outbursts, although potentially counterproductive, are nonetheless a characteristic of being human. A sense of humor, warmth in executing leadership responsibilities, and the strength to admit—and learn from—mistakes are other universal traits.

In the health care setting, where illness and death are ever-present, these survival characteristics can be helpful attributes. Maintaining a lighter side can be achieved through sharing a witty anecdote, relating a tasteful joke, or laughing at your own foibles. However, pick your spots and times carefully, always mindful of others' feelings, cultural or social sensitivities, and the decorum of the workplace.

Remember that performance is inspired as much by who you are as what you are. That is to say, your title and authority will automatically garner you a certain amount of respect. Yet your personality and people skills will also be closely monitored and factored into how your staff and the larger organization view your leadership style.

Ability to admit to errors demonstrates human fallibility, not weakness. It also shows that you are grounded in reality, thus further establishing your credibility.

Much has been said about the ability to listen to the concerns of customer-patients, staff, and administrators. Take care not only to listen but to hear. Listening shows compassion and involvement in the group process. Hearing and understanding show perception.

All these characteristics—sense of humor, warmth, fallibility, and so forth—can get you started in constructing (or building on) your leadership matrix. The matrix criteria can serve as a blueprint for your initial actions in your new leadership role.

Your leadership matrix can also incorporate negative characteristics. For example, you might consider making a negative matrix, replete with leaders who failed in their efforts and the reasons (right-hand column) they failed. This negative matrix will help you maintain a balanced perspective.

Continuous Leadership Development

In addition to the initial strategies detailed throughout this chapter, it is vital that you continuously seek new applications of leadership and new insights into leadership style, and continuously upgrade your leadership effectiveness. With those objectives in mind, I will provide you with some guidelines for ensuring that your leadership style develops progressively and your effectiveness grows over time.

• *Try to get as much feedback as possible on your leadership effectiveness.* Use the sources in Figure 8.1, your family, peers, and trusted subordinates, to give you feedback on your leadership effectiveness. Remember that you are the ultimate expert on how effective you are. If you are truly introspective, you will find that these discussions are more of a validation of what you thought as opposed to a revelation. Though you might gain some new insights, you basically are seeking information on what you did right and what you did wrong relative to your leadership efforts. Get suggestions from all these individuals and try to incorporate any good ideas into your future efforts.

• *Give clear direction at all times to all individuals on your staff.* Try to specify exactly what is expected and provide as much insight as appropriate on why something should be done. Sharing this information with employees builds trust and allows you to have the precious two-way communication that is essential for any successful leader. Use appropriate follow-up methods to ensure that progress is being made and provide as much additional instruction as possible as employees strive to achieve their goals. This enhances communication and trust, two commodities that are always helpful.

- *Give people an appropriate amount of freedom, particularly individuals on your staff.* Assume that staff members know what they are doing until they prove otherwise. Providing too much direction or constraining performance can create the perception that you are unnecessarily overbearing or not trusting of your staff. Closely monitor performance, provide inspiration, and measure the goal attainment of all individuals on your staff.

- *Balance positive and negative information realistically.* You will on occasion have to give your staff bad news. Provide this information on a timely basis, try to identify an up-side (if there is one), and deal with problems realistically. On these occasions, verbally stress your confidence that your work group can handle adversity and bounce back from negative circumstance. Strong leaders participate in adversity as much as in prosperity.

- *Try to keep perspectives on all issues.* The true measure of leaders, in the opinion of many, is their reaction to things that are above and beyond the call of duty or beyond the norm. Try to maintain a balanced view of things, and exhibit the courage and strength necessary to handle tough situations.

- *Learn from every situation.* If there is one thing that is readily available in the health care environment, it is opportunity to learn every day. Collect as much information as possible, process that information, and incorporate it into your leadership efforts. Remember that the best way of learning things is to ask appropriate questions. These could be questions that you ask yourself about what you have learned from a situation, questions you ask your peers and your supervisor about their insights and experiences. The more you learn, the greater your frame of reference becomes and the better leader you become.

- *In all cases, be yourself.* Whatever makes sense to you should inspire the judgments you make. Whatever you are comfortable communicating or exhibiting in your words and actions should rule the way you communicate ideas, thoughts, and objectives. Your actions and words are being closely examined by your staff because they provide the impetus and inspiration for staff's activities. Therefore, in the long run, whatever is most natural and comfortable for you will be the most progressive precedent to set.

- *Pace your activities both inside and outside the workplace.* Do not try to accomplish everything at once, and make time to enjoy your new capacity rather than unnecessarily allowing it to be a burden. Strike a balance between the things that you like to do and the things that you have to do.

• *Trust your instincts.* Your instincts and intelligence are what got you the management job to begin with. As a leader, your good intentions, frame of reference, and basic values will be the greatest strengths you have to offer those who want you to succeed.

Perhaps the most important point is that the organization wants you to succeed, your staff wants you to succeed (if for no other reason than it will make their life easier), and of course you want to succeed. This innate desire, coupled with all of the factors discussed throughout this chapter, will allow you to become a strong, positive leader. After spending some time in the best classroom available—the health care management forum—you will find yourself learning, growing, and enjoying the opportunity of helping others provide stellar health care to those in need.

Chapter Nine

Case Study
Carolina Hospital Student Health Center

The following is a fictitious case study based on a compendium of actual events and individuals from my consulting experiences. The case study will illustrate some practical applications of leadership from the first eight chapters of this book and provide insight into the experiences and positive strategies used by a new health care manager in the first three months of tenure. The chapter should provide a realistic perspective on the problem-solving and strategy-formulation skills vital to success in the initial stages of your management career.

The Carolina Hospital Student Health Center (the Center) was established in 1989 as a free-standing facility on the campus of Carolina State College. Located in the Coastal South, the college has grown dramatically over the past thirty years due to an exploding population in response to the service and computer industry's relocation and market expansion. Enrollment at the public college has grown from twelve hundred students in 1973 to seventy-five hundred full-time, undergraduate students for whom health services were needed to handle routine preventive medicine, counseling, sports medicine, and a variety of other services.

Carolina Hospital is a large, nonprofit, public facility located in Carolina City. To meet the demands of the college community, the hospital established the Center on the college's campus. Although it is considered an integral part of the hospital from an operations standpoint, the Center is geographically removed from the hospital grounds and is located in a one-story brick building on the college campus. The building, constructed five years ago, was provided by the college and was funded by donations from several wealthy alumni. Two of these alumni served on the Center's board of directors, which also includes the president of Carolina Hospital, Kim Losurdo, and two members of the hospital's regular board of directors.

The mission of the board of directors is to act as guiding force for the Center. The board advises the Center's director on policy formation, reviews budgets and other fiscal matters, and generally serves as an advisory panel for activities within the student health center.

The staff include twenty-seven full-time employees and nine part-time employees (see organization structure in Figure 9.1). The Center has three main departments. The first, the medical department, is under the direction of Dr. Gus Sylvester, a staff member at Carolina Hospital who spends three days a week at the health center. The department is responsible for provision of medical services. Dr. Sylvester performs routine check-ups, provides expertise in cases ranging from common colds to broken bones, and basically directs the technical side of health care services.

The operations department, supervised by Tony Shayne, is responsible for physical maintenance of the building, as well as other nonmedical services (admissions, record keeping, and other administrative activities). A medical records specialist by profession, Shayne works largely in the admissions-reception area. He has worked for Carolina Hospital for nineteen years and has been the Center's operations supervisor since its inception in 1989.

The medical support department, headed by Carlene Neville, attends to ancillary services that help facilitate delivery of clinical services. The Center's support staff include a physical therapist; nurses; several counselors who specialize in mental health, drug rehabilitation, and family planning; and some of the skilled and nonskilled part-time employees (a dietitian, two social workers, and several clerk-typists). Neville, a nurse by training, has been in her current position for two years. Previously she was a staff nurse at a major Chicago public hospital, a position she held for ten years.

When the Center opened in 1989, its first director was Larry Kelly. Prior to his appointment, Kelly had been an assistant man-

Figure 9.1. Organizational Chart:
Carolina Hospital Student Health Center.

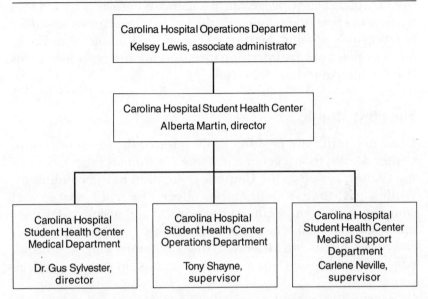

ager in the hospital's large rehabilitation department. He had two years of supervisory experience, following a seven-year career as a physical therapist. Because he had completed extensive graduate work in the area of health administration, with specific focus on sports medicine, he was considered a natural for the new director's position. Kelly resigned three years later.

The reasons for Kelly's departure are unclear. His stated reason was the desire to return to physical therapy on a full-time basis. However, during his tenure at the Center he received only marginal performance evaluations. Both the board and the associate administrator of operations (to whom Kelly reported) were less than enchanted with his performance.

The associate administrator of operations, Kelsey Lewis, conducted an extensive internal search in selecting a replacement for Kelly. After interviewing several candidates, she named Alberta Martin as the Center's new director.

Alberta Martin is a registered nurse who has worked for Carolina Hospital for the past six years. In addition to having demonstrated stellar performance as a staff nurse, she has completed all of the required courses for a bachelor's degree in public administration from Carolina State College. She is a native of Carolina City and lives ten minutes from the campus. Of the various candidates assessed for the director's position, Martin was clearly the leading candidate in terms of potential, past performance, and her interview with Lewis and the human resource director.

The First Month

Upon assuming the position of director of the Student Health Center, Martin took a general inventory of student expectations of the Center, as well as the Center's reputation in the community. While a part-time student at the college, she had heard several comments about the Center, both positive and negative. Furthermore, she had established a network of contacts among her fellow classmates and lifelong friends in the community who were knowledgeable about the Center and its relationship with the college community.

Martin discovered a variety of expectations for the Center across the college community. A typical expectation was that the Center should be an entity that can provide comprehensive service; that is, solve virtually any medical problem on demand. This is a big order—possibly an unrealistic one in terms of available resources. Martin is fully aware of the tremendous public scrutiny (both on campus and across the community) focused on the hospital's reputation. She knows the community consensus is that Carolina Hospital is or should be a public provider of health care services supported by property taxes and other local revenue sources. Although for the most part unrealistic, this perception nevertheless dominates the thinking of the average resident and the typical student. Martin understands that this perception translates into a student customer-patient who will expect top-quality health care services at minimal or no cost immediately upon demand.

In reviewing internal factors, Martin discovers that morale is not particularly high among the Center's employees. The staff appear less enthusiastic than her colleagues at Carolina Hospital do; in fact, many appear apathetic, thus confirming her suspicion of a fundamental lack of leadership within the health center. Furthermore, she has discovered a noticeable difference in attitude between employees who previously worked at Carolina Hospital and those who did not. This difference is evidenced by how workers interact with one another and communicate while undertaking their job responsibilities. This is also a problem that Martin will seek to resolve in the coming months.

During her first week, Martin randomly jots down in a notebook her observations and events that seem significant in terms of everyday conduct at the Center. Her objective is to understand how the clinic operates, how customer-patients are treated, and what the pool of human resources is in terms of staff strengths and weaknesses. To further this effort, she asks questions of the staff and walks around the facility at least once every hour to observe staff conduct and the Center's operations.

On the first day of her second week, Martin meets with Kelsey Lewis to discuss her new role. In this meeting they discuss Lewis's expectations for the Center. Lewis reviews her observations of what the former director did right and wrong and presents to Martin specific expectations she has for the clinic. Martin asks for a set of goals and a preliminary performance-evaluation form that lists the goals and expectations for the job and spells out how success will be evaluated in her first year as director.

Later in the second week, Martin arranges to meet with her three reporting supervisors. Because of a medical emergency, Dr. Sylvester is unable to attend, and the meeting proceeds with Shayne, the operations supervisor, and Neville, the medical support supervisor. In this open-ended meeting, Martin enlists their help in setting a course of direction for the student health center. Referring to the fact that this is her first management role, she admits to being somewhat overwhelmed by her responsibilities and the level of daily activity that takes place at the Center. She asks Shayne and Neville for their help in ascertaining resources needed to reach those goals. Martin contracts with them to hold a monthly supervisors' meeting as well as a monthly department meeting for the entire staff.

During the meeting, Martin noticed that Neville takes the lead in presenting ideas. She has known Neville for several years, having worked with her at Carolina Hospital when both were staff nurses. Furthermore, they attended the same high school in Carolina City (although Neville was two years ahead of Martin). Based on this history, Martin assumes Neville is effective and needs no special support from her. However, Martin has no prior history with Shayne; this might explain why Shayne is less talkative in the initial meetings. To elicit more communication from Shayne, Martin decides to start with his department in her organizational review of the facility.

On the day following this first staff meeting, Martin has a one-on-one meeting with Dr. Sylvester, who pledges his support in making the Center a better and more productive health care facility. His key concern seems to be better integration of services and the need for additional equipment. Sylvester agrees to jot down in a notebook his specific ideas for these two concerns and discuss them with Martin at a later date. Seizing this opportunity, she schedules a meeting with him for the end of the month. Martin also asks Sylvester to consider whether the three days a week he spends at the Center is sufficient given the increase in student enrollment and the Center's escalating responsibilities. Sylvester replies that he believes three days is adequate and will let Martin know if there is a change in this perception.

Martin spends her third week conducting meetings with all the Center's employees. Over three successive days, she conducts meetings with half of each key department, scheduling them to be compatible with the projected departmental workload. For example, knowing that Monday morning is somewhat slow for the operations department but very busy for the medical department, she meets Monday morning for two hours with half of the operations personnel. On Monday afternoon, she meets with the other half of the operations staff. On Tuesday morning, she meets with half of the medical department. In the afternoon, she meets with half of the medical support staff. On Wednesday, she meets with the two remaining halves of these two departments. By scheduling strategically, she minimizes interruptions of workflow, thus encouraging workers to participate freely in the meetings.

These meetings become more than an occasion for simple introductions. Following individual introductions and a basic presentation of her expectations for the Center, Martin asks for ideas from the group that might help formulate a strategic plan for the entire year. Five basic problems emerge:

1. *There seems to be very little employee identification with Carolina Hospital.* Many employees previously were on staff at Carolina Hospital but now feel removed from the hospital environment. Any information they receive about the hospital—whether in regard to a new medical service or to the annual picnic—is secondhand. Because of this they feel little or no affiliation with the hospital or, in the words of one employee, they feel that the hospital "really doesn't care about us."

Martin asks why this is important to them, and the employees' answers are predictable. Many of them still have friends at (and thus strong allegiances to) the hospital and wish to maintain those relationships on both a social and business basis. Second, they feel a lack of support in certain areas and that any support provided by the hospital is done only as an afterthought. Finally, many of them want to maintain identity with Carolina Hospital because its reputation in the community is solid and would contribute to establishing a strong reputation for the Center, which is still regarded in the community as a new entity even though it has been in business four years.

2. *Many employees cited lack of a strategic plan.* The former director never established or presented a plan to the employees. They never participated in devising one for their departments and consequently have no vision for the Center.

Martin asks the employees to start a list of their perceptions of what the Center should be. She initiates this list by writing on a chalkboard two objectives synthesized across the three key departments. These two objectives are (1) to provide prompt, professional medical service as needed and (2) to provide students with a wide range of services. By encouraging all employees to add to this list, Martin hopes to generate some new ideas she can incorporate in her strategic plan for the health center.

3. *No job descriptions are in place.* This concern is raised in all the meetings and among all thirty-six employees. Because no job descriptions were ever established, no performance evaluations have been completed since the Center's inception in 1989. As a

result, salary increases were based strictly on cost-of-living adjustments and basic compensation policy information provided by the hospital's human resource staff.

Based on her experience serving on the hospital's human resource advisory council, Martin is confident that this concern can be addressed easily, and she assures the employees she will look into this area. Descriptions are essential to any personnel administration, not only from a legal viewpoint but also from a business viewpoint. Upon concluding these meetings she calls the hospital's human resource director. She knows that Kim Losurdo, president of the hospital and an advocate of promotion from within, is vitally concerned about human resource administration and professional development. Therefore, she gambles on getting support for implementing a sound personnel management system. (She speculates that failure to address this important matter might be one of the reasons Kelly fell short in his role.)

4. *Salaries throughout the Center are perceived to be lower than market standards.* In each meeting, employees voiced concern that their salaries were not up to market standards in the Carolina City metropolitan area. This was raised successfully by a nurse, a custodian, a medical records specialist, and a part-time clerk.

While facilitating these meetings, Martin asked whether this was a general concern held by all members of the staff. She got a mixed reaction, from shrugs to nods of assent; a few heads in disagreement. Once again, she promised to enlist the help of the human resource department to solve this apparent dilemma.

5. *Communications were deficient throughout the Center.* This concern echoes universally throughout health care management. Individuals felt as though directives were not communicated appropriately, that they had little idea of what other departments did, and that many issues on campus that affected the Center were not presented in a timely and effective manner.

Alberta Martin asked the employees to give specific observations regarding poor communication. She received several suggestions. These included generating a health center newsletter, more meetings for dissemination of specific information, and increased dialogue between the college and the health center to get a better idea of major campus events and inclusion of health personnel in the college's information loop. Martin thanked the employees and pledged to look into the suggestions at the earliest opportunity.

Upon entering the final week of her first month on the job, Martin already has an appreciation for the challenges of management. She has learned that communication is key to the most important aspect of management, that of managing *people*. She has appropriately involved all the players on her team: her immediate supervisor, her three reporting supervisors, and all members of her diverse staff.

Alberta Martin has a challenging agenda. None of her three reporting supervisors seems to harbor resentment over not getting the job. Though she has a positive frame of reference regarding Neville, Martin is still not completely sure of all of the managers' abilities and wonders what their various levels of commitment are to the Center's success.

In the initial month of her tenure Martin established a support network consisting of one of her college professors, two colleagues form Carolina Hospital, and a high school friend who is a supervisor of three record stores in Carolina City. These four individuals acted as a sounding board for many of her ideas, graciously providing insight as she undertakes her new responsibilities. However, Martin recognizes that the decisions and actions to be undertaken must be based ultimately on her own instincts and intelligence.

The Second Month

As Alberta Martin settles into her second month on the job, she realizes that many management responsibilities demand quick reaction and sound judgment more than planning and proactivity. She is confronted with a variety of problems and opportunities that must be acted on by her and key members of her staff.

To begin with, Martin has had several informal conversations with members of the community, both on campus and throughout Carolina City, and is surprised to discover that a significant number of people have no information about the Carolina Hospital Student Health Center. They do not know where the Center is located and, in some cases, do not even know of its existence. Furthermore, many students have gone directly to Carolina Hospital—or to its main competitor, St. Gregory's Hospital—for emergency or even routine health care services.

This lack of representation in the customer-patient population is an obvious concern to Alberta Martin. She takes three approaches to resolving this problem. First, it is essential that the Center have a strong image within the community, particularly on campus. Second, a decline in utilization of services raises questions about the Center's financial viability if students choose St. Gregory's over the Center (or over Carolina Hospital). Therefore, she realizes that she must take immediate action to promote the Center's visibility and credibility. To accomplish the objective, she implements the use of InfoCards at the registration desk. With the support of Tony Shayne and his staff, she has devised a three-by-five card listing three questions:

1. How did you learn about the Carolina Hospital Student Health Center?
2. To your knowledge, do most of your fellow students and friends know about the Center?
3. Please list on the back how the Center might better serve student needs and how more people might learn about the services provided at the Center.

Issuing these cards is a logical starting point in that it provides a data bank of readily available information from individuals who may be interested in the Center's success.

In her second approach to solving the problem, Martin enlists the support of the hospital's public relations department to provide a brochure describing the health center. (A colorless, condensed brochure was developed four years ago by Larry Kelly and his staff but without favorable results.) At the suggestion of the hospital's public relations specialist, both the college's logo and the hospital's logo are displayed prominently on the brochure's front page. After three months' work, staff volunteers wrote a six-paragraph overview of the Center and its activities. Following completion of this effort, Martin holds an informal dinner to thank the volunteers and arranges to have copies of the brochure distributed to various heavy traffic areas on the campus (student cafeteria, recreation center, athletic box office). She also gets the admissions staff to include the brochure in its application package to prospective students and in its orientation package for new students. Furthermore, Martin agrees to have one of her supervisors appear at student orientation programs for freshman and transfer students.

A third approach to promoting visibility and community awareness used by Martin is networking through one of her contacts to get the word out. This contact is George Webster, her high school friend who manages the three World Class Records retail outlets in the Carolina City area. Knowing that these stores are favorites among the student population, Martin arranges a meeting with an ancillary manager named Alexandra Hensler, George Webster, Kelsey Lewis, and herself to discuss the possibility of cosponsoring a "dance-a-thon" as a muscular dystrophy fundraiser. By cosponsoring this event with World Class Records, Martin has set in place a plan to publicize the Center's services in support of a worthy cause and with a benefactor who routinely deals with a large percentage of the student population. Lewis fully supports this idea, and Webster graciously accepts a large shipment of brochures for prominent display at the cash register counters of all three stores.

Martin has discovered that no procedure manual exists for the Student Health Center. In discussing this with her three reporting supervisors, she learns that Kelly (her predecessor) assigned this task to Dr. Sylvester. Sylvester says that he has gathered the medical-specific material required by the state and other regulatory agencies but has not had time to complete the rest of the project.

Martin asks Sylvester to give her all the material compiled for the manual's medical section. She then asks Shayne and Neville to compile basic text for the operations section and medical support section, respectively. She volunteers to convert the material into a first draft to be approved by all regulatory and governing bodies.

Martin's motivation in taking on this responsibility is twofold: to ensure manual completion and to gauge the supervisors' motivation and knowledge of their specific areas. The latter also will provide her with an overview of their centric responsibilities. As a result, she will be able to develop supervisor job descriptions, understand their department functions, and learn how each department's services affect the overall operations throughout the Center.

In her sixth week on the job, Martin is approached by Tony Shayne with a plan for establishing a new collection system for customer-patients who have outstanding bills. This has been a long-standing problem because many students use their parents' insurance plans, have no insurance, or use a mix of health insurance payment plans. Martin encourages Shayne to review his plan with Carolina Hospital's audit director.

Following his conversation with the audit control director, Shayne makes several refinements to his plan and resubmits it to Martin. Before making a decision on whether to implement the plan, though, she asks him three questions:

1. What benefits will this plan provide to the organization?
2. How will this plan specifically assist in the collecting of outstanding payments?
3. What problems do you foresee in implementing this system?

Shayne has ready and acceptable answers to the first two questions but states that he expects problems in implementing the new system, specifically with his two accounts receivable clerks. Shayne, a generally somewhat reticent communicator, is hesitant to explain further.

After asking some questions, Martin realizes Shayne is supportive of the new program and thinks that it will be a major improvement. His apprehension lies in his fear that Walt Linial, one of the accounts receivable clerks, might "shoot holes in the program" from the outset. Considering this, Martin decides to implement the new program and take the lead in presenting it to the clerks with Shayne present. This will not only ease the implementation but also help Shayne handle adverse reaction quickly and effectively.

During the presentation meeting, Martin observes that the two clerks are very vocal; Walt Linial is also somewhat arrogant. Martin shifts her questions to Linial, emphasizing the goal of providing solutions as opposed to restating problems. She pointedly tells him that the decision has already been made to implement the new system, and that his expertise is needed to make the system work, not determine what new problems might exist in its implementation. Furthermore, she announces that she fully expects Shayne and the two accounts receivable clerks to implement the new system within two months and she wants to be apprised of progress every two weeks.

After the two accounts receivable clerks leave, Martin tells Shayne that she understands the problems he might encounter with Linial, a twenty-year employee who seems to be a know-it-all. She advises Shayne to monitor the implementation progress closely, reminds him to keep her informed, and tells him not to hesitate to ask if he needs her assistance in dealing with Linial. Most important, she assures Shayne that the plan is a good one and thanks him for his efforts in developing it.

Another problem that becomes evident in Martin's second month is the increasing perception that the Center's yearly performance objectives were not defined clearly. Apart from the fiscal performance expected by the board of directors and by her supervisor Kelsey Lewis, no objectives were ever set for the Center. Therefore, Martin had no goals for the organization to attain and consequently no basis for establishing performance expectations among her staff.

To resolve this problem, she devised a set of goals based on her preliminary discussion with Kelsey Lewis (see preceding section). These goals were directives and were finalized into a set of objectives that were realistic and meaningful enough to serve as a guide for members of all three departments.

In addition, the board's advisory information was valuable in establishing a context from which the procedures manual could be drawn. By now, Martin has concluded that her predecessor, Larry Kelly, fundamentally managed by crisis; that is, he never established specific plans and managed daily situations reactively. Although Martin has had to allow the Center to run itself in her initial seven weeks as manager, by doing so she has given herself opportunity to learn the operation and to install several management dynamics—monthly meetings, mechanisms for bonding with her board and supervisor, and the establishment of procedures—that in turn facilitate programs and plans for progressive development of the Center.

By her seventh week, Martin also has a better understanding of the supervisors who report to her. Dr. Gus Sylvester appears capable and dedicated to providing high-quality medical services. However, his time is limited by his responsibilities as staff physician at Carolina Hospital, his private practice, and his involvement in community activities.

By means of her InfoCards as well as though simple observation, Martin has learned that additional medical services are needed. As a nurse, she knows that students need the same variety of health care services as are available in other health care environments. Drug abuse prevention, AIDS awareness, pregnancy-related issues, and a host of other concerns are as pertinent to the college student patient population as to any other health care consumer group. Consequently, she recognizes that more diversity of medical services should be offered.

With this in mind, Martin and Dr. Sylvester discuss the possibility of additional medical expertise. Sylvester's staff is a team Martin has identified as all veterans. The nurses who assist and report directly to Sylvester have been with him for most of their careers and have developed an ease of communication that allows them to operate flawlessly as a team. The last thing Martin wants to do is upset this delicate balance, but both she and Sylvester acknowledge a need for more medical personnel.

To meet this objective, they list specific services most needed at the Center. After reviewing this list, they agree that the addition of a pathologist, an obstetrician, and another general practitioner would be ideal. After discussing this with Kelsey Lewis, Martin discovers an opportunity to use physicians on staff at Carolina Hospital, particularly several specialists who are undergoing their internships as part of an ongoing program at the hospital. Martin encourages Sylvester to arrange interviews with selected candidates for these three part-time positions. Both will participate in the appraisal process.

The key benefit to these new physicians is opportunity to work with Sylvester's veteran staff. To maintain the balance of talents and personalities that already acts as a positive force within Sylvester's staff, Martin encourages the candidates to spend some time with his staff to further ensure a good match in terms of expertise and personality.

Upon entering her eighth week, Martin realizes that she has worked closely with Tony Shayne (instituting a new accounts receivable program) and with Dr. Sylvester (adding to the Center's medical expertise). Her time with Carlene Neville, however, has been somewhat limited, so she schedules a luncheon meeting at a local restaurant. The reason for this venue is that with fifteen people reporting to her, Neville has the largest staff among the three supervisors and is often called from meetings to attend to a pressing problem or other crisis. Martin wants Neville's undivided attention, so she holds this meeting at an off-site location.

Martin asks Neville to tell her generally about areas in which she might need additional support or resources. Neville responds that she and her staff feel overwhelmed by their work load. Moreover, Neville feels as though her responsibilities have broadened considerably since the Center opened and that the inclusion of medical records, rehabilitation services, and sports medicine have added to the pressure of her daily responsibilities. She needs Martin's assistance in easing the pace and pressure inherent to her responsibilities.

Martin assures Neville that she was unaware of this situation, but that she has observed firsthand that everyone in Neville's department certainly appears to be fully occupied throughout their work shifts. She proposes three questions for Neville to consider, and the two agree to meet exactly one week later at the same restaurant for a follow-up conversation. These questions are as follows:

1. How might the workload be reduced in your department without jeopardizing service provision?
2. How might department morale and team unity be enhanced?
3. Other than workload, what are some sources of stress and how might this stress be reduced?

In using the word *stress* as a key, in a way similar to how *communication* is used in management discussions, Martin encourages Neville to come up with an action plan that will assist in fully using the various talents and abilities of staff members. She is relying strongly on Neville's expertise to solve these problems, while pledging her support to make some positive change happen. Furthermore, she is charging Neville with the specific responsibility of solving the problems relative to her department and establishing a dialogue that will become a precedent for all future work-related conversations.

Following their conversation, Martin realizes that she could have had this conversation at the outset of her tenure but that she had assumed that Neville had no problems. She has learned two important lessons in health care management: One, never assume anything (she assumed Neville was operating at a 100 percent effectiveness rate whereas in reality she needed the same management support that most supervisors require). Two, just because someone was successful in the past, success in the present environment is not guaranteed. It is the responsibility of a health care manager to render assistance proactively, constantly, and individually to all staff members.

At the conclusion of the second month of Martin's tenure as director, she has established a relationship with all three of her supervisors, generated positive discussion among her staff and board of directors and with her boss, and she has set in place the basis of a specific action plan and performance goals for the entire organization. Furthermore, she has exhibited an ability to make decisions and execute action and has charged all three supervisors with developing their work groups into teams. As she enters her third month, she is ready to make the transition from rookie manager to full-fledged leader.

The Third Month

Alberta Martin begins her ninth week on the job with another meeting with Kelsey Lewis. The two have established a routine of meeting during the first week of each month to discuss issues pertinent to the Center's operations. These include new plans for the Center, a review of the past month's activities, and any specific problems that might have surfaced over the past month.

The objective of these meetings is threefold. First, the expectations that Lewis has for Martin as a manager and for the Center as a whole can be reviewed and discussed on a regular basis. Second, the meetings provide a natural forum for Lewis to serve as a mentor by giving Martin the benefit of her own experience, perceptions, and managerial expertise. Third, two heads are better than one. As in any health care management setting, the Center can always benefit from shared points of view. Both Kelsey Lewis and Alberta Martin are ideally positioned to exchange points of view to further progressive solutions and programs for the Student Health Center.

Another event that takes place in the ninth week is Martin's follow-up lunch meeting with Carlene Neville. After considering the questions posed to her in the previous week, Neville has come up with several answers. She cites dealing with the unique temperament of college students as one source of employee stress. Many of her employees have never dealt with college students before and are ill prepared to relate to them, particularly in crises.

Martin asks Neville's opinion about the correlation between employees' ability to deal with this age group and their level of technical performance. Neville acknowledges that there is a direct correlation between certain employees' poor interpersonal skills and their difficulty in executing their professional responsibilities. She cites three who come to mind. They work in three distinct technical areas, perform at an unacceptable level, and are very confrontational when dealing with the patients. Martin advises that these individuals should be transferred back to the hospital, terminated, or dealt with through the performance evaluation process that will be instituted within the next month, based on concerns raised in Martin's initial meetings with the employees. Neville will soon have a tool with which to address these inadequacies.

By the close of their follow-up luncheon meeting, Martin has learned a number of things. Another source of stress, according to Neville, is the clashes that occur between her and Dr. Sylvester. As a former nurse, Martin asks whether this conflict is part of the turf battles known to occur between nurses and physicians. Neville believes that the problem runs deeper; that it exists because of duplication of services provided by both departments and because of poor communication due to Sylvester's limited hours spent each week at the facility.

To address the communication problem (and by extension, the problem with duplication of services) Martin implements an orientation process for the three new part-time physicians. Over the course of two days they will spend an hour with each department of the Student Health Center. This process affords opportunity for

Neville and Sylvester to work together in presenting the needs of each department, and to address the specific needs of the medical records section, the sports medicine section, the drug awareness section, and so on. This effort also instills a sense of team unity while reducing workload.

To deal with the duplication of services, Martin creates, in conjunction with the orientation program, a forum for veteran and rookie physicians and nurses to discuss and eventually eliminate this problem. After four forums, conducted by Martin with Neville and Sylvester's leadership participation, a new strategic plan is implemented to eliminate duplication of medical and nursing services, and the orientation program is fine-tuned accordingly.

Martin determines by her tenth week that a group staff activity could boost morale, reinforce common objectives, and create opportunity to address some other concerns. With this in mind, she schedules a one-day workshop to be conducted on two successive days (again ensuring full staffing and full participation). She schedules the workshops during spring recess, when the Center's patient volume is at low ebb.

Each one-day session (six hours per session) will have three basic components, as defined by needs and desires stated in Martin's first two months on the job. The first component, lasting one hour, will be a review of the goals and objectives for the Student Health Center. By now, these goals and objectives have been distilled to include a mission statement and a list of ten objectives for the year. These objectives were submitted by the employees, reviewed by Martin and her three reporting supervisors, and ratified by Kelsey Lewis. Each participant will receive a copy of these clearly stated objectives as well as the mission statement, printed on one side of a pyramid-shaped desk ornament that also has the college and hospital logos etched on each of the two remaining sides of the pyramid. This "pyramid of success" will be the motivating first segment of the session.

The second part of the workshop will be divided into two presentations that underscore the solution to problems posed by the employees in their initial meetings with Martin. Recall that two key problems were lack of strong identification with the hospital and lack of job descriptions. In this two-hour segment, both problems will be resolved.

For the first hour, Martin has arranged for one of the college's recruiters, Mike Flanagan, to present a slide presentation about the history of Carolina State College, its future goals and aspirations, and a review of its special features. Flanagan has been authorized by the president of the college, at the request of Kim Losurdo and Kelsey Lewis, to present each staff member with a membership card in the college's Cougar Club. The Cougars have tremendous athletic programs in men's and women's sports, and membership allows a sizable discount on athletic events and college productions (plays, movies, and concerts). This strategy will strengthen the bond between the Center's employees and the larger college community.

The second hour of this segment consists of a program presented by the hospital's director of human resources, Ashley Seton. She will discuss how to complete the form that helps employees construct a job description. This will begin the job description process, which is to be completed by the supervisors at the end of the workshop. Seton will also give a presentation on the hospital's benefits package and answer any questions on hospital events, policies, and new employee programs.

Seton closes by giving each participant complimentary copies of the latest Carolina Hospital newsletter and discusses the feasibility of printing a Center newsletter or including a section dedicated specifically to the Carolina Student Health Center. The employees unanimously elect for a section in the existing newsletter and form a four-person committee responsible for submitting information for newsletter coverage.

These first two segments of the program take up the entire morning. After a one-hour lunch, a stress-management program conducted by a clinical psychologist employed by the hospital fills the remaining three hours. Using a commercially produced stress-management workbook, each employee completes the practicum, including focused exercises contained in the book. This program addresses specific concerns about stress, provides an educational dimension of the forum, and gives the clinician an opportunity for further work with staff.

As she enters the final half of her third month on the job, Alberta Martin's main objective is to bring closure to any remaining loose ends. She closely monitors implementation of the new programs all three of her managers have suggested. Dr. Sylvester has hired his three new part-time physicians and is supervising their orientation process.

Tony Shayne's new accounts receivable program is still meeting with resistance from Walt Linial. To solve this problem, Martin begins her eleventh week with a meeting with Shayne and Linial. At Martin's direction, Shayne has documented several episodes in which Linial failed to perform his duties. In a prior counseling session, upon reviewing his documentation, Martin and Shayne agreed on a statement of expectations for better performance and a clear outline of the ultimate outcome of probation or termination should poor performance continue. Martin has thus prepared Shayne to take the lead in this discussion. Although somewhat nervous, Shayne conducts this session effectively, and Linial leaves the meeting with clear notice of his choices.

Also in the eleventh week, Neville and Martin meet to review all job descriptions for Neville's staff. In doing so, Neville notices that the same three employees she identified as problem cases did not complete their job-description work sheets. In individual counseling sessions, Neville and Martin "suggest" that each complete the job-description work sheets by the end of the following week, and they do so.

Another revelation is that four of Neville's employees are doing a lot more work than she thought originally—and without fair market compensation. Martin assures Neville that this will be considered in the salary review process, which she has started with Ashley Seton and will be completed within a month.

As she enters her twelfth week on the job, Martin is aware of having made a transition from neophyte to (at least) experienced novice. She has learned a great deal and has established some sound precedents that will lead to strong regular practices and procedures. By taking timely action on several key issues, she has assured her staff that she will be an active leader and can empathize with their problems and needs. More important, she will pursue solutions to problems and keep in mind the best interest of the Center.

By asking her managers the right questions, Alberta Martin has gotten a great deal of information to assist her initial efforts as a manager. In asking questions she has established relationships based on dialogues and creative thought on her part, as well as on the part of her three supervisors. This dynamic enhances the team orientation that she needs to instill among all of her staff members.

As Martin moves into the second quarter of her management responsibilities, her primary focus will be to build on her initial momentum by continuing to ask the right questions, exemplifying leadership, executing decisions and actions promptly, and encouraging individual performers to act as a cohesive team. In doing so, not only is furtherance of her own management development ensured, but also the progress and positive development of the Carolina Hospital Student Health Center will be fully maximized. Every key member of the organization will feel as though his or her contribution is vital to the success of the organization. As a result, that success will become a reality.

Part Two

Management Strategies

Chapter Ten

Encouraging Creativity

Doing more with less is a frequently echoed health care mandate that demands strong creative contributions from each team member. Although everyone on your team is probably creative, methods to stimulate creativity and a progression of creative management techniques help maximize this essential resource. To be progressive and to achieve its goals and objectives, a health care organization must tap the creativity of all workers throughout its ranks. Unfortunately, in many health care environments, creative ability goes untapped. For example, some organizations are highly structured and do not encourage or reward creativity. Other organizations encourage creativity but do not progressively reward creative contribution. For a health care organization to survive and thrive, it is essential that all members attempt to make creative contributions that generate positive results and further the organization's goal of high-quality and affordable patient care.

As a newly appointed health care manager, you have a prime opportunity to foster a creative environment within your department and to set precedent with the plans you implement and the policies you incorporate into your management approach. Creativity not only helps organizational achievement, it also acts as a positive catalyst within a department, as it improves morale and fosters a sense of participatory allegiance.

The opportunity to be creative inspires participation from all members of the staff and demonstrates to them that what they bring to the effort is valued and vital to the organization's success. Creativity is essential to the growth and development of all members of the organization. To grow and develop on the job, your staff must stretch its wings and venture into new areas and explore new methods of achieving results. As mentioned, creativity is a primary health care mandate. With customer-patients placing new demands on providers and needing services that heretofore were either nonexistent or unavailable, it is critical for each member of the health care organization to offer ideas that might meet these consumer demands.

In this chapter I explore the prerequisites for creating an environment, examine the fundamentals required to encourage creativity throughout your department, and, most important, provide you with specific strategies for boosting creativity and garnering new ideas and approaches from your staff—all with a view toward how you as a new manager can apply these strategies to your own personal development while using them to institute new programs.

Establishing a Creative Work Environment

To develop a creative team process, the work environment must be conducive to breeding new ideas and new approaches on the part of workers. Furthermore, your team members must know that their creative thought will be valued and rewarded so that they do not feel afraid or intimidated to present creative solutions. This of course is easier said than done, for reasons I discuss in the following sections. In developing the notion of encouraging creativity, I present group and individual strategies that will help facilitate the creative process.

The team creative process begins with identifying individuals among your superstar and steady employees who will be helpful in establishing the proper climate for creativity. With this objective in mind, review the following specific list of your more likely, positive, creative contributors:

- The true superstar
- The new team member
- The previously disenchanted individual
- The technical expert (or *techie*)
- The "untapped steady"

Once again, although running the risk of stereotyping, you are simply categorizing personality types who will help you establish a creative environment. These are the likely depositors into your creative idea bank, and they strongly support your efforts. Many of these individuals have been hungry for the chance to provide creative input, and your new presence represents for them an opportunity to liberate their ideas. These individuals will be like strong thoroughbreds who merely must be guided and directed toward the finish line in your "run for the roses."

The True Superstar

True superstars are the positive leaders in your department who possess most of the technical knowledge and consistently demonstrate stellar professional ability. Their very presence and approach to the daily undertaking of their work responsibilities indicate that superstars are employees who would "run through the wall" for the organization. They will become your demonstrable role models for the work group and will always be ready and willing to present new, creative input that will lead to positive action.

Draw on these individuals heavily in the creative process. Ask for their opinions and input first in your work discussions and have them summarize their objectives and intentions at the end of the meeting. This will also underscore the type of performer you value on your staff. Furthermore, make certain that you clue these people in, without playing favorites, prior to any creative meetings. For example, upon a chance encounter with a superstar the day before a creative input meeting, give her some specific objectives to think about and ask that she be ready to share input at the upcoming meeting. Superstars provide a stellar contribution to your staff and hence deserve the reward of special consideration. Again without showing favoritism, show respect for their ideas and give them the maximum opportunity to contribute, which they richly deserve.

The New Team Member

The new team member can also be a prime contributor to the creative process. For example, new members recently arrived from other institutions may have a wealth of ideas on new applications for their work activities. They also may have several ideas of what worked or did not work at their previous institution. Hence, they might have some new angles that can benefit your staff and help spark forward thinking in your creativity meetings. You also might have new department members from other parts of the organization. They also will have new ideas and approaches, and a sense for what did or did not work in their previous department. Once again, tap these sources for their creative input. Their immediate participation will help make them part of the team right away, and they and veteran team members will get to know one another at once. You will hope that they will get off on the right foot in establishing their work roles within the department and will be positively drawn to your other strong players.

The Previously Disenchanted Individual

A less obvious but likely creative contributor is the previously disenchanted individual. In many cases, new managers take on responsibility for a department that is in trouble. That is, you may have gotten your job because your predecessor had a large hand in the department's poor track record. In many scenarios, new health care managers are replacements for predecessors who were totally ineffective, too authoritarian, or simply were not two-way communicators. Individuals who worked under such leadership may have been strong performers but became disenchanted and disengaged from the staff performance process. They fundamentally did their own thing, without regard to departmental progress or team contribution. They probably were strong performers and well-motivated individuals prior to your predecessor's arrival.

Once again, you have a prime opportunity to use the creative process to achieve overall greater staff performance. By allowing these disenchanted players the opportunity to contribute and provide input, you are recognizing their abilities and demonstrating clearly your esteem for their performance. In many cases, they will respond by returning to their previous high-level motivation. Remember also to examine the dynamics of their job descriptions and daily work responsibilities. One technique in this regard is to spend a day with each individual in your department at the outset of your management tenure. Constantly ask questions to learn as much as possible not only about the work role but also about the individual. This establishes an excellent precedent for dialogue and allows you to spur their creative and innovative thinking right from the outset.

Workers with a negative attitude for any number of other legitimate reasons might also fall into the category of the disenchanted. For example, their job may have been restructured for good reasons, the lines of report may have changed, or they may be suffering inordinate stress created by workplace circumstances that may now be smoothing out. In each case, once you have identified the person as disenchanted, concentrate initially not so much on the circumstances that created their outlook but on applying your efforts toward positive action.

For an individual who has a negative attitude, once you have initiated positive action, identify what created the negative attitude. If it is something that is job related, consider restructuring or reorienting the job role and the basic job description. If it is something that does not pertain to work but rather is generated by the individual's personal life, you might want to get an assist from your personnel department or an employee assistance program. If the negative attitude was specifically pertinent to the actions of your predecessor, simply ask this individual for a chance to prove yourself as a manager, thereby enlisting his support and participation. If the individual fails to respond to any of these actions, you no longer have a potentially supportive team member—you have a nonplayer performance problem.

The Technical Expert

As discussed throughout this book, most of your staff are technically proficient, or *techies*. For these individuals, their work interest is founded in the technical application of their jobs. They have a strident affection for these technical angles, even though they sometimes may appear to live in their own little world. Their work is defined by the parameters of their technical aptitude and the responsibilities that specifically use their technical expertise. A strong health care manager plays to the strengths of these individuals while ensuring that they continually have opportunities to participate fully in the work of the team.

The "Untapped Steady"

Techies can also fall into the category of the "untapped steady," an individual who endeavors to put in a good day's work for a fair day's wage but could be enticed to give a little more if approached appropriately. Like techies, untapped steadies are interested in the organization but heretofore have never been specifically challenged to make creative contributions. Involve them in the group process, specifically charge them with idea innovation directives, and, regardless of category, make the process as engaging and enjoyable as possible.

Stimulating Innovation

It is essential to use some techniques immediately upon entering the management ranks to establish a creative environment. In this section I discuss several techniques you can incorporate to make the creative process part of your everyday positive work actions.

Playing to Individual Strengths

Remember to play to individual strengths. That is, encourage an individual who has a strong technical proficiency to come up with technical ideas and newer specialty innovations that might bear on the entire department. Widen your scope as you do this; for example, ask a radiology technician how she might improve laboratory performance outcomes by using existing resources and providing stronger service. Then, based on that person's own activities, ask what might be done to encourage stronger intradepartmental cohesion—that is, how department members can better support each other's efforts.

This process can be initiated via a "spend-a-day-with" program. Upon assuming your management responsibilities, try to spend a day with each individual on your staff. Try to learn the specific objectives of each department member, and the specific dimensions of his or her work role. This activity will also help you in the creative process, as you will gain ideas on how to reorganize the department, restructure certain jobs, and use all the resources in your department more fully.

In undertaking this endeavor, present each individual with a brainstorming notebook. Ask each to record any ideas that answer the following questions:

- What can I do to make a stronger contribution?
- What resources would I ideally like to have to get my job done?
- What new and different approaches have I heard about or read about relative to my technical area?
- What new and different approaches have I heard about that might assist us in becoming a better department or better organization?
- What wild and crazy ideas have I considered and think might actually work and generate positive results?

With this notebook approach, you are formalizing the creative process. Each individual will see clearly that idea generation will not be your exclusive domain but a team effort in which everyone's participation is encouraged and valued. To follow up on this technique, try to hold meetings at least monthly, but certainly quarterly to review all new ideas generated and allow everyone the opportunity to offer their ideas and present any suggestions that might bring about positive action.

Asking Questions and Gathering Ideas

As discussed repeatedly throughout this book, it is vital to ask questions throughout the creative process. Numerous questions have been provided that you can use in a variety of management situations. Always ask questions on both an individual and a group basis. This not only allows you to get answers that are pertinent and valuable to your own management activity; it also encourages all members of your staff to ask questions. As posed by a popular media advertising campaign several years ago, great companies always ask, *What if . . . ?* In a similar vein, the biggest question you can ask in the creativity process is, *What would happen if . . . ?* Always present ideas, and try to get the upside and downside of incorporating any new ideas or new programs into your daily activities. After all, if you do not ask the question, you will never get the answer, and you might be missing something that could be valuable to your departmental activities.

Many organizations take asking questions one step further by holding what are commonly called *blue-sky meetings*. In blue-sky meetings individuals are charged with looking at the short-term and long-term perspective of their department, and while considering their department's future, they are asked to ascertain specifically what mission and objectives the department should be pursuing. In following this strategy, they try to innovate plans that accommodate these new suggestions. If you use innovation notebooks and give each individual in your department an idea notebook, you have a ready-made resource to use in these meetings. You can supplement this effort by simply asking, *If you had a magic wand, what would you make it do—besides making the hospital disappear or creating a perfect world?* This is yet another way of generating new ideas and allowing people to expand thinking in a free-flowing manner.

Encourage individuals to consider all sources in their idea generation. This would extend not only to other departments within your organization but also to any ideas that they might have heard or read about in the media. It can also include ideas from organizations that they are involved with, aside from their health care employer. For example, they might belong to a community, civic, or religious organization that used a successful management or customer satisfaction system.

Sometimes, customer-patients are also neighbors of the organization's employees. Therefore, individuals in your department probably have access to a vast repository of ideas on how to improve service and, certainly, on common perceptions of the institution held in the community. Some of your staff members might have heard comments about your health care facility and specifically about your department as compared with other provider organizations and departments. This can also be a tremendous source of ideas and potential new applications. Finally, their previous job experience and the input they hear from peers within the organization might be yet another untapped resource in idea generation, which can be collected in their idea notebooks and presented in your meetings.

Most individuals in your department attend some sort of education and development programs. They could be programs presented by a technical or a civic organization, or they could be in-service education within your institution. In all these activities, your staff hears the perceptions and ideas of other individuals. Once again, they should bring significant input back to your idea generation meetings, and record in their idea books specific comments that might be helpful. For example, a dietitian might attend a national association meeting and come back with ideas on a food program used by a hospital in another state.

Individuals attend retreats and workshops that might have very little to with their technical areas, as these functions engender their participation by virtue of their membership in community organizations. Once again, some useful ideas could be generated. Furthermore, in some health care organizations, managers go on retreats to discuss basic issues and receive the benefits of professional education. This is yet another source for new creative ideas.

Regardless of what idea sources are used, it is incumbent upon you as a manager to identify the value of acknowledging and recording potentially useful ideas. No idea is a poor one—it is simply that some ideas have more merit and potential application to the workplace than others. Therefore, it is important to emphasize consideration of all sources in idea generation, encourage all members of your staff to present these ideas, and reward individuals who contribute new ideas through recognition and other merit systems.

Using the I-Formula

To provide you with an even more concrete framework for bringing imagination and ingenuity into your workplace, I present the I-formula, which I devised for use by military officers in the late 1970s. It has since been adapted and used successfully by thousands of health care managers. It is a simple approach to making imagination and creativity an everyday part of the health care workplace. In this section I review all elements of the I-formula, explain the importance of each element, and present case study examples of a health care manager's application of the formula in dispatching his own responsibilities and a case analysis of a health care manager who used the formula for her staff.

Figure 10.1 illustrates the basic elements of the I-formula. The formula is structured in four phases: need, design, action, and establishment. Each phase is further divided into six subphases, for a total of twenty-four I-components.

Phase One: Identifying the Need

A creative process begins with a need, or an opportunity to improve the status quo. The need phase begins with an inspiration.

Inspiration

Inspiration is the motivation to create a new process or a new application. Without proper inspiration, the creative process cannot

Figure 10.1. I-Formula: Conceptual Overview.

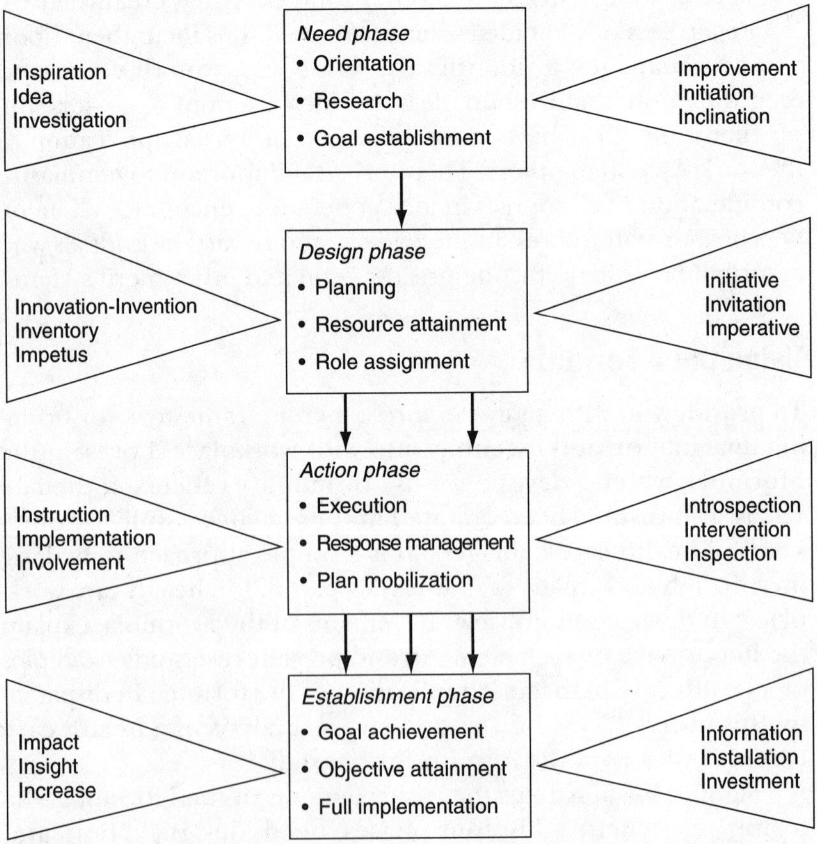

Inspiration Idea Investigation	**Need phase** • Orientation • Research • Goal establishment	Improvement Initiation Inclination
Innovation-Invention Inventory Impetus	**Design phase** • Planning • Resource attainment • Role assignment	Initiative Invitation Imperative
Instruction Implementation Involvement	**Action phase** • Execution • Response management • Plan mobilization	Introspection Intervention Inspection
Impact Insight Increase	**Establishment phase** • Goal achievement • Objective attainment • Full implementation	Information Installation Investment

take place; with inspiration, a clear goal is defined and individuals can begin to contribute pragmatically to the creative process. Although the inspiration for addressing a need should be defined and communicated by you as manager, it can be suggested by any member of your staff or any other participant in the action area, such as a supervisor, colleague, or customer-patient.

To illustrate the I-formula, let's follow the progressive use of this strategy by two health care managers, Kyle French and Alyse Beatrice, who hold very different positions in two health care organizations. French, a personnel director at a small-town clinic, has been told by her boss that turnover is an increasing problem among the clinic's staff of sixty. The inspiration, provided by the clinic director, is to identify the root of turnover and to stop its negative effects.

Beatrice is the chief operating officer (COO) of a long-term rehabilitation facility. She has decided to come up with a new guest relations program that will accurately collect the perceptions of discharged customer-patients.

Idea

The second segment of the need phase, the idea, is a potential solution, or set of solutions, that might meet the need specified in the inspiration. Once again, the idea should be generated by members of your staff and ratified and clarified by you, the manager. For Kyle French, the human resource director, some potential solutions include engaging an outside consultant such as the Gabrielle Reynolds Firm, running an attitude survey, or conducting exit interviews. For Alyse Beatrice, the ideas range from customer-patient surveys, demographic analysis, and a wide range of other solutions.

Investigation

The third segment of the need phase is investigation, which is extremely important at this point, when all viable options are considered based on potential effectiveness, maximum use of available resources, and overall potential to produce a high-quality final product. The investigation should be conducted by the most expert members of the staff with the leadership of the department manager; it should use all the talent available. The investigation must be accurate, comprehensive, and realistic in scope. Otherwise, the entire process can be a failure.

After considering a wide variety of options, Kyle French has decided to conduct exit interviews. He feels that use of questionnaires by individual managers will be cost-efficient and user-friendly and will generate the data necessary to ascertain the root of the turnover problem in his organization. Alyse Beatrice has decided that her segment of the health care industry relies on the personal touch. Therefore, she will use a follow-up call system, which (as will be shown) is also cost-efficient, user-friendly, and seems to be the best bet to achieving the desired results.

Improvement

The fourth segment of the need phase is perhaps the most important. If no improvement can be measured or directly recognized by implementing a new process, the entire process is a waste of valuable time and effort on the part of the health care staff. Although individuals like to be creative and arrive at new and different solutions, a distinct improvement must be made. To draw an analogy, the best pharmaceutical companies are those that not only perform research but develop new drugs. To carry this one step further, the difference between research and development is that development yields new and better products.

Initiation

The fifth segment of the need phase is initiation. At this point, individuals will present their ideas to other appropriate members of the organization: members of their staff, peers, and superiors. In this context, the word *initiation* has two applications. First, effort will be made to initiate the participation of all members of the staff and the organization so that they can contribute their thoughts and offer suggestions on how to improve the process at hand. Second, initiation refers to a period set aside for orientation of all appropriate organization members to the problem at hand to at least provide them with knowledge and offer membership into the creative process.

Kyle French has scheduled a fifteen-minute meeting with all members of the hospital's executive team in the interest of getting their ideas. He will also make some preliminary comments as to how they might participate in benefits they might gain from the process.

Alyse Beatrice, however, has decided to talk informally to all members of the long-term rehabilitation facility staff individually so that she can customize her presentation and ask specific questions of each member as appropriate to the process. Because she has five managers reporting to her, she will make sure that each member of the team has a discrete opportunity to participate in the process and to discus perceptions with their leader. Both managers are new to this process, as French was previously a personnel recruiter and Beatrice was a nurse team leader, and both recognize that communication is the key not only to creativity, but also to performance.

Inclination

The final segment of the need phase is inclination, the sum of personal preferences for action that will spell out the initial plan of action. For example, French has decided to use a set of six questions he has drawn from various human resource textbooks that can be used in exit interviews. Beatrice's inclination is to experiment with some survey questions herself, and make some personal calls to previously discharged residents in the hope that these questions can be fine-tuned for use by other members of the organization.

Phase Two: Designing the Action Plan

The second phase of the I-formula, the design phase, begins with innovation and invention. The attempt now is to formalize plans and design a specific action plan for accomplishing the goal, which is to arrive at a new and creative process that meets an organizational need.

Innovation-Invention

Innovation refers to the use of existing resources to come up with a new process; invention mandates using unavailable (or nonexistent) resources to create (invent) a new process or product. A reality of health care is that an innovator is preferred over an inventor. The reasons for this are simple. With resources shrinking and available revenue in a state of constant decline, no health care provider truly has all the resources desired. Most, however, have all the resources *needed*. Therefore, an innovative style is preferred to an inventive style, as the innovator will have infinitely more opportunities to accomplish something.

Inventory

Tightly aligned with innovation-invention is inventory. Inventory refers to taking stock of all existing resources at hand, considering all players involved, and incorporating this inventory into the plan design.

Both case study individuals have decided on innovation over invention. French realizes that he simply needs a copier to make copies of the sets of questions he has for the exit interviews. Beatrice decides to use a process that just needs the participation of her staff and a clear understanding of the objectives.

Impetus

A most important, but commonly overlooked, factor in the design process is impetus—the spark that starts the fire, often referred to in marketing terms as the hook. You must consider what will get potential stakeholders' attention so that they will want to become involved with your process and support the overall effort. If no impetus is provided, people will fail to see the importance of your actions and will not participate in its successful attainment. Furthermore, with time being an extremely limited commodity in health care organizations, any investment of time must be met with a guarantee of a strong return.

Turnover has plagued all members of Kyle French's organization, so any solution that will alleviate this problem will be met with strong support and a positive outlook. For Alyse Beatrice, however, the challenge is more formidable. She has several benefits that can be achieved by her efforts, including increased customer-patient satisfaction and an array of secondary data that will be gathered in her study that will help improve the overall quality of her facility and in turn the financial stability of her organization. However, she is using an element of intrigue in her efforts. Recognizing that people are naturally curious about how they are doing, she is using this human factor as part of her impetus strategy. She will simply ask members of her staff, *Wouldn't it be interesting to find out what our customer-patients really think about us?* Any motivated player on her team will answer this with a ready affirmative, and thus she will have both the attention and positive support of all members of her staff.

Initiative

Initiative is the basic drive to see the design process through to its logical end and to take ownership of the new process. In both cases, the players are clearly in charge of the action and will generate all the forms necessary to complete the action, assigning responsibility as appropriate.

Invitation

Two factors are closely related to initiative. One is invitation, whereby people are invited to become involved in the process. Kyle French will invite three key department leaders to initially participate in his turnover study and exit interview process. Alyse Beatrice will invite any two of her five direct reports to participate on a voluntary basis in the first round of customer-patient action calls.

Imperative

Invitation can also be supplemented with imperative. In certain cases, it is very important to get the backing of your leader and superiors in a new creative process. In some cases, this might mean your soliciting the involvement of your CEO or other executive players. In most cases, you should seek to get the support of your immediate superior so that the mentoring process can be further solidified and you can get the necessary authority (clout) needed to make your new process happen.

Both case study individuals have garnered the participation and support of their senior executives in the process. In Kyle French's case, the CEO has agreed to send a letter to all members of the staff explaining the turnover problem, delineating its deleterious effects on the entire organization, and detailing the general aspects of the plan. In Alyse Beatrice's case, the CEO has raised the topic of customer-patient opinions and perceptions. As can be seen, the participation of senior members in the process provides an imperative to all individuals to become interested in the process. Moreover, it clearly demonstrates that the organization is interested in the outcome of these projects, has deemed them to be important, and has set a very clear expectation that everyone will participate and contribute toward their success.

Phase Three: Implementing the Action Plan

Upon completing the need and design phase you now move into the all-important action phase. If the two phases have been followed strictly, and each segment has been met with a certain amount of ingenuity and productivity, the action should be productive.

Instruction

Now that your plan has been established and a need identified and addressed, you must instruct individuals on what their participation will be relative to the new action. Many health care managers fail to orient and instruct individuals on new processes. Accordingly, fear of the unknown works in concert with fear of change in negating the creativity process. It is extremely important to educate all individuals not only about what is to be done, but also how to do it.

For example, Kyle French has set up meetings with his three colleagues on the management staff who are going to use the exit interviews. He not only is instructing them on the purpose of the exit interviews, but also about the questions, and how to register responses appropriately. Furthermore, he will discuss possible outcomes and the possible perceptions (such as dissatisfaction with low wages, disgruntlement with superiors) that might be held by individuals leaving the organization.

Likewise, Alyse Beatrice is instructing all five of her charges on how to get customer-patient feedback via her ten-part system. Because all five of her staff members were interested in participating in the process, she is using this positive interest to get all her managers involved. She is instructing them on when to make follow-up phone calls and what questioning procedure to use in the follow-up phone calls, and she is assigning a basic objective of ten random calls per month to be conducted by each of the five managers.

Implementation

Initial implementations are referred to in the business world as pilot projects or test runs. The likelihood of achieving success across 100 percent of your organization on the first attempt at a new process is next to nil. However, many great ideas are lost due to this misguided expectation of first-run success. It is therefore essential to attempt to achieve success in a smaller area of the organization so that you can fine-tune your process and also engage the feedback of initial users who are meeting with success. Natural momentum can be built upon the success of the few individuals using your process, which could elicit the interest of the majority of the rest of the organization.

Looking at the example of Kyle French, we can see a prototypical example of this dynamic at work. Two of Kyle's colleagues, Craig Presley and Lauren Robertson, are department managers who have used the exit interviews. Following use of the questions on a couple of occasions, both individuals have suggestions for rephrasing the questions to get a more comprehensive response. Lauren has suggested putting the questions in a format that allows the manager to fill in the responses as they are relayed by the outgoing employee. Furthermore, she has found it valuable to simply give the questions to a disgruntled employee, and allow him or her the opportunity to write down responses and mail them as convenient. These are two very good suggestions that French can now incorporate into his process and use as he expands his efforts.

Involvement

Involvement rests on getting the full participation of all suitable parties throughout the organization who might benefit from your process. Once an implementation has been made and is fine-tuned and used successfully, involvement should be a fairly natural progression in the process. Involvement can use not only members of the organization, but outside individuals such as colleagues at other health care organizations, professional contacts, or customer-patients.

Alyse Beatrice's five team members have now made their follow-up calls over three months. Given the span of these 150 calls, she has collected a tremendous amount of information that will provide her with needed primary and secondary data about her organization and its effectiveness. However, to collate all the information, she is now seeking the involvement of a nursing school friend who has computer ability. Her friend, who works for a public organization, has graciously donated a couple of hours to Beatrice's nonprofit organization to show her a software package that will help her collate responses and present data in a logical fashion. Furthermore, she has secured the involvement of a member of the organization's board of directors who owns a printing business. This individual will print up the questionnaires and Info-Cards, which can then be used by members of her staff and incorporated into the new computer scheme of tabulating and assessing information.

Introspection

It is important at this point for the manager to sit back and assess the action taken to date. This introspection is a period you can use for validating your creative process. Ask these five questions:

1. Is the process moving toward meeting the stated need?
2. What major lessons have been learned already in the process?
3. Am I using all my resources successfully and efficiently?
4. What improvements can be made immediately on the process?
5. What will some of the long-range benefits of the process be?

Intervention

After answering these questions, you are now ready to accept intervention as needed. Intervention is any participation on your part to add creativity to the process and to constantly develop the positive nature of the effort.

Intervention need not be dramatic. For example, Kyle French needs only to ensure the participation of other managers and not take any further personal action himself. However, Alyse Beatrice has a good opportunity to increase intervention in her efforts. First, upon introspection, she has determined that follow-up calls on her behalf as facility COO will be quite useful. For example, two particular previous customer-patients were quite upset at the lack of consideration they felt they experienced upon calling the facility following their discharge. In such cases, Beatrice has decided to follow up with a phone call herself, in which she identifies herself as the COO of the facility, states that she understands the problem, and pledges to try to provide some practical positive action. In doing so in these two cases, she has alleviated the complaints and, what is more important, has increased the satisfaction level of these two previous customer-patients by her progressive action.

Furthermore, Beatrice has decided that the participation of the board of directors is key to the success of the program. This suggestion, fully supported by her boss (the CEO), entails having each member of the board make five calls a month to previous customer-patients in the interest of determining their level of satisfaction with the facility and its services. The entire organization recognizes that the board's participation in this process will add another point of view to the process and is a very creative method of assuring the customer-patients that the organization truly cares about their welfare and is vitally interested in constantly improving its efforts and services.

Inspection

The action phase concludes with an inspection. A comprehensive inspection should include answers to the following ten pertinent questions:

1. On a scale of 1 to 5, with 5 being high, how would we rate our action at this point?
2. If the score is lower than 3, should we go back to the drawing board, starting with the need process?
3. If the score is higher than 3, how can we make it a solid 5?
4. What major organizational benefits are being realized by the process?
5. What additional resources might be needed to make the process even more fruitful?
6. Are our expectations being met realistically?
7. Is this new process contributing to the values and ideals of the organization in a progressive manner?
8. Should others be involved in the process?
9. Should other actions be taken to improve the process?
10. Given the best of all circumstances, how can we make this process part of the realistic day-to-day action of the facility?

If you are satisfied with your inspection checklist, you are ready to proceed to the final phase of the I-formula, the establishment of long-term change.

Phase Four: Establishing Long-Term Change

The objective of the establishment phase is to provide a sound answer to question 10 of the preceding list by making the process an ongoing part of the organization's activity.

Impact

At this point you are measuring the impact the new process has had on the organization. Reviewing both case studies, Kyle French has now been able to fine-tune his exit interview process to the point that all managers in his small hospital are using the questions when an employee leaves the organization. Not only has this made the managers aware of the dilemma caused by turnover, it has sent a subtle signal to the employees that management is concerned about the turnover.

In Alyse Beatrice's case, customer-patients who are at the facility currently are aware that managers will be calling following their release, and are naturally now looking at services more closely. In addition, all members of the organization—particularly those reporting to Beatrice's five managers—are keenly aware that their efforts are being closely evaluated. The impact of this action is twofold. First, individuals are taking more pride in what they are doing, and are appreciative of the good feedback they are getting relative to their work efforts. Second, Beatrice is aware of the fact that in the future, individuals will expect the opportunity to provide feedback upon their discharge.

Insight

Now that the new creative process has been established and used by appropriate members of the health care organization, insight and opinion should be collected from all users. For example, Beatrice has asked all members of her team for suggestions on how to make the process better and, in fact, has used all the questions appearing in this section. As a result, she has gotten the new idea of providing InfoCards to all discharged customer-patients. This includes giving individuals a questionnaire when they leave the facility, which augments the random phone calls.

Increase (Positive Gain)

Increase relates to any improved productivity evidenced or generated by the new process. The insight provided by Kyle French's efforts is that employees are leaving the facility strictly because the benefits and wages do not compare favorably with the marketplace. Consequently, he has conducted a wage survey and has gotten the board of directors, with his supervisor's help, to approve a wage increase and a strengthening of the comprehensive benefits package. A year from now, the turnover rate will have gone down, length of employment for the typical employee will have increased, and some other positive gains will have been generated by his efforts.

Information

Information is any kind of data or significant communication generated by a new creative process. In Alyse Beatrice's case, a wealth of information has been provided relative to customer-patient concerns that has helped set criteria for what constitutes a successful stay at her long-term facility. Through this information, another usage of the word *informed* comes into play. As word gets out through the grapevine in both organizations, both case players are enjoying certain benefits.

For Kyle French, once word got out about the exit interviews and the benefits that are an effect of the exit interviews, top management of the organization authorized him to compile a set of questions that could be used during selection interviews, which would help identify and select individuals who could likely be retained. In Beatrice's case, once all five of her managers used the customer-patient follow-up call system, all the staff began to use the process—staff nurses, therapists, and even physicians affiliated with the facility.

Installation

These two systems will now be installed into the organization, much in the manner that a new physical facility is incorporated into a larger structure. Installation occurs if the answers to each of the following ten questions is a resounding *yes:*

1. Did the process meet a specific need?
2. Is the process user-friendly?
3. Did the process generate clear results?
4. Is the process viable?
5. Does the process underscore the ideals and values of the organization?
6. Does the process have a long-term benefit?
7. If the process has a short-term benefit, should we use it again?
8. Was customer-patient service improved by the process?
9. Were employee relations and motivation improved by the process?
10. Did the process help make the organization more productive and progressive?

For both French and Beatrice, the answer to all these questions was *yes*. Although for educational purposes these two cases were very positive and idealistic in scope, both examples were taken from real-world situations from my experience over the past two years. What is important is to understand the elements of the I-formula and to use its components effectively and efficiently as you try to bring creativity into your workplace.

Investment

The final essential I-element is investment. This factor should be a natural result of the entire I-formula process, as the proven initial success of the new product garnered from the entire effort should encourage potential stakeholders in investing resources, and indeed a stake in the new entity as it takes shape and becomes part of the health care organization's daily fabric. The investment of time, energy, personnel, budget finances, and other precious resources is a formidable stake for a health care manager to put up in any semblance, so a clear, cogent presentation of results potentially available to your peers is the key to getting the long-term support needed to grow your new process or product.

In the case of the exit interview process implemented by French and Beatrice, the word-of-mouth promotion that they have received from colleagues who have already benefited from the new process is the greatest attribute in garnering investment in the process from other managers. Furthermore, by specifying the benefits of the process along with the minimal investment of time and energy required by a reviewing manager, the prospect of using the exit interview process becomes low-investment, high-return for any manager in the organization.

Other Factors Critical to Long-Term Change

Three additional I-factors (not shown in Figure 10.1) should be considered in looking at the total spectrum of team creativity. First, recognize that *inertia,* the failure to move forward (that is, the state of remaining stagnant) unfortunately has taken hold in many health care organizations and departments. Hence, initially you may meet some resistance whenever you try anything creative. You must be the prime motivating factor, and by using the tenets of this chapter you can gain the support of all appropriate parties to move things forward toward a progressive new goal. Two other factors, *importance* and *interest,* must also be underscored. Make sure that your new process is important, and get everyone interested in the process. By engaging the work interest of others, motivating their participation, and achieving some important new goals, you are bringing much-needed innovation and ingenuity to the health care workplace. Not only will this benefit you; it will also serve the most important person in the health care organization—the customer-patient.

Conclusion

Creativity from all team members and resultant progressive action are vital lynchpins between potential and realized success. By optimizing the potential of all team members appropriately, garnering their creative input, and creating a synergy between individual talents and contributions to form a comprehensive and progressive work unit, you will ensure that a substantial contribution to your organization will be generated by your staff. Furthermore, the customer-patient needs of your operating environment will be met by a cohesive group of motivated, constantly developing professionals.

Chapter Eleven

Selecting and Hiring Top Performers

In your new responsibilities as a health care manager, one of your most important goals is to build and motivate a top-notch staff. The selection, motivation, and constant upgrading of performance is one of the most important concerns of a health care manager—certainly one of the most debated. The approaches and strategies you use to select new members of your team can easily spell the difference between your own success and failure as a manager. When you select a top performer, you have an individual whom the entire team can draw inspiration from and rely on for steady or stellar performance.

Conversely, when you select an individual who is not a top performer, the negative results can be staggering. To begin with, the job position for which the new individual was hired will not be properly filled and will present a performance gap on your team. Second, the poor habits and low motivation of this nonperformer will take root as a negative contagion throughout the work group. Third, and perhaps most pejorative, the effort that you undertake to motivate such individuals, and finally to terminate their employment, will be extremely time-consuming and in many cases will become one of the most negative episodes of your management career.

To avoid all the negative aspects of hiring a poor performer, you need to understand immediately the selection process, the interviewing elements, and the important aspects of orientating a new employee. Unfortunately, many health care managers have not mastered these essential elements. As a result, they are constantly plagued by the trauma created by poor performers. However, health care managers who have successfully mastered the selection and orientation process not only diminish the chance that they will have to terminate poor performers or address performance problems, they also enhance all their management responsibilities by having the luxury of working with well-motivated, talented people.

Although far from being an exact science, the process of hiring and selecting new employees can take on some structure, complete with strategies and proven approaches for success. In this chapter I progressively develop the entire hiring process from start to finish and present you with as much information as possible to make your initial selections progressive ones. I examine the positive aspects of hiring and orientation and point out the most common mistakes made in the process. You need to look not only at what you should be doing, but also at what you should not be doing when undertaking this vital endeavor.

The Preselection Process

The first mistake many managers make in conducting their first interviews is to jump into the process without preparation. Frequently this happens because a new manager is immediately presented with a department that has several openings and a short time in which to fill them. Consequently, the new manager may review resumes without any forethought as to the type of individual he is looking for or the long-range consequences of the selection decision. In the next five subsections I outline five recommended stages to incorporate into a preselection process:

1. Compiling a wish list
2. Compiling a list of expectations
3. Reviewing the job description
4. Reviewing recruitment tactics
5. Reviewing resumes

Compiling a Wish List

As shown in Figure 11.1, the preselection process should begin with compilation of a wish list, a type of brainstorming exercise. In this step, review everything you know about the position you need to fill (your own personal knowledge, the success-failure ratio of prior efforts to fill the position, and any input that can help determine critical needs for the position). For example, with regard to determining critical needs, you might ask others who have worked in that job position or supervised a similar position for insight into what makes for a successful performer in that particular job.

Your outcomes in compiling this wish list should be both quantitative and qualitative. This means you should look from several standpoints at what the jobholder needs to do the job. For example:

- Job requirements (past, present, and future)
- Past success and failures associated with the position
- Potential expansion of the position
- Collective insights (from self, staff, and peers)
- Quantitative-technical requisites (things that can be measured by numbers); for example, use figures such as the jobholder's number of years in the field, total years' education, number of technical degrees and accreditation licenses, and number of years employed in your specific technical area
- Qualitative factors (work personality, attitude, and ethic)

Qualitative outcomes incorporate factors that are not clearly measurable numerically but are nonetheless essential to the job. Some industrial psychologists maintain that whereas quantitative information indicates whether the individual can do the job, qualitative information indicates how they will do the job. For example, if you are filling the position of staff pharmacist, you would look at a candidate's number of degrees, the number of years she has been a pharmacist, the number of licenses held in your particular state (and number of years licensed overall), and the number of years worked in the unique setting of a hospital pharmacy. Qualitative indicators might include attitude—whether she demonstrates flexibility, assertiveness, persistence, and a basic work ethic. Qualitative factors might also include the people skills needed for interpersonal relations; that is, communication skills, abilities to listen and perceive information, and innate ability to create a positive presence and conduct herself with a professional bearing while on duty.

Figure 11.1. The Employee Acquisition Process.

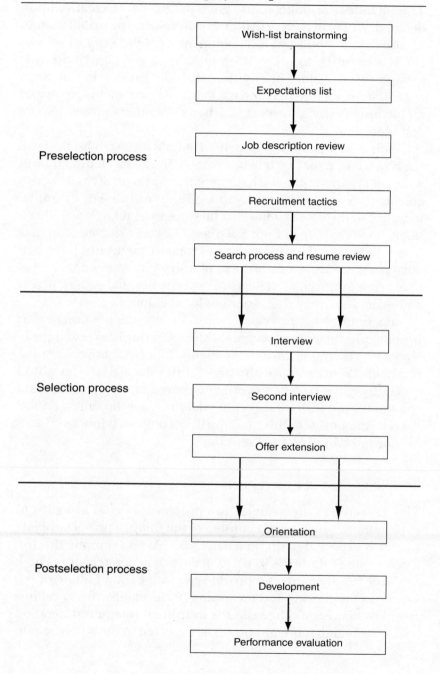

A candidate's managerial aptitude would also be important. This includes the ability to use good judgment, be creative upon demand, and plan daily activities. Furthermore, you would want to ensure that an applicant is a team player, able to support others, act as a resource to other team members, and contribute to a group process. Values orientation, including strong loyalty to an organization, a sense of compassion for the customer-patient, and an intrinsic desire to respect the dignity of others should also be considered.

With these parameters in mind, compile your wish list by dividing a piece of paper into two columns. In the left-hand column write all the quantitative characteristics you seek. Remember to consider why someone failed in a given position. For example, to return to the case of a hospital pharmacist again, you would certainly hope that she did not fail due to lack of a degree or appropriate licensure. However, the pharmacist might not have had adequate knowledge of a hospital pharmacy as opposed to a retail pharmacy, for instance. Therefore, specify hospital experience as a pressing requirement in your left-hand column.

In a similar vein, perhaps a jobholder in a staff position at your hospital pharmacy is not a good listener. If this has caused problems with relating to customer-patients, filling prescriptions accurately, and setting up for the night-shift pharmacist, you would specify listening skills as a pressing requirement in the right-hand column of your wish list. Listening skills not only become a critical need in the position, this quality will become an important focus in your interview and final selection.

Compiling a List of Expectations

The next step in the preselection process is to establish a list of expectations, which simply consists of the things a prospective job-holder is expected to do on a daily basis. As you compile this list, a good rule of thumb is to try to make this a "top ten" list. These ten basic job elements can provide you with a sound frame of reference in monitoring and measuring performance. Try to list in a free-flow manner all the tasks the individual is required to do on a daily basis and, more important, is expected to do as part of normal job conduct. If a job description is already on file for this position, you can use it as a starting point.

Another potential resource for compiling a list of expectations is your own observation of the position. Given your personal knowledge of the position, add to the list of daily expectations. Talk to others who might correspond with this person in daily work roles to elicit their expectations for the position. Finally, look at the big-picture ramifications. Ask yourself, *What does this person do to support the entire organization?* The answer can give you additional information to include on the list of expectations.

Some other keys can be used when compiling a list of job expectations. As you analyze the particular job position, for example, try to use time proportions to determine the major activities of the position. List all elements of the job that take up at least 10 percent of a "typical" day (allowing for the unpredictable nature of the health care setting). In the case of the hospital pharmacist, for example, imagine that a typical one spends at least 40 percent of the day actually filling prescriptions. Therefore, "filling prescriptions" would go on the expectations list. List all work activities that are undertaken daily and are part and parcel of the basic job profile. Furthermore, consider which work actions are most critical to overall department activity.

Use a variety of sources in compiling your analysis. Not only should you gain the input of others, but once you have set up your list of expectations, ask others in your organization to review the list; for example, your supervisor, colleagues, and past holders of this or a similar job position. Outside review will provide you with a final checkpoint to ensure that your list is valid. Remember, use current top players as guides, as anyone currently in the position who constantly provides stellar performance and seems to do all the right things in the job position is a useful model.

Reviewing the Job Description

If one is already on file, the job description can be extremely helpful in the preselection process. However, the description might not be accurate, or it might not reflect all the activities required in the job. Furthermore, the elements of the job might have changed to the point that the job description is only 50 percent (or less) accurate. As a result, you might have to review the job description and perhaps restructure it in terms of content and application. Contact your human resource department for specific guidance and ideas for updating and upgrading the job descriptions of your team members.

At this point, however, some things are pertinent to the job description process that applies to your preselection efforts. For example, once you have established your wish list and your list of expectations, it is certainly fruitful to review the job description. To begin with, compare your wish list and expectations to the job description to ascertain the accuracy of the content and whether there is anything in it that might be helpful in determining the critical aspects of the position as you undertake the selection process. You will hope that the job description will have several characteristics that will be helpful in the preselection process. If it does not have the characteristics described below, you might consider working with your human resource department in strengthening the job description content.

First, the job description should have maximum clarity of language. It should be free of jargon (except for relevant technical language suited to the position), and the elements should be printed clearly and accurately so all members of the organization—regardless of their technical proficiency or proclivity—can understand fundamentally what the job entails. In addition, all elements of the job description should begin with action verbs that delineate all the things the individual is responsible for, as well as the expectations of the job. Inclusion of appropriate verbs that give a clear indication of the work activity is also important. Examples of action verbs are *monitors, inspects, dispenses, manages, directs, initiates, reviews,* and any other verb that clearly indicates the job responsibility.

Second, a good job description should strive to establish a maximum of ten major factors. If more than ten exist on the job description, you might want to use the rule of applying a 10 percent quotient to each factor. This means that each job responsibility should be considered in terms of the amount of time spent on a particular application. If the time is less than 5 percent or the job responsibility is very complex, establish subcategories for each job description characteristic. To illustrate this, consider the position of a staff nurse, for whom a major responsibility would be, for example, "to manage direct patient care." Obviously, much is involved in this particular responsibility. Therefore, the description "manages direct patient care" would be listed as number 1. Any subcategories of the responsibility (such as checking charts, bathing the patient, and responding to patient complaints) might be listed subcategorically by using the letters *a, b,* and *c.* This helps streamline the job description process and makes it a more comprehensive guide as you review resumes and conduct the preselection process.

Third, anything specifically unique or critical to the job position should also be listed as part of the job description. This is anything the jobholder is required to do that separates the jobholder from others in the department; that is, unique responsibilities that historically have been handled by the individual who holds that particular job position and that certainly required additional education or experience. For example, assume that the candidate for hospital staff pharmacist would be in charge of ensuring hospital compliance with state regulatory agencies concerning controlled pharmaceuticals. Obviously, part of the job description should be a statement along the lines of "prepares for all state inspections and ensures total compliance with state mandates." Not only should this be included on the job description, it should also be part of your wish list in terms of the quantitative ability to conduct such inspections (that is, previous experience, a particular educational designation and background, or perhaps even a specific license or professional accreditation). Furthermore, the qualitative aspect of your wish list should also be the ability to do precise work, prepare for inspections, and have the patience and communication skills required to work with government agencies.

Reviewing Recruitment Tactics

You are now ready to undertake the search phase of the preselection process. This means that you will now turn your efforts to work with your human resource department, professional contacts, your supervisor, and anyone else who might be able to assist you in the recruitment of someone who will match the criteria you establish in the first three phases of preselection. This is no easy task.

Recruitment is certainly one of the most difficult endeavors for the modern-day health care manager. The reason for this is the unfortunate shortage of qualified personnel in virtually all health care positions. (The 1990s saw immense shortages in both the United States and Canada in the ranks of nurses, pharmacists, physical therapists, dietitians, and several other professional categories.) This means you must work assiduously toward generating a good roster of candidates and use as many recruitment sources as possible.

Several recruitment resources are available for your use and are enumerated in one of my earlier publications (*Handbook of Personnel Selection and Performance Evaluation in Health Care* [San Francisco: Jossey-Bass, 1988]). There are ten recruitment resources you should become familiar with as a newly appointed health care manager: human resource department contacts, job fairs, school liaisons, employment referral system, professional contacts, agencies, media coverage, informal staff referrals, internal candidates, and community-based recruitment.

Human Resource Department Contacts

Your human resource department probably has a network of contacts throughout the recruitment field and certainly a resume bank on hand of resumes from individuals who have contacted the department for employment opportunities or who were past candidates for positions at your health care organization. Furthermore, your human resource director can assist you in identifying key recruitment sources and make specific contacts for you in this effort.

Job Fairs

Job fairs can be good sources of meeting contacts and identifying potential talent for your staff. Whenever possible, try to attend job fairs in your specific technical area. This will help you build a data bank of talent in your specialty; you might even find qualified applicants for other areas of your organization. Keep in mind that many job fair attendees are simply shopping around and are not interested in immediate employment. However, collecting resumes and obtaining information on potential candidates is a continuous process and one that should be undertaken at every opportunity.

School Liaisons

Many health care professionals maintain contact with the school (or schools) they graduated from, whether a nursing school, four-year university, or other accredited academic institution. Call your alma mater, either the placement office or one or two of your favorite teachers, and ask whether any up-and-coming talent might be suitable for your open position. Furthermore, they might know alumni in the field who might either be suitable candidates for your position or know someone who might be. If you are trying to fill an entry-level position or an unskilled job role, you might contact a guidance counselor at a local high school or vocational school and inquire about likely candidates.

Employment Referral System

Most organizations have an employee referral system that assists in recruitment. Basically, this is a system whereby employees refer qualified individuals to the personnel office for openings in the organization, which are posted in a central area by the human resource department. If your organization does not have an employee referral system, or if you work in a small health care organization, you might want to discuss with your supervisor the possibility of providing a monetary reward to an employee who recommends a candidate for an open position who is subsequently hired. Employee referral systems give individuals the opportunity to participate in their organization's selection process, have a hand in selecting their fellow workers, and earn some extra money.

Professional Contacts

Many new health care managers have regional and national professional contacts. If you were previously a physical therapist, for example, you probably worked at another hospital or in another health care organization that employs other physical therapists. You can call these institutions and check with your former colleagues as to the availability of potential candidates and inquire into their knowledge of sharp people in your field who might be looking for a job. If you belong to a professional organization of physical therapists, you might very well have contacts in that organization who could also help generate a list of potential candidates.

Agencies

Many health care recruiters frown on placement and search agencies, basically because of a perception that agencies represent the largest expenditure of all recruitment sources. What's more, the yield may be less than satisfactory. Do not contact an agency without the assistance of your human resource department or your immediate supervisor. They both know who the good agencies are, their proven track records, and which ones have demonstrated consistent ability to provide the desired quality of talent. If you do work with an agency, spend as much time as possible with the primary recruiter in reviewing your wish list, list of expectations, and revised job description. This will help you in the long run, for it will screen out unqualified candidates, thus saving time, money, and energy.

Media Coverage

Health care institutions run employment ads regularly. Media advertising can be somewhat expensive and unfortunately does not provide consistently good results, but if you run an ad, again solicit the support of your human resource director and supervisor. Make certain that your ad is run to the best advantage possible—that it receives good placement within the newspaper or magazine, has a catchy logo, and contains a three-to-five-sentence depiction of the job, the salary range, and the name of a specific contact person (yours or someone else's). These elements will eliminate people who are simply job shopping or who are not in the salary range established for the position.

Informal Staff Referrals

Members on your team probably know of someone who might be qualified for the open position. However, unless they are asked, they may assume you are not interested in their recommendations. Furthermore, because they are busy and preoccupied with their own job responsibilities, if your predecessor has not established a policy of obtaining their input in the recruitment process, they will simply assume that input on candidates is not their concern. Therefore, make a concerted effort to ask your department staff for recommendations. Simply ask, *Do you know someone who might fit this description?* Encourage them to participate by telling them that in many cases they probably know better than you who might be a successful applicant.

Internal Candidates

A qualified applicant for your open position may be somewhere within your organization, perhaps in another department or at an affiliated facility. By working with your human resource department you might be able to identify these potential candidates. Some individuals might have applied directly to your department (either during your predecessor's tenure or since your own assumption of command). Furthermore, there might be outside individuals who have written to you in the past or contacted your human resource department about job positions. Maintain a file in which you have your wish list, list of expectations, and job descriptions. Also maintain one file for each position in your department, so that every resume received (even if a position is not currently open) can go into this folder. If the position becomes open, you have a file folder of immediate possibilities, complete with preselection data.

Community-Based Recruitment

Smaller health care providers, particularly in rural areas or in distinct neighborhoods (of large East Coast cities, for example) use community-based recruitment. These institutions take a three-to-five-sentence depiction of the open position, the point of contact, and salary range, and make copies on their organization's stationary. They post these copies on bulletin boards in five key areas within the community: (1) supermarkets and convenience stores (which have high traffic and prominent bulletin boards); (2) libraries and other community centers (which again have high traffic and common bulletin boards); (3) post offices (which always have bulletin boards or areas for posting notices); (4) places of worship (which commonly have posting areas); (5) cleaners or uniform stores (an often-overlooked opportunity: Health care people wear uniforms!).

When using community-based recruitment, be sure to get permission from the appropriate authority at each posting area. Getting their permission is also an opportunity for you to gain their support and participation in the search effort by reviewing the contents of your notice and discussing any potential applicants they might know among their customers or congregation. In my experience, the business and religious anchors in the community have all been positive allies in the health care recruitment process.

Reviewing Resumes

The fifth and final phase of the preselection process is reviewing resumes. Having established criteria for the position, and having drawn on the ten resources of recruitment to generate a flow of applicants, you can now review resumes to determine who among the applicants will be selected for an in-person interview.

Your main objective in reviewing resumes is to determine whether the person can do the job. The purpose of the subsequent interview is to determine what type of person the candidate is and how they would do the job. Therefore, when reviewing resumes, you must bear in mind several issues that need to be evaluated and assessed closely while you compile your interview roster.

Start with your wish list, list of expectations, and job description to try to establish a match with the resumes. Remember that throughout the entire process of selecting a new employee you will never (or at least very seldom) find a "perfect" match. Avoid being fooled by the product of a good resume-writing service or business-writing acumen. Put these "perfect" specimens into a "possible" pile and continue your review.

Try to sort the resumes by your criteria, and organize the candidates into three basic categories. The first category should be individuals who are not qualified. If you establish three separate piles on your desk, or use three separate file folders, this would be the pile to the left-hand side of your desk or the file folder on the bottom of the three folders. Unqualified individuals are applicants who simply do not have the quantitative skills you established on your wish list and list of expectations. For example, they either do not have the required degree(s) or years of experience (or specific experience) required. Send each one a courteous letter thanking him or her for the application or resume, then return it to the human resource office to be considered for other positions. Remember, you are reviewing resumes and, in many cases, applications (depending on your organization's human resource policies), so always clip both together as you go through the review process (as well as the actual interview process).

The second category is made up of possible candidates, defined as individuals who definitely have the quantitative skills sought and might have additional factors that merit consideration. For example, for the position of staff pharmacist, an individual in the "possible" category would have all the necessary degrees, including the specific professional accreditation to prepare for state compliance reviews, and a good range of years of professional experience. Furthermore, this candidate might have good experience working as part of a team, as evident by information on the resume and by the number of employment years at the current or a previous health care organization.

The third category consists of probable candidates. Most likely this will be your smallest pile. These are individuals who seem almost perfect for the position. Again, using the hospital pharmacist example, assume that you received a resume from an individual who not only has all the quantitative characteristics, but has completed several successful state reviews, worked as a team leader, participated as part of a quality management process throughout the entire organization and perhaps in several employee relations committees, and currently works at a hospital nearly equal in size and scope to yours. Assume further that he works with youth groups on the weekends (as indicated in the personal interest section of the resume) and therefore probably has terrific people skills. This candidate goes into your probable file and will almost certainly merit interview consideration.

After you have completed this process and sent thank-you letters, send the unqualified pile to your human resource department. Then try to establish a "short-list" roster of a maximum of seven interview candidates. Beginning with your probable group, rank them in numerical order, based on your insight and your summary perception from the preselection process. If you have fewer than seven candidates in this category, go to your possible group to complete your list of seven candidates, send the remaining candidates, if any, from the possible group to your human resource department for consideration for another job. Alternatively, file them in your position folder, which you are keeping with the job description, wish list, and list of expectations.

There are several things to remember as you review the resumes initially and, more important, as you establish your list of "the magnificent seven." First, you are not using the resumes to make your hiring decision; you are reviewing resumes simply to decide whom to interview. Furthermore, the resume is a selling tool for the candidate. With this in mind, be assured that often the best candidate is not necessarily the one with the best resume.

Do not fall into the seductive trap of reading too much into a resume. Try to take the information at face value—that is, remember that the resume is simply a summary of qualifications, not an in-depth insight into the applicant's personality. A good rule of thumb is to review resumes strictly based on quantitative characteristics, with only an initial thought to qualitative characteristics. Although there is no accepted rule of thumb, any resumes that are more than two pages might be a bit too lengthy. This must be taken in context, however. For example, if you are reviewing the curriculum vitae of a research scientist, ten pages might be too short. The best rule of thumb in this case is to consider what is appropriate for the position, based on what your instincts tell you.

Do not allow yourself to be overwhelmed by this review process or consider its parameters to be absolute. In establishing a list of seven, you are simply coming up with the best seven candidates, those who will be the first to be interviewed. This is just a commonsense exercise; the candidate who appears to be the best candidate should be the first you interview so that he or she sets a basis of comparison throughout the selection process. Allow the first candidate to pick the time and location for the interview, based on the options you present.

Finally, the resume-review process simply helps you establish a pool of candidates. This pool of qualified candidates will be interviewed, and in many cases one will be your candidate of choice. If none of the candidates in this initial pool measure up completely to your satisfaction, you will simply establish another pool. Once again, you are trying to strike a balance between the "perfect" candidate and a "somewhat suitable" candidate in a realistic manner.

In progressing through the next section, you will see more clearly how this process works.

The Selection Process

Following completion of the preselection process, you are now ready to conduct interviews of qualified candidates. The selection process begins with scheduling candidates for interviews. Using the list of candidates you have selected for interviewing based on resume submission, set up an interviewing slate by scheduling interviews based on candidates' rank order; that is, according to your most preferred candidate's first preference for desired interview time.

For an hourly or nonskilled position, twenty minutes is an acceptable maximum time for an interview. For a professional technician or other nonsupervisory health care professional, such as a nurse or therapist, thirty minutes is acceptable. For a manager or supervisor, allow at least forty-five minutes. Depending on your own preference, you can interview several candidates back to back, so you interview them in succession within a given time frame. For example, you might interview three candidates within two and one-half hours, allowing each candidate a half-hour interview and leaving yourself time between interviews for assessment and review.

However, remember that scheduling candidates closely or undertaking a large slate of candidates can cause the candidates to run together. This means that a large number of interviews within a limited time frame can cause the candidates to appear similar in your evaluation and keep you from maintaining a fresh perspective on each candidate. A good guideline for interviews is to conduct no more than three a day in order to maintain this important fresh perspective.

Preparing for an Interview

When preparing for an interview, be certain to have on hand the candidate's resume, a notepad, and a set of prepared questions. A good starting point for this effort is to use the questions in Appendix B to structure a set of questions appropriate for the interview. A professional touch can be added by using a file folder bearing your organization's logo and placing the resume and your questions on the right-hand side of the folder. With this folder and notepad combination, your information will be well organized, thus giving the candidate the impression that he or she is interviewing for a position entailing a high regard for professional demeanor within a well-structured organization.

In preparing the structure of the interview, select questions from Appendix B, which will give you the maximum information you need to match the candidate's skills and personality to the qualitative criteria that you established on your wish list. Each question in the appendix will generate at least two to five minutes of response time if used properly. Therefore, ten to fifteen questions should be more than enough to conduct a thirty-minute interview. Remember also to review the resume one final time prior to the interview to make certain that you have areas targeted for questioning and that you have a strong grasp of the candidate's background.

Opening the Interview

Having made these preparations, you are now ready to conduct the interview. Be sure to adhere to the following guidelines throughout the interview to make it an effective tool. To begin with, remember that the candidate's feelings and self-esteem should be respected above all else at all times. The candidate will make a clear decision about your organization based on experience gained from the interview. Fundamentally, the candidate is interviewing you and your organization as much as you are interviewing the candidate. Therefore, even if you are having a bad day, it is essential that you maintain professional courtesy and positive demeanor.

Strive to put candidates at ease and maintain maximum comfort conducive to candidates' acting naturally. Many industrial psychologists debate whether an interviewer should conduct the interview from behind a desk or in a setting where interviewer and interviewee sit in two chairs facing each other in close proximity. Do whatever is most comfortable for you. A candidate will sense your behavioral clues and react accordingly. So if you appear nervous, the candidate will become edgy; if you appear comfortable, the candidate will be at ease. The more comfortable candidates are, the more they will reveal and the clearer your determination about their comprehensive abilities and potential will be. Therefore, set up your office in any manner that will facilitate your comfort and, certainly, that of the candidates.

An interview should be a pleasant exchange of ideas, not an interrogation. The problem with the so-called stress interviews, so fashionable in the late 1970s, was that they only monitored one psychological reaction—how a candidate handled stress. They assessed this characteristic at the cost of getting a good look at the candidate's qualifications for the position. If the interview is a pleasant exchange of ideas, a professional conversation, and opportunity for both the interviewer and interviewee to learn more about their mutual fit, the interview has met its objective. The interview, then, should give you a microcosmic view of the candidate's professional life. There is nothing mystical about the interview. It is not an in-depth psychological assessment. However, it is your main tool in selecting an important team member.

In achieving this end, begin the interview with a pleasant, professional introduction and initiate some appropriate light conversation. There are three topics you can always discuss with a candidate to begin an interview correctly and to set the stage for a professional conversation:

1. You can always talk about the weather, a topic everyone has some knowledge of and is willing to discuss.
2. You can talk about the traffic, and how the candidate traveled to your facility or whether the directions provided were adequate. Discussion of a common traffic problem can also establish some empathy while getting the candidate into a conversational mood.
3. You can extract a nonthreatening piece of information from the resume to help initiate conversation. For example, the fact that the candidate attended the same college you did can provide an opener.

At the initial meeting, take note of how the candidate introduces himself or herself. Use whatever title is used in the introduction, such as Doctor, Mrs., Ms., Mr., a religious title, or simply a preferred nickname or first name. Once again, the key is comfort. Whatever form of address the candidate uses is probably the name or title preferred. Use this appropriately throughout the interview, as it will increase familiarity and again underscore the fact that this is a professional conversation, not an inquisition.

Also important at the outset is notifying the candidate that you will be taking notes. As you open the interview, thank the candidate for coming, explain that you will be asking a series of questions concerning his or her background and potential for the job, and that you will be taking notes. In almost every case, a candidate will not object to note taking. If there is objection, ask why and record the reason mentally as you consider the candidate. It is my contention that any candidate who objects to note taking by the interviewer probably has something to hide, is paranoid, or is psychologically maladjusted for the demands of the health care environment. Finally, use the outset of the interview to explain to the candidate not only the time parameters of the interview but also that there will be time at the end of the interview to ask questions.

Questioning the Candidate

As you begin your questioning, remember to start off with the prototypical life-story question: *Tell me about yourself, beginning with. . . .* The open-ended segment of this question should be filled starting with the point at which he or she entered the health care work force, or began secondary education in college or professional school. For example, you might ask the candidate, *Tell me about yourself, starting with your graduation from* [name of college]. Usually a candidate is well prepared for this question, and it increases the comfort level following the light conversation. It also signals to the candidate that you have now assumed control of the interview and that it is time to start presenting his or her ideas and credentials. Recognizing that the interview is a selling process (by no means a negative connotation), the interviewee will now begin the sales campaign. This also gives you a comprehensive overview of the candidate's background, from which you can begin your specific questioning at the conclusion of the response.

As the interview progresses, remember to ask as many questions as needed to elicit the responses you need to make a clear determination about the candidate's suitability. In addition to the questions in the back of this book, use a rejoining process. The rejoining process uses both verbal and nonverbal triggers. For example, after asking one of the questions from Appendix B, follow up with the candidate by using verbal rejoinders such as, *Tell me more about that. Give me another example. What else was involved? Why?* Using these rejoinders will make the candidate's response fuller in scope, add to the context of the interview, and provide you with specific information essential to your evaluation of the candidate.

It is important to use verbal rejoinders whenever the candidate appears to be stalled in a particular area, is hesitant about answers, or has given an abbreviated answer. Use verbal rejoinders freely to trigger new lines of response, get additional information in a specific area, or clarify the candidate's response.

Nonverbal rejoinders can be equally important in this regard. Nonverbal rejoinders include eye contact, facial gestures, hand gestures, and any other nonverbal communication that might encourage the candidate. It is essential that you not lead the candidate toward a desired end, so do not react emotionally in either a verbal or nonverbal manner. Rather, maintain steady eye contact throughout the course of the interview, and clearly demonstrate that you are vitally interested in what the candidate is saying, but without judging any information provided.

The key words *pleasant* and *professional* should be your guiding lights in using nonverbal communication throughout the interview. As you conduct the interview, keep in mind your role as the organization's representative. *To the candidate, you are, in essence, the organization.* Remember that the interview is a public relations tool in this regard, for a potential candidate is also a potential customer-patient. Therefore, you want to give candidates as many opportunities as possible to answer a question fully, and you must be patient in allowing them to respond. Along these lines, let the candidate do most of the talking; a good guideline is to allow the candidate at least 80 to 85 percent of the proverbial interview "air time," with you doing 15 to 20 percent of the talking (see Figure 11.2). Candidates who talk 90 to 95 percent of the time are probably going into areas about which you do not need information, or you are not guiding them strongly enough toward your objectives. If you are talking 30 percent of the time, however, either the candidates are not seizing the opportunity to present their background assertively, or you are not allowing them the opportunity to do so. There is one certainty about the interview process: If candidates cannot sell themselves successfully to you—that is, if you are not convinced of the value of their potential and past background—they will not be able to convince you of their worthiness for the position once you have hired them. Therefore, be fair in giving them enough air time, but recognize that if they cannot properly present themselves to you, they will not be able to do so to customer-patients or other members of the organizational team.

In questioning candidates, try to avoid close-ended questions, case study questions, or legally sensitive questions. Close-ended

Figure 11.2. Interview "Air Time" Guidelines.

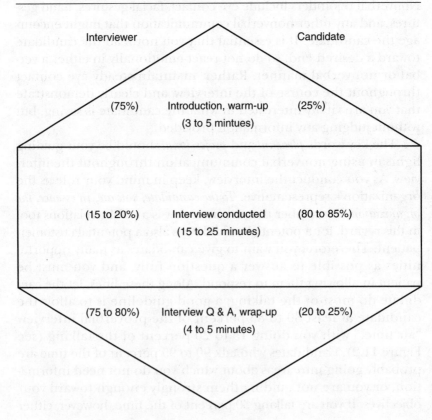

Interviewer   Candidate

(75%)   Introduction, warm-up   (25%)
                    (3 to 5 mintues)

(15 to 20%)   Interview conducted   (80 to 85%)
                        (15 to 25 minutes)

(75 to 80%)   Interview Q & A, wrap-up   (20 to 25%)
                          (4 to 5 minutes)

questions require a simple yes-or-no response, thus adding little to the interview and providing you with little useful information. Such questions also demonstrate to candidates that you have not put a lot of forethought into the interview, thus leading them to question later whether you, as a potential manager, have a creditable depth of thought. In case study questions, you present a situation to candidates and have them answer in an academic fashion what they would do if presented with the dynamics of the case. These questions also have limited value because candidates merely demonstrate that they can solve a pertinent situation in theory. A better way of getting this information is to ask a question along the lines of *Tell me about the most difficult operational problem you had to resolve.* This forces candidates to provide their own case and gives you a realistic, not a theoretical, perspective on ability.

Never use questions that might wander into legally sensitive areas. To ensure that you do not violate equal opportunity laws, ask your human resource department to provide you with a list of Title VII mandates and other pertinent labor law requirements. Better yet, ask your human resource director to brief you on legally sound questions and the phrasing of questions. In general, direct questions about a candidate's religious beliefs, race, sexual preference, family status, marital status, or age are strictly prohibited by federal law. However, once a candidate volunteers a certain amount of information, the material becomes open ground if it is relative to job performance. For example, if a single mother volunteers the fact that she has three children at home, her family status can become an essential occupational issue. (All the questions in Appendix B are legally and structurally sound.)

However, there is a more tactful and progressive way of handling this very important issue. Assume that you are a nursing manager seeking to hire a staff nurse who will work alternately on both the night and day shifts. One of your more qualified applicants is a young woman who has a family at home. Although you are not certain of this, you suspect it and are justly concerned that this individual will not be receptive to working on the night shift. Rather than waiting for this candidate to volunteer information on marital or family status, simply make the following statement: *This particular job requires alternating on the night and day shifts, often with no more than a half-day's notice in terms of when you might be working. Does that present any problems?* This is a legal way of asking the question, and the candidate who answers *yes* might disqualify himself or herself from consideration by providing a forthright response. The candidate who answers *no* and reinforces the answer by stating that he or she has worked in similar circumstances in many other organizations with successful results would be a very qualified candidate and has alleviated any concerns you had about this bona fide occupational qualification (or BFOQ; see Chapter Twelve).

No arbitrator or labor judge has the right to prosecute you if you asked a question in an interview that you were unaware of as being illegal, or were asking simply because it related to a bona fide occupational qualification. The *intent* of your question is what is most important. If you ask candidates if they speak Spanish, for example, because a majority of your customer-patients speak Spanish as a first language, this is a question asked with good intentions. If you ask candidates whether they are of Spanish descent or speak Spanish because you dislike Spanish Americans, however, you will be justly prosecuted in the labor law courts. Many health care managers require assistance in this area, and even some senior health care executives are under the impression that they cannot ask any questions in these areas. Remember that the intent of the question is the foremost legal consideration, and your guiding light should be whether you are trying to determine the candidate's ability to meet a true, established occupational qualification.

Conducting and Completing the Interview

As you conduct the interview, remember that you are examining candidate evidence in three key areas. The first area is interview behavior. For example, if you need a worker who has a high degree of energy, try to gauge the candidate's energy level in the interview process. An individual who has a positive outlook and is somewhat animated and enthusiastic probably would have a suitable energy level for the position that you are trying to fill.

The second area is work philosophy and beliefs. Candidates at all levels of a health care organization will state their commitment to the health care mission and the customer-patient. Determine whether this commitment has been underscored with action in the past, and also try to note any other beliefs and convictions they hold relevant to the job position at hand.

The third area of candidate evidence lies in past performance and accomplishment. Beyond the resume, try to get a complete sense of the candidate's experience and expertise-based accomplishments in previous work roles and the duration of their professional and academic career. A good candidate will cite accomplishments and professional achievements, and give you a wealth of specific episodes of contribution to the good of a health care organization.

Use all three areas of evidence in combination; do not isolate any one or delve into one area of evidence at the expense of another. For example, the interviewer who simply looks at candidate behavior in the interview and discounts philosophy and beliefs and achievements and accomplishments risks hiring someone who is a good interviewer but not a particularly strong performer. The following list offers a summary of interview assessment keys for easy reference:

Interview Assessment Keys

Candidate comfort	Action orientation
Presentational flow	Growth potential
Balanced dialogue	Promotability
Genuineness	Overall potential
Past performance	Work personality
Philosophies, beliefs	Team orientation
Interview behavior	Positive attitude
Professional presence	Health care knowledge
Accomplishments, achievements	

With this in mind, try to avoid the *five-minute actor factor*. This catch phrase, which I use extensively in my management seminars for health care professionals, refers to the ability of a candidate to look spectacular in the first five minutes of an interview. Such a candidate might have been seeking employment for the past six months and therefore is in good interview shape. He or she has all the right answers and makes a terrific first impression. However, upon closer evaluation throughout the duration of the interview, the responses might not be as spectacular or terrific as they appeared at first glance.

Let us take an example of the five-minute actor factor in reverse. Assume that an individual has worked for the past eleven years—their entire professional experience—at a competing institution across town from your organization. To get to the interview with you this morning, the candidate had to feign a doctor's appointment, an alibi that makes the person, basically honest by nature, very uncomfortable. Having arrived at your office in a somewhat flustered state, this individual might very well take five minutes to calm down and get into the groove. If you fall victim to the five-minute actor factor, your initial impression of this individual might not be a very good one. However, if you listen to the person, ask a wealth of questions, allow him or her to get comfortable, and get an overall impression in the half-hour interview, you might decide that this is a very loyal, progressive individual with terrific technical proficiency. In other words, do not let your first impression become your last one, no matter how tempting it might be.

Remember, interrupt the candidate only when necessary, and then with tact and brevity. Only when you might have missed some information or simply did not hear or understand the candidate clearly should you interrupt a statement. Unnecessary interruption of a candidate might lead to an abbreviated answer or a change in the course of the answer. Make certain that you downplay excessive negative information and control positive excessive rambling by using another question or rejoinder. Do not allow the candidate to go so far off track that this irrelevant information takes precedence over the objectives you are trying to achieve in the interview. You are relegating control of the interview to the candidate to respond; you are not giving carte blanche with the interview time.

This raises an interesting point. On the rare occasion you might get a candidate who is 100 percent unqualified for the position. This candidate might have a falsified resume or is clearly not a match for your organization, a determination you have made halfway into the thirty-minute interview. At this juncture, simply begin to ask the candidate all the questions you are asking the other candidates and that you have drawn from Appendix B but without follow-up questions or rejoinders. This will abbreviate the interview, still allow the candidate the opportunity to answer all the questions posed to other candidates, and maintain the integrity of your interviewing process. A structured system ensures that every candidate who applies for a certain position will be asked the same questions. This not only allows you opportunity to compare certain responses to an established set of questions, it also gives every candidate an equal opportunity for the position. In the case of the totally mismatched candidate, the process will be abbreviated, yet the candidate will still have opportunity to make a comeback because you are asking open-ended questions. Fundamentally, if your initial judgment of the candidate was incorrect, he or she will still have a suitable opportunity to prove you wrong and make a more positive impression. Even if this is the case, they probably will not look as strong as other candidates who use the first fifteen minutes to make a more positive, sincere impression.

Postpone all final judgment of the candidate until after the interview. Once you have completed your questioning process and have held tightly to your thirty-minute time parameter, allow candidates five minutes to ask a few questions about the organization, the specific job position, or anything else that might be of importance to them. You can learn as much about a candidate from the questions asked at the end of the interview as you will learn from asking questions throughout the interview. Many health care managers have used the positive approach of taking the candidate for a quick tour of the facility, or at least the departmental work area, at the end of the interview. This provides additional opportunity for the candidate to ask questions and supply information with which you can further assess the candidate.

Answer all questions about benefits and salaries appropriately by simply reiterating the salary scale published in the ad or quoted as part of the job description. Any information you might provide about the organization such as an annual report, employee newsletter, or any other publication might be beneficial to the interviewing process.

Thank the candidates at the conclusion of the interview. Tell them that you will be in touch with all candidates within two weeks. With this in mind, send an appropriate, tactful letter of rejection to all marginal candidates within two weeks. Otherwise, they will ring your phone exactly two weeks and one minute later. Keep all good resumes on file for at least one year. Even candidates who do not get the job should be put in your position folder along with the job description, your wish list, and your list of expectations so that they can be considered for future positions.

Always keep your responsibility as an organizational gatekeeper at the forefront of your interviewing strategy and approach. Remember, not only are the candidates nervous, but you may be nervous too as you interview someone for the first time. This is natural and should not cause alarm on your part. Therefore, as already mentioned, prepare fully for the interview, make the candidate feel as comfortable as possible, and conduct the interview in a professional, courteous manner. In doing so, you are not only representing your organization in a professional manner, but you are also laying the foundation for a successful manager–team member relationship with the candidate fortunate enough to get the job.

At the conclusion of the interview, simply record your overall perceptions of the candidate's strengths and potential weaknesses. Do this by reviewing your notes and listing in a two-column format the candidate's negative and positive attributes. This will give you a strong frame of reference for making your decision. Do this with each candidate you have interviewed, and then rank each one from strongest candidate progressively down to the weakest.

Making the Selection

The next phase in adding new talent to your work team is making the selection. This process, as well as that of orienting the new employee, can be greatly assisted by the efforts of your human resource department, as well as your immediate manager or director. Some general guidelines might assist your efforts.

To begin with, when making a final decision on which candidate to hire, the best advice is to trust your instincts and common sense. As you review the candidate, use the following questions as guidelines in picking the best possible candidate:

- Which candidate seemed to exemplify the ideals and values of the organization?
- Which candidate seemed to have the best general background?

- Which candidate seemed to have the specific technical capabilities and most experience in the particular area needed for this job?
- Which candidate would mesh nicely with the rest of my existing team?
- Which candidate might be a leader among team members?
- Which candidate had the most potential performance liabilities?
- Which candidate did I feel most comfortable with?
- Which candidate did I feel least comfortable with?
- Which candidate would I be most likely to trust?
- Which candidate would I be least likely to trust?
- Which candidate seemed to be the most willing to grow?
- Which candidate was looking for a career opportunity, not just a job?
- Which candidate seemed to be the most genuine and confident in the presentation?
- Which candidate seemed to be selling me a bill of goods?
- All things considered, which candidate did I really like best?

The answers to these questions can be very telling. Remember that the interview is the major tool in the assessment of new job applicants. It is more important than checking references, for example, or an aptitude test or other selection devices. Although it is certainly important to check references, what you have seen in the interview should provide the most important data in making your selection.

Even though you should certainly seek the guidance and input of your supervisor and human resource manager in making your decision, the ultimate responsibility rests on your shoulders. This is exactly as it should be, for you are the one who must live with the people you hire, in a close-knit work environment. You will have the most exposure to them, the authority in helping them achieve and prosper on the job, and responsibility for directing and planning their performance. Therefore, forthrightly answer all the questions in this section and, most of all, trust your own instincts in making a final decision.

Many health care managers still believe that references are very important in assessing a candidate's viability. I and many other prominent industrial psychologists, however, believe that facets of the Privacy Act abused during the Clinton administration negated the impact of references. Fundamentally, individuals who provide references are restricted to giving the person's name, position title, length of employment, and approximate salary range. This information is limited. Another example might demonstrate an important point of the selection process. Suppose an individual approached you saying that he has the perfect job, in the ideal location for you, complete with a contract for $1 million dollars per year. The only way for you to get this job, however, is to provide a sterling set of references within the next two weeks. Would you have a problem doing this? Of course not.

Modern-day American labor law restricts the reference process to the same parameters. Therefore, reference content must be taken with a proverbial grain of salt. When you do receive a reference, however, it might not be a bad idea to contact the individual who provided it and ask questions similar to the interview questions in Appendix B. For example, ask about the applicant's ability to work as part of a team, his or her basic value structure, and some tough situations that the individual successfully handled. This might provide you with more in-depth background information about the candidate. However, if the reference is unwilling to give you additional information, or is hesitant and restrictive in the comments, this might give you another indication about the candidate's background.

A simple fact of health care life is that not everyone gets along with his or her boss, or a person may make a poor career decision. Therefore, candidates might be unable to provide comprehensive references simply because they were in a bad situation. Again, in this rather different scenario, the reference might have limited applicability. In all cases, it is important to use the reference simply as a validation of what you might already have decided about a candidate, not as a revelation; certainly, in no case should it be the main factor in your decision.

If you have reviewed all the candidates and you are absolutely convinced that no one you interviewed is suitable, you must establish a new pool of candidates. Although this rarely happens, it can be a very costly step and will take a tremendous amount of your time. Remember what was said at the outset of this chapter: You should not seek to find a perfect person or perfect match for the position, simply the best qualified given the criteria for the job.

Once you have arrived at your candidate of choice, it is time to make the offer. Using the expertise of your human resource department, prepare to make a phone conversation supplemented by an offer letter, which will acknowledge your positive impression in the interview, extend an offer to the candidate for employment, and seek both his or her acceptance and a potential start date. If the candidate desires a higher salary than what you offer, promise to get back to the candidate by a stated time. Then discuss with your human resource professional or your immediate supervisor (depending on which is most appropriate) the options you might have in restructuring the salary. Once you arrive at a figure, do not waver. If the candidate is not impressed with your second offer, you are probably better off looking for another candidate, particularly if you are offering fair market value.

The Postselection Process

The postselection process begins with the employee's orientation and extends through tenure on your staff to include skill development and performance evaluation. The orientation should include a number of elements for ensuring that the employee gets off to a good start, listed as follows for easy reference:

Potential Orientation Activities

Clear job expectations	Wage-benefit information
Exposure to other team members	Insurance forms and information
Organizational mandates and standards	Major project overviews
Performance evaluation system	Three- to six-month performance goals
Personnel department liaison	Insight into department work goals
Department work conduct	Organization and department history

| Customer-patient profile | Assistance in personal relocation |
| Future plans for department and organization | Assistance in any personal need acquisition |

Once the candidate has accepted the position and agreed on a start date, begin the orientation process on a personal basis. Have your new employee meet you in your office on the first day. Arrange beforehand for no interruptions during the first hour. You want to have the opportunity for an exclusive interchange with your new employee. Discuss your expectations of the job, and give him or her copies of the job description and your expectations list. Furthermore, spell out the specific goals and aspirations you have for the job. Finally, underscore your support for the employee's success and offer encouragement to seek out your assistance or guidance at any time.

Next, introduce your new team member to the rest of your staff. In this effort, try to schedule a set time with each staff member to give the new employee opportunity to ask questions and gain an understanding of what everyone in the department does on a daily basis. Ensure that all members of your team realize that there is no second opportunity to make a first impression. Accordingly, they should set aside this exclusive time for the new employee to ask questions and to ensure that the actions of their new teammate will be in alliance with their own.

Involve your human resource department in the orientation process. A number of insurance forms and other paperwork must be completed. Make sure that a personnel representative is available to do this and that this business is scheduled appropriately. Benefits are an essential element of the health care professional's compensation package. Encourage your human resource colleagues to give the new employee as much support as possible in benefits enrollment by explaining forms and ensuring understanding of the benefits package.

Another essential part of orientation is imparting basic knowledge about the orientation. Introduce your new team member to your immediate supervisor, particularly if your supervisor did not participate in the interviewing process. If it has not been done already, take the new employee on a tour of the entire facility and encourage questions about anything that expands on his or her initial perception of the organization.

Finally, make sure the new employee is aware of the performance objectives for the first month and the type of performance evaluation tool used at your facility. As discussed in Chapter Twelve, this is an important guiding tool for your own management activities and will assist greatly in providing clear direction to the employee.

Conclusion

In this chapter I have reviewed an array of suggestions and guidelines for one of the most important management duties: the selection and initial orientation of new employees. Many large organizations in the health care world and in other industries pride themselves on spending millions of dollars on training programs, compensation programs, and state-of-the-art facilities. All of this money is misspent if individuals hired for the organization are miscast. By following the guidelines in this chapter, as well as your intellectual skills, intrinsic instincts, and basic common sense, you will be able to achieve success in this extremely important management responsibility.

Chapter Twelve

Performance Evaluation

One of the most difficult responsibilities of a health care manager is the assessment and conduct of performance evaluations. Taking qualitative, subjective perceptions of performance and ascribing a quantitative, objective rating is generally a difficult and complex task. This task becomes important specifically as most performance evaluations are tied to the individual staff member's salary and potential salary increases. Even with the bromides of continuous quality improvement efforts, which suggest that criterion-based systems with merit increases are somehow detrimental to staff performance, performance evaluation is still an important and visible part of every health care organization's management structure.

In this chapter I review specific guidelines for performance documentation and suggest how to construct a performance evaluation. I also discuss how to set performance goals proactively and enhance performance in an ongoing fashion. Regardless of whether your organization uses a criterion-based performance-evaluation tool or a basic summary of achievement and performance, it is essential to master the elements of performance documentation, performance assessment, and the dynamics of delivering a performance appraisal early in your management career. For people who want direction and desire challenge in their everyday responsibilities, it is essential to have a sound, creditable system of performance evaluation in place.

Performance evaluation should begin on a new employee's first day on the job. Evaluation of current employees starts on the first day of the performance cycle (for example, the beginning of the new year or the day immediately following the last evaluation). This "Day 1" approach will be advocated throughout this chapter and explained in detail. Furthermore, it is incumbent on the manager to establish a sound system of documentation relative to all employee performance, as certain elements of performance evaluation must be enforced throughout the entire grading cycle. Delivery of the performance evaluation, complete with a plan for future performance, must be enumerated and presented to the staff member. I will also examine the twenty essential dimensions of performance evaluation, and their use, as keys to enhancing stellar staff performance. I conclude the chapter by discussing actual delivery of the performance evaluation, exploring potential problem areas, and considering ways to use the performance evaluation to its fullest potential as a vital management tool.

Design and Implementation of a Documentation System

Documentation, the linchpin to successful performance evaluation, is the process of objectively taking mandates and recording performance and performance levels. Managers and executives at all levels of a health care organization rely on documentation in a litigious climate where organizational mandates require full proof that accepted standards of performance have been met. Without it, the compilation of a comprehensive performance evaluation is next to impossible. Your documentation tool will be your performance logbook.

Performance Documentation Logbook

Sound documentation starts with investing in a simple spiral-bound notebook in which you can record the dates and events (significant incidents or critical contributions) pertinent to each staff member. The performance logbook should also note counseling sessions between you and each employee in which you provided constructive, corrective direction for poor performance or positive reinforcement for good performance. This book should not be used for finger pointing but rather as a guide to chronicle individual staff performance objectively.

Documentation that is irrelevant or too broad is useless. Here are nine examples of poor documentation (from actual management notebooks):

1. "Has a bad attitude"
2. "Didn't listen to what I said"
3. "Dresses like a clown"
4. "A racist snob"
5. "Never documents well on charts"
6. "Showed up late a couple of times"
7. "Even though I told him how to do it, he didn't do it"
8. "Has a bad memory, poor attention span, and lacks confidence"
9. "Disappears for long breaks"

Example 1, although common, is useless because not only is the attitude not described, its effect is not set forth so that an employee can learn from a specific critique and begin to demonstrate acceptable behavior. When discussing attitude, consider the dimensions of adaptability, aggressiveness, perseverance, and work ethic; then note the particular effect that the absence or presence of these characteristics had relative to performance. Furthermore, be sure to *date all entries.*

Example 2 ("didn't listen to what I said") refers to an employee who failed to follow a work direction and complete an assigned task. The manager should have been more specific in terms of what direction was provided, when it was provided, and in what way the employee failed. Without documenting particulars, it is impossible to specify how to improve performance.

Example 3 ("dresses like a clown") relates to appearance. The manager should have researched the organization's dress code policy and specified *how* the employee failed to comply with it. Anything else is an invasion of the employee's privacy.

Example 4 ("a racist snob") is particularly troublesome, for it violates Title VII of federal regulations governing equal rights in employment, and it violates labor law. In this case, the manager came to a subjective conclusion that the employee in question did not enjoy working with a particular ethnic group. Because of the sensitive nature of this episode, the documentation must be clear-cut, explain the effect on performance, and enumerate the specific guidance given the employee for corrective action. Inadequate documentation jeopardized the potential for positive employee performance. The manager also opened the proverbial can of worms by inserting the difficult question of race relations where it may not have been the prevailing issue.

Example 5 ("never documents well on charts") uses two words that render the documentation specious. The first word, *never*, is nonspecific and arguable. For example, if the employee failed ninety-nine times to complete a particular task—in this case documenting on a particular chart—the employee could probably present the one time in a hundred occurrences that she did document well, thus neutralizing the "never" contention for this claim. The second word, *chart*, is without an adjective. The type of charts the employee was required to use, their importance, and the number are all essential information that should have been included in the entry.

A similar problem occurs in example 6 ("showed up late a couple of times"). Two important time elements are unspecified. The first is the number of times the person in fact "showed up late." The second time element relates to how late the person was on those particular occasions. Depending on a facility's policy, there are major differences, for example, between being fifteen minutes late and being one hour late. Lateness parameters must be specified on the documentation, and the next entry should indicate that the employee was counseled relative to the specific negative behavior.

In example 7 ("even though I told him how to do it . . ."), the manager provided specific direction on how to complete a particular task, but the employee failed to comply with the instructions and thus failed to complete the task. This documentation could have been strengthened by the *who, what, where, why, and how* approach. That is to say, *what* direction was implied, *which* method the employee should have used to complete the task, *how* it should have been done, *what* parameters were used to measure the performance, and *why* the assignment was important. The broad nature of the entry allows no chance for the employee to improve performance, or even to understand why the task was not performed to expectation.

In a similar vein, example 8 ("has a bad memory, poor attention span . . .") fails to provide direction. Furthermore, all the characteristics—memory, attention span, and confidence—are subjective, personal characteristics and in this entry have little relevance to job conduct. The risk of this example is that the employee can wind up being not only confused, but extremely de-motivated by receiving such personal, meaningless feedback.

Example 9, "disappears for long breaks," would be a positive notation for a circus performer for whom "disappearing" was part of the job. Use of the word *disappear*, however, is problematic, as is the lack of definition for what constitutes "long breaks."

Finally, notice that none of these entries were positive in nature or provided any positive direction or corrective discussion on how the employee might improve performance. Compare the following list to the preceding one.

1. 3/4/xx: Counseled D. Smith on 15-minute tardiness occurring on 2/28, 3/2, and 3/3
2. 3/15/xx: Discussed resolution of tardiness issue with D. Smith and expressed appreciation for voluntary overtime by Smith on 3/11
3. 3/21/xx: Set a performance goal of 25 percent increase in accounts receivable collected by O. Flanagan in the next quarter
4. 4/2/xx: Counseled M. Street on completing only twelve job description reviews (fifteen was set goal) during last quarter; emphasized importance and gave verbal warning; told M. S. that written warning will be issued if next quarter goal of fifteen is not met.
5. 5/2/xx: Reviewed charting deficiencies that occurred in three charts on 4/28, 4/29, and 5/1

Notice that all of the entries are dated. This is particularly meaningful in examples 1 and 2, in which a performance problem was identified, crystallized for the employee, and then resolved within a two-week period. Furthermore, the manager made a point of noting the employee's good performance, as well as the corrective action, in entry 2 dated March 15. This information will assist the manager not only in ongoing charting of performance, but also at performance-evaluation time when the manager considers the entries for the scope of employee performance. Aside from dates, note other quantitative measures such as the time frame and percentage increase specified in example 3, which again is concrete and direct in providing feedback and direction to the employee.

Example 4, dated April 2, is almost textbook perfect. The performance goal is quantified, time parameters are noted, and a performance plan is set forth (along with consequences if the plan is not followed by the employee). This documentation would be particularly useful in the unfortunate event that the employee's performance level plummeted to the point that termination or other disciplinary action was mandated.

Example 5, dated May 2, notes deficiencies in what appear to be everyday responsibilities and lists specific dates of infractions. This entry does not, however, describe what types of charts were involved.

Documentation Rules

From the comparison of poor documentation examples and good ones, we can list several rules of thumb that should be followed when recording documentation in your logbook:

- Always date entries.
- Use time, money, percentage, and numbers—quantitative data—as much as possible.
- Use clear, concise language.
- Use examples, evidence, episodes, and explanations as much as possible to present a clear picture of performance.
- Use sound references. (As will be discussed in the next section, use sources that are creditable and will be considered valid by the particular staff member.)
- Emphasize quality as well as quantity; explain the big picture to the employee.
- Counsel the employee on a timely basis. Do not store up information to use only at performance-evaluation time, but make feedback and direction a continuous process.
- Document counseling sessions for your reference as well as for the progressive development of the employee.

- Avoid use of subjective or biased language that might cause more problems than it solves (for example, racially based epithets).
- Enforce disciplinary measures as needed, and discuss any emergent performance-evaluation problems with your supervisor or human resource manager as appropriate.
- Record good (that is, detailed and concise) examples of behavior, critical contributions, and significant incidents that were handled positively or negatively. Review of these events with the employee provides positive reinforcement or corrective counseling appropriate to the situation.

Your documentation logbook contains your own professional notes and cannot be used or subpoenaed in court. Many health care managers fear that what they write in their logbooks might be used against them in a court of law. This is not the case, as the only documentation used in a court labor proceeding is the official performance evaluation filed with the health care organization. You use your professional notes—not anyone else. Use them to increase employees' constructive performance and in turn provide stellar health care to your customer-patients.

Performance-Evaluation Resources

Sound data sources are essential in documenting performance and compiling a performance evaluation. These sources provide the basis on which you will form perceptions about an employee's performance and document specific performance achievements or shortcomings. In the following sections I point out credible sources of performance evaluation and observation that you can use to collect performance data on an ongoing basis.

Firsthand Knowledge

The first, and perhaps most valid, source of performance observation is your own firsthand knowledge. This source might include personal observations, conversations you have had with the employee, or written reports submitted directly to you from the employee. Firsthand knowledge is a particularly strong data source because it is usually not subject to argument (the employee usually participated in the action from which the firsthand knowledge is derived). However, firsthand knowledge tends to be a bit subjective if not recorded correctly or observed fully. For example, if you observe an employee arriving late and do not record it, the evidence is lost. If you only "hear" that an employee is always late, but do not observe it yourself, your evidence is specious at best and litigious at worst. For this reason, it is doubly important to use your logbook fully and to observe the entire scope of performance, not just particular aspects.

Job Description Compliance

Your first step in hiring people, and then evaluating their performance, is to study the job description and ensure that it is valid, current, and at least 80 percent reflective of the major duties of the position. An effective method for ensuring validity of job descriptions is to have current employees compile a top-ten list of what they do on a regular basis. Then sit down with employees and assign the percentage of time that they spend on each task in a typical workday. Next have employees assign a weighted value to each task. A weighted value is a number between one and a hundred assigned to the task according to its relative importance. Most managers adopt this system using multiples of ten. For example, a pharmacist might have a weighted value of forty assigned to a task such as filling prescriptions and a weighted value of ten assigned to inventory record keeping.

The multiple of the percentage and the weighted value result in a number that represents the relative importance of a given task. By reviewing this list closely with the employee, you not only ensure that the job description is valid, you also make sure the employee has a full understanding of the job expectations.

All specific duties should be covered on the job description, and this guide should be used throughout the course of the grading period. The entire range of responsibilities should be enumerated and specified for employee job conduct. You and the employees should maintain copies of the job description and use them as references in all employee discussions. Furthermore, the job description should be used in combination with the performance evaluation throughout the year, particularly at the annual performance evaluation.

Goal Attainment

Attainment of management-by-objective goals refers to the goals agreed on by the employee and manager at the beginning of the year. In a system that uses incentive compensation, these goals will be specified for the employee at the beginning of the year. In a system that does not formally identify specific goals for completion, the manager and employee should design a list of goals above and beyond the context of the job description. Both types of goals give the manager and the employee a clear idea of what will be expected throughout the year and make the manager's job a little easier in terms of comparing the achievement of these goals against the employee's actual performance.

Working Numbers

Another area of performance observation should be the category of working numbers. Any job in a health care organization has significant numbers that reflect job performance. Job performance can be measured by percentage, time, money, or other particular numbers. For example, a laboratory technician must complete a certain number of assays in a given time slot at a particular percentage of efficiency. A human resource recruiter is tasked with recruiting a set number of candidates within a set monetary budget and with a certain percentage of retention. Whatever the working numbers are in a given job, as a manager you must set objectives, document performance, and educate the employee toward fully achieving the set parameters of performance.

Monthly Reports

Most employees in a health care organization are charged with presenting a written or oral report at monthly meetings either individually, with their supervisor, or within the context of a departmental monthly review. Results should be documented throughout the course of the year. Also, any upward or downward trends should be documented and recorded in your logbook. These trends should be reviewed with the employee and ideas for improvement should be solicited, whether performance is poor or stellar. Monthly reports should be examined closely by you and the employee, and opportunities for improvement should be explored continually. A good rule of thumb is for you to sit down with each employee on a monthly basis for at least ten to fifteen minutes to discuss the current month's performance and ensure that the next month will see additional progress or, if needed, corrective action.

Peer Input

Because most modern health care organizations pride themselves on "doing more with less," many employees work along interdepartmental lines. Therefore, peer input is an observation resource that yields data from managers in other departments who have knowledge of the employee's performance. The obvious risk with peer input is that your fellow manager's evaluation of the individual's performance may be subjective. Another risk is that the manager may have limited knowledge as to the employee's technical acumen. Therefore, this input must be viewed as secondhand and used in conjunction with other, more reliable sources. Make sure that the interrelations and interpersonal skills of your staff members are strong and that they are perceived as team members throughout the organization. Accordingly, limit peer input to the employee's cooperation, relations with her peers in your colleague's department, and the employee's technical proficiency in solving problems and providing positive outcomes.

Organizational Input

Another secondhand source of performance observation, but one that is usually valid, is organizational input. This refers to any communication you might receive from the organization relative to the employee's performance. For example, receipt of a letter citing the employee for a particular achievement (or level of achievement) should be entered into your logbook and subsequently incorporated into the performance evaluation. Letters of recognition also might come from patients who were in the employee's care and felt that the performance was either positively or negatively outstanding. Such feedback can also include phone calls and other forms of communication from both internal and external customers, such as department heads or payers. Again, organizational input must be used in conjunction with other aspects of performance and other sources.

Unit Performance

Unit performance refers to the employee's contribution to overall departmental objectives. This includes relationships with overall department members, the degree of technical expertise provided to others, and peer relations in the department. Any information that indicates the level of performance, particularly as it applies to contribution toward group goal attainment, is worthwhile and should be recorded in your logbook.

Critical Contributions

Significant incidents and constructive contributions of a critical nature should be entered in your logbook. This category of resources covers activities "above and beyond the call of duty" that the employee has either contributed in terms of performance or failed to attain. Critical contributions should be closely noted, clearly examined and reviewed with the employee, and set forth as part of the employee's overall performance objectives. In that much of health care delivery is in fact above and beyond the call of duty, this is a particularly important category that not only reflects on organizational performance but also on an individual's overall performance development. Performance enhancement is a recurring theme throughout this book but must be considered with special emphasis within the context of documentation criteria. Accordingly, be certain to record and use for employee education all examples of critical contributions and significant incidents handled by the individual employee.

Work Approach

Anything that reflects employees' attitude orientation, people skills, managerial aptitude, and team orientation should be recorded. This means not only what employees do, but also how they do it. Any performance examples in these categories should be documented, explained to the employee, and reinforced either positively or negatively according to the guidelines.

In summary, I recommend that you use all documentation and performance observation sources as described. Try to get a comprehensive picture of employees' performance to construct a performance review, as well as reinforce the continuous, educational nature of the performance-evaluation process. By using all the tools described here, you will take the first step toward ensuring that the performance evaluation is not only an equitable tool, but also a constructive and progressive one.

Remember, each source may carry with it certain risks and liabilities. Remain objective in the collection of performance data, trust your own instincts as you observe performance, and match actual performance against the requirements specified in the job description and other position data. Finally, use any performance information in a timely fashion, document quickly, and use the first available opportunity to provide feedback and direction to your employees. Doing so will inspire your entire work group to strive for high-quality performance and provide employees with the direction needed to improve performance from both an individual and group perspective.

Critical Factors of Performance Evaluation

In the scope of performance evaluation from initial documentation through presentation of the performance appraisal, twenty essential factors of performance evaluation come into play. In this section I review each factor, explain its significance to the performance-evaluation cycle, and present practical suggestions on making the factor part of your performance-evaluation strategy. Note that these factors are also the contributing elements for a criterion-based performance-evaluation process. By incorporating the factors into your performance-evaluation approach, you will ensure that the process becomes a meaningful and progressive management instrument.

Factor 1. The performance evaluation must be comprehensive in scope. The evaluation, as well as the documentation and performance observation leading to the evaluation, must be all-encompassing and take in the entire breadth of performance. In addition to assessment of performance in all aspects of the job position, there should be evaluation of organizational values or work personality traits essential to doing the job. By failing to be comprehensive, you risk the employee's focusing on just one aspect of job performance at the neglect of other essential job elements.

Factor 2. The performance evaluation must be seen as a process intended to elicit stellar performance and encourage professional growth and development. With this in mind, sections in the performance evaluation should cover critical incidents relative to the job, job-related training and development activities, and other motivational data. This perspective helps provide the employee with a full view of the job position, and it provides comprehensive insight into how important improvements might be made within the scope of the job position.

Factor 3. Performance evaluation must be an ongoing process. As discussed throughout this chapter, the performance-evaluation cycle should commence on an employee's first day or on the first day of the performance cycle (the day following the last review). Performance should be evaluated continually, feedback should be provided on an ongoing basis, and the opportunity for work discussion should be available at all times. Unless the evaluation process is continual, you risk the liability that performance will not improve over the course of the year. You also risk that all aspects of performance will be "saved up" until the end of the cycle, thus creating a breach of trust between you and the employee. You might focus only on a one-time sequence as opposed to the entire year; for example, focus only on the past three months of the yearly cycle, as opposed to the entire year.

Factor 4. The performance evaluation must be individualized. This means that the individual aspects of the job, as well as the particular talents and skills of the employee under review, must be assessed. Nothing demeans the validity of an evaluation more than identical evaluations on different individuals in the same job position. This sort of evaluation destroys manager credibility and sends a distinct message to the employees that the performance evaluation is no more than a paper exercise not to be taken seriously. Therefore, examine each employee's individual attributes, potential, and performance within the job role to ensure the validity of the evaluation. Eliminate "identical" evaluations by using your documentation logbook, specifically paying attention to critical incidents (positive or negative) and significant contributions made by each employee.

Factor 5. The performance evaluation should take individual situations into consideration. Each job role should take into consideration the situation in which the employee operates and performs every day. Certain employees find themselves in work situations where "a little bit goes a long way." Other employees in the same job role might find themselves in situations where "you have to go a long way to get a little." Therefore, the intensity of situations, the level of difficulty that prevails, the degree and effect of change, the occurrence of critical incidents, and other dynamics should be considered when looking at each job situation and evaluating performance based on job aspects. For example, two housekeepers can work in the same department. However, if one housekeeper worked in a situation where major construction was under way throughout the year and the other housekeeper under more static conditions (for example, in the lobby or other construction-free areas), you must take into consideration these situational differences. Your sensitivity to environmental conditions when evaluating performance will convey a sense of fairness in the evaluation process while encouraging the employee to achieve even under adverse circumstances.

Factor 6. The performance evaluation has the potential to be a motivational tool. For strong players, the evaluation affords two opportunities to give positive motivation. One is by providing high performance ratings. The other is by allowing employees to offer input on how they can enhance performance even further. For steady players (those who achieve at a satisfactory level), the evaluation can be a shot in the arm and a step toward reaching a higher performance level. For poor performers, the performance evaluation can be an opportunity for you to present, in an exclusive one-on-one interchange, new parameters for performance and give notice of consequence(s) for failure to improve. With strong documentation and the techniques for delivering a performance appraisal described later in this chapter, you can clarify requirements and consequences for underachievers.

Factor 7. The performance evaluation and job description should be prioritized. Most (if not all) health care jobs can be prioritized according to the relative importance of responsibilities. This can be accomplished by listing the job requirements on a scale from one to ten, with one as the most important and ten as the least important.

Another way of prioritizing job elements is the weighted-value approach described earlier in the chapter. Write the weighted value of each job element on a sheet of paper in the margin to the right of the performance expectation. Considering a total weighted-value quotient of a hundred, the most important facet of the job might be a forty weight, and each of the least important facets might be a ten weight. In this fashion, you can explain which are the most important facets of the job, highlight those elements of the employee's performance, and still maintain the integrity of the evaluation by explaining that all elements of the job description are important on some level. Whether you use a listing technique or a weighted-value technique, it is important to express a sense of priority so that the employee's job focus is appropriate and well calibrated.

Factor 8. All terms used in the performance evaluation and on the form itself should be easily understood by, and meaningful to, the employee. A very important aspect of performance evaluation is that it must be understandable. Unfortunately, many forms are obscured by "psychobabble" or incomprehensible or misleading language that fails to delineate the job position clearly. Examples of meaningless verbiage are "professional maturity," "tough-mindedness," or "circumspective responsibility." Ensure that the employee understands the terminology and applicability of the scoring mechanism as it relates to his or her job and potential pay raises. From an overall perspective, the form and the evaluation process should be user-friendly.

An unclear form promotes distrust and destroys any credibility the process might have. Additionally, an unclear form eliminates opportunity to use the performance evaluation as an education tool—the employee simply does not understand what the manager is trying to get at. During the discussion as well as the review process itself, use language that is clear, concise, and relevant to the employee's particular job scope.

Factor 9. A good performance appraisal should provide employees insight on what the organization expects from the employee and what standards and measurements are being used to judge performance. The evaluation should clarify employees' expectations of the job, and it should make clear your own expectations and desires. Moreover, it should spell out what you deem as stellar performance and enlighten employees on how they might improve performance and methods.

From another perspective, the performance evaluation can be an education for you by providing insight into how effectively you are managing your assigned human resources. It should also indicate your skill in giving clear direction and, perhaps, how employees perceive your leadership style. Specifically asking employees for feedback on your leadership and management efforts is a good idea with stellar and steady employees but perhaps not a good tactic with poor performers, who might seize the opportunity to criticize your performance unfairly. Often, poor performers will use the opportunity to blame you for their own inadequacies. In any case, if done correctly, the performance evaluation should enlighten the manager as well as the employee.

Factor 10. The performance evaluation should be a tool for long-term employee development. The performance appraisal form should include a section for a development plan. A good strategy is to ask employees to cite areas in which they can improve, and list activities or training opportunities they desire to improve skills or acquire new ones. Chapter Fifteen suggests an arsenal of ideas in this area. With Chapter Fifteen as a guide, establish a training plan along with conducting a performance appraisal with each employee's input. Many health care organizations pride themselves on promoting from within and through provision of growth opportunities for their employees. This claim becomes mere lip service if it is not substantiated by a strong development plan that is part of the performance-appraisal form.

Factor 11. The performance evaluation should also provide short-term direction for the following year's performance. In addition to encouraging long-term development, a strong set of objectives should be established for the coming rating period. Be proactive in establishing what the job objectives will be for the coming year, and present this projection at the performance-evaluation session. You will give the employee a clear picture of your expectations for the following year and underscore the ongoing nature of the performance evaluation.

Part of the health care manager's initiative is to ensure that employees reach their highest possible level of potential and performance. To do this, the evaluation must be used as a directional tool, with goals, directives, and guidelines that will help employees reach their highest level of performance in the following year.

Factor 12. The performance evaluation form should be user-friendly and comprehensible. The performance evaluation carries with it a certain responsibility. As manager you are responsible to the employee to provide a clear picture of what is expected and how the employee performed in the past grading period. The organization has a responsibility to managers to provide a strong and meaningful instrument. If you are uncomfortable using the performance-evaluation form, contact your human resource department for instruction on delivering the performance evaluation. If you feel the system is impractical, it might be a good idea to discuss with fellow managers and human resource staff ways to improve the instrument.

Factor 13. The performance evaluation must be viable in scope and application. The performance evaluation should be a communication exercise in which all parties participate so that the goals listed for the following year are realistic and practical, goals that everyone can live with. Applying this standard, review the performance evaluation prior to its delivery to make sure that goals are realistic and attainable, yet challenging to the employee. Overtaxed employees risk burnout, whereas underchallenged employees neither take full advantage of their potential nor demonstrate maximum work interest. The way to ensure balance is to review the past year's record of achievement and increase goals by using a "10 percent solution"; that is, increase percentage goals by 10 percent, cut the time spent on each activity by 10 percent, or increase significant numbers by 10 percent. Remember that this is a general guideline; the proper quotient must be ascertained according to your own instincts and the work situation.

Factor 14. The performance evaluation should be measurable. The evaluation should use clear-cut quantitative measures and rating scales that are understandable and relevant to employees. Otherwise, employees lack a standard or benchmark to which they can aspire or against which to compare their performance last year. For employees who want to be challenged and want to increase their performance, clear measurements should give them motivation. Without this goal they may slack off from long-term objectives or fill the motivational void with self-directed goals. In using quantitative measures, discuss with the employee whether the measurements are realistic and seek their opinion on what constitutes fair measurement. This discussion will once again increase the performance evaluation's educational value to you.

Factor 15. Financial considerations must be taken into account in a performance-evaluation sequence. Evaluations should distinguish between individuals who receive a cost-of-living increase and those who do not, as well as separate those who will be retained from those who should be terminated. In organizations whose quality-improvement programs assign the ratings "above expectations," "meet expectations," or "below expectations," raises are given to those who exceed expectations, cost-of-living adjustments are given to those who meet expectations, and disciplinary probation is the fate of individuals who fall below expectations. This is one example of a system whereby the overall performance rating should relate directly to the amount of pay increase the individual received, or any other available monetary increase.

From another perspective, financial considerations should be taken into account in view of goals. Five questions can be asked in this regard:

1. Did the employee use unnecessary resources in accomplishing objectives?
2. Did the employee incur costs to the organization needlessly in carrying out work efforts?

3. Did the employee generate cost-saving techniques?
4. Did the employee devise new ideas that helped the organization save money?
5. Is the employee cost-conscious in the pursuit of everyday activities?

By looking at these financial parameters, you can ensure that your organization's fiscal resources are not being wasted and that every employee is truly doing more with less. By starting with your own department, you set a precedent that will allow you to take maximum advantage of whatever financial resources you have at hand.

Factor 16. The performance evaluation should be legal in content and scope. No undue bias or prejudice should be introduced into the evaluation. As with selecting and hiring new employees, bona fide occupational qualification (BFOQ) is the key guideline under Title VII. The individual's performance—not ethnic origin, gender, religion, or any other protected category—should be the only consideration. If you have any questions as to the fairness or legality of an entry on the form, review it with your human resource department. Do not be afraid to cite something you think is performance-based; the inclination among most health care managers is not to cite something that should be on the performance evaluation. If you think an entry is truly an occupational qualification, review it with your human resource department prior to including it.

Factor 17. The performance evaluation should be objective. Use objective information collected from your documentation efforts, and use a preponderance of evidence, rather than opinion, to make your case on negative, neutral, and positive performance. Again, use clear-cut, technical language as much as possible, but make sure that it is understandable.

Factor 18. The performance evaluation should be cumulative. The need for evaluation is continual, in that it shows rises or falls in performance levels throughout the grading period. Remember to look at both positive and negative trends.

Factor 19. All information on the performance evaluation should be drawn from factual evidence backed up by your logbook. If you have done a good job compiling your documentation logbook, the evaluations should rest on fact. The more factual they are, replete with points of evidence throughout the course of the year, the more validity they will have for employees, and the more employees will learn from the exercise.

Factor 20. The performance evaluation should be ethical. It should be fair, respectful of the employee's dignity, and maintain allegiance to the organization. There should be no hidden secondary agendas when presenting the evaluation. The individual employee should be given the opportunity to discuss any aspects of their performance and have maximum opportunity for input. However, as manager you are ultimately in control, and you must guide the performance appraisal accordingly.

In attending to the twenty critical factors of performance evaluation, you will have moved closer to a successful performance evaluation. Keep them uppermost in your thinking as you gather performance data and deliver performance evaluations. By embracing these tenets, you can conduct a meaningful exercise that will be a building block for departmental and individual development.

Delivering the Performance Appraisal

By keeping a documentation logbook and incorporating the twenty performance-evaluation factors into your evaluation process, you have worked toward making the process an optimum management tool. Here are eight guidelines for delivering an appraisal effectively.

1. *Make sure the physical environment is conducive to performing an evaluation.* Sit at your desk, a table, or wherever you are most comfortable; close the door; and avoid interruptions while delivering the evaluation. The occasion should be an exclusive interchange and one that gives the employee a feeling of privacy.

2. *Provide the employee with a copy of the evaluation.* She can use it as a guide, follow the discussion throughout the entire process, and keep the copy as a planning tool for future performance.

3. *Manage emotionalism.* If an employee becomes emotional during the evaluation, usually because of a negative reaction, ask

whether the employee would like to take a break or reschedule the evaluation. If the employee elects postponement, allow him to keep the copy; then schedule a follow-up meeting within a week's time and deliver the appraisal fully at that time. If the employee again becomes emotional, either get assistance from your manager or the human resource department, or simply conduct the review in monologue fashion. The latter strategy should be used when you suspect the employee is reacting poorly to the performance evaluation as an excuse for poor performance or as a means to avoid the evaluation completely.

4. *Use a direct and objective style.* Use clear terms, state your case objectively, and avoid personalizing the evaluation. Try to stay on an even keel, using emotion only as appropriate. At the same time, feel free to express dissatisfaction to an employee who is not performing acceptably or pride in an employee who is performing at an outstanding level. Be natural, direct, and comfortable in your delivery.

5. *Prepare fully for the evaluation.* Ensure that the form is filled out correctly and completely, requiring only the employee's signature. Consider how you want to present the performance evaluation, and simply conduct a review of what you have written on the evaluation.

6. *Use a point-by-point strategy.* Work through the evaluation from beginning to end. Stop frequently to ask whether the employee has any questions or would like elaboration on any part of the information given so far.

7. *Set a specific time limit for the appraisal and try to stay within it.* For example, an hourly employee might take a half hour to complete a performance appraisal, whereas a skilled worker might need forty-five minutes. Try to stay within these parameters, and keep that standard for all employees so as to promote a sense of fairness and equity.

8. *Give closure.* Ensure that the employee signs the performance-evaluation form and that all questions are answered. Remember, not all employees will be thrilled with their reviews. If you have followed the guidelines discussed in this chapter, you can rest assured that a fair and reasonable effort was made and that it is now the employee's responsibility to improve on performance.

The performance-evaluation process is rarely mastered on the first attempt. As always in dealing with people, there are no right and wrong answers. However, by using the strategies presented in this chapter, relying on your own common sense, and trusting your instincts, you will be off to a very good start in making the process a meaningful management exercise, one that will have the potential of becoming a building-block for all individuals on your staff.

Chapter Thirteen

Negotiation Strategies

Most new health care managers are not born negotiators, skilled negotiators, or educated negotiators. This potential shortcoming—shared by new health care executives of every ilk—can be detrimental to the new health care manager. In the course of a given day, the new health care manager might negotiate a fee-for-services contract, establish new performance standards for a nonperforming employee, or set a new schedule for an operating room. All these interactions, like many of the interpersonal interactions managed by an effective physician leader, call for negotiation skill, strategy, and savvy.

Few medical school curriculums contain practicums on effective negotiation. Likewise, few graduate programs in health care administration offer courses on negotiation skills. The background of a typical new health care manager, however, does provide certain informal opportunities to acquire negotiation skills in learning to negotiate a favorable grade during their organic chemistry class during their undergraduate career, standards and curfews for teenage children, and certain privileges with their health care administrator.

In this chapter, therefore, I use the natural foundation of negotiation skills possessed by every new health care manager to build a set of dynamic strategies that will assist you in undertaking your leadership responsibilities. By examining the techniques delineated in this chapter and adapting the strategies that most naturally complement your already acquired negotiation skills, you can devise a comprehensive strategic approach to all future negotiations for maximum results.

Basic Concepts of Negotiation

Since the early 1950s, much has been written in management textbooks and popular management literature concerning negotiation skills. As corporate America became the driving engine of the American economy in the early 1950s, many managers became enamored with an almost mystical approach to negotiation. The approach basically combined popular psychology with intimidation, thus resulting in programs such as "winning through intimidation," in which one side dominated another side to get a favorable result in negotiation, and the "win-win" approach to negotiation, in which both negotiation parties received full value for their efforts.

Let's briefly review these two types of negotiation and see how they evolved into perhaps the most effective negotiation strategy— *logical negotiation*. In negotiation through intimidation—the *win-lose approach*—the dominant negotiation party's behavior can be perceived as abusive in their attempt to intimidate the opponent through an emotionally driven approach to negotiation. If this abusing party is negotiating an agreement that will have long-term impact, the intimidating negotiator risks negative fallout throughout the relationship through subtle "revenge" tactics used by the opposite negotiating party and an array of other nefarious recourse actions that can, in the long run, jeopardize the entire business relationship. Although negotiation through intimidation can occasionally be an effective tactic if used sparingly, in the long term it can cause bitterness, rancor, and unnecessary retribution. In essence, it is not negotiation in the purest sense.

Negotiation in the purest sense is when two parties enter into a discourse that results in a mutually beneficial agreement. This is the rudimentary objective of win-win negotiation. In win-win negotiation, both parties receive an optimum objective. Win-win negotiation is based largely on psychological ploys. Fundamentally, an individual attempts to use one or a combination of several basic appeals:

1. *Appeal to ego.* One uses an array of compliments, "ego-stroking," and other self-esteem gratification techniques to reach a favorable settlement. Using expressions like, "a smart individual

like you," "someone who is a real player in the market," or "a super-intelligent manager like yourself," as preambles to statements helps to build an appeal-to-ego strategy. Once again, this strategy might be effective in the short term, but over the long term it can be seen as manipulative, less than genuine, and basically phony.

2. *Appeal to authority.* In this case, an individual will use an authority such as a state regulation board, the board of directors, or other proverbial "powers that be" as the driving factor in why a negotiation settlement should be reached quickly and favorably. Once again, this tactic is not only somewhat disingenuous, as it connotes a power play by the negotiator who uses it, but is also an abdication of authority relative to the basic responsibility of the individuals present at the negotiation table.

3. *Appeal to the norm.* This appeal is in evidence when one negotiator cites the need for commonality or normalcy as a driving force for reaching a settlement. Statements such as, *Most physicians would take this deal, Every hospital in the state does it,* are examples of appeal-to-norm strategies. This technique might be effective in some cases, where standards and practices are the prominent feature of the need to reach a negotiated settlement, but in all cases it is a less-than-effective strategy.

4. *Appeal to emotion.* Anger, pride, friendship, gravity (such as *If we don't do this, the hospital will close!*), and other emotional drivers are used to trigger a negotiated settlement in an appeal-to-emotion ploy. This is a perilous tactic for a health care leader in any capacity to use. Fundamentally, most people who have had any sort of tenure in health care are "tough cookies" who have witnessed a wide array of emotionalism displayed by patients and employees on any given day. Therefore, they become exceptionally tough skinned in gauging emotion, and are not likely to be motivated by someone crying, yelling, threatening, conjoining, or displaying any other type of emotional behavior that is not specifically related to the negotiation objective at hand.

5. *Appeal to a vision.* The negotiator presents a picture of what the final negotiating outcome might be. This is perhaps the only effective strategy among the appeal-process negotiation ploys. In painting a picture of a harmonious work place, effective emergency room, progressive medical service organization, or any other favorable vision of health care excellence, the new health care negotia-

tor can create a vision that is equally alluring to their opponent as to themselves. The vision can be not only the objective for the negotiation but also the driving motivation for reaching a settlement. However, the vision must be one that is equally shared and desired by both negotiation parties, otherwise the tactic is doomed to fail.

6. *Appeal to mission.* For instance, a negotiator constantly cites the mission of the hospital, health care organization, or physician practice as the driving force for reaching a negotiated settlement. This can be an effective appeal only if coupled with the vision appeal and other artful negotiation. For example, I once used the mission of the hospital as the driving force during a bitter union negotiation with a Midwestern hospital. After I told my opponent, the union president, that both sides should be interested in making sure that the patient is taken care of, the union president replied, "I'm here for the patient too—to get as much of their money as I can through union wages and dues!" As evidenced in this example, different individuals might have varying opinions on how the overall general mission of the hospital holds specific relevance to their specific needs!

7. *Appeal to personal relationships.* Friendship, collegiality, past history, and other personal notes are used as catalysts for obtaining a progressive settlement. Though a certain amount of strength of interpersonal relationship can be drawn on in any negotiation, the effective negotiator will not rely strictly on personal friendship as the centerpiece for negotiation. Simply put, if an individual uses personal friendship as a mainstay of negotiation, her opponent can simply say, *Friendship is one thing, business is another—let's get down to the brass tacks of reaching a good agreement.*

Many elements of the psychological win-win approach can be incorporated into a more effective strategy of the *mutual-benefit logical approach* to negotiation.

The rudiments of the logical approach are based on several parameters. First, preparation is a major key of the mutual benefit approach to negotiation. If you are prepared and your opponent is not, or is not as well prepared as you are, the odds will increase in your favor that you will prevail in the negotiation. Preparation takes several forms in logical negotiation, as I demonstrate throughout this chapter. Nuances such as knowing your opponent, preparing your bargaining position, preparing counterarguments, and planning overall negotiation strategies are essential to a well-prepared negotiation sequence.

Second, knowledge of your opponent is crucial to the success of an effective negotiation. By understanding your opponent's position, analyzing potential methods and approaches of your opponent, and counteracting your opponent's forays in the negotiation process, the likelihood of a negotiation victory is enhanced. Once again, preparation is key, and the requirement that the negotiator does the homework is paramount to success.

The third parameter of mutually beneficial negotiation is to establish a negotiation range, as pictured in Figure 13.1. It is vital for the prepared negotiator to understand the differences between wants and needs and to negotiate within the "needs" zone, as depicted in Figure 13.1. Often two negotiating parties reach an immediate impasse when both sides endeavor to move the other party toward the "want" position. This often ends not only in an impasse, but also in a failed negotiation. However, within the parameters of the need range there exists the opportunity for a well-negotiated settlement that will be favorable to both parties; hence the name *mutual-benefit approach,* as both sides will receive benefit from the negotiation.

Notwithstanding the mutually beneficial flavor of this type of negotiation, one party can certainly gain more within the need category than another. Therefore, it is essential to identify the range of specific needs that might be obtained through a negotiation. Primary as well as secondary needs should be identified. The artful negotiator will assign specific power ratings to the

Figure 13.1. The Range of Negotiation.

Part A	Negotiation Range	Part B
Wants of A	Needs of both A and B	Wants of B

planning process. With this type of preparation, the negotiator is certain to be able to trade secondary needs in order receive primary needs, negotiate more forcefully and intently on primary needs, and allow the opponent, if necessary, to "steal" secondary need items in the interest of gaining consensus on a positive primary item.

The fourth essential parameter of mutually beneficial negotiation is that of communilogical management. *Communilogical* (that is, a fusion of communication, logic, and psychology) aspects of negotiation cannot be underestimated. As discussed throughout the chapter, there are many essential communilogical keys that should be embraced throughout the communication process. For example, the construction of a negotiation team with a balance of listeners, talkers, presenters, and perceivers; the ability to ensure understanding throughout the negotiation process; and the proper utilization of caucuses and other communication dynamics throughout the negotiation process.

Certain aspects of both the intimidation win-lose and psychological win-win processes can be incorporated in the mutually beneficial negotiation strategy. Intimidation, for example, is a factor at a negotiation table when the new health care manager is more prepared for the negotiation than his opponent. Appeal to ego can be used effectively if the communilogical keys are in force throughout the negotiation process. To cite another example, the perception of a win-win outcome in the eyes of the opponent might be achieved if mutually beneficial negotiation is pursued vigorously, accurately, and effectively.

The Preparation Phase

As you as negotiator prepare to enter the bargaining process, review several preparation keys in order to reach maximum readiness.

Self-Assessment

To begin with, take a few minutes to conduct a self-assessment and make certain that you possess certain personal attributes that will become vital throughout the negotiation process:

1. A sense of integrity and purpose (including honesty, candor, and trust), which can be built upon and reinforced throughout the negotiation process and the long-term relationship that results from the negotiation.
2. Certain interpersonal skills, with an objective of being conscious and aware of the power of interpersonal skills throughout the negotiation process, including the ability to
   Communicate effectively
   Present information accurately, cogently, and confidently
   Observe how your opponent is presenting positions
      and certain arguments
   Listen accurately to what is being said
   Perceive why your opponent is taking a certain position
      or presenting a certain case
3. Fortitude, including courage of convictions, strength of character, and, perhaps most important, the ability to say *no* at the proper time throughout a negotiation. Fortitude can be reinforced through good preparation and analysis of your opponent's negotiation position and presentation.
4. Adaptability, including the ability to be flexible to demands for increased information throughout the negotiation process. If a team negotiation is taking place, all members should be able to act not only flexibly, but also fluidly and adapt offensively to each of the strengths, weaknesses, and tendencies throughout the negotiation process.
5. Stress-positive resistance. That is, you must not be easily rattled and nervous or, at the other extreme, complacent or lackadaisical throughout the negotiation process. In fact, in some cases, it is important that you elicit stress from the opponent, for example, by asking a critical question, imploring them to present facts and figures, and basically charging them with the accountability of proving their cases.

Analyzing Your Opponent's Position

Another essential part of preparation is understanding your opponent's position. This includes not only their stated negotiation position, but also an array of other factors that become intrinsic to the negotiation process. These factors include the following:

• The role that your opponent likes to play: the heavy, the intimidator, the people-pleaser, the good cop–bad cop, or any other of an array of dramatic or psychological roles. In addition, certain communilogical roles can also be a part of the process. For example, some negotiators like to be listeners, whereas others like to be questioners and interrogators. Some like to be leaders in the process, whereas others attempt to be reconciliators. By knowing your opponent's role, you will be able to counteract the psychological impact of their role by simply being prepared for it and reacting appropriately.

• The previous history of your opponent, particularly the recent history. This can include the recent financial position of a health care institution with which you are negotiating, or the recent promotion of a health care administrator who is negotiating your fee-of-services contract. Recent history can even be more specific: a spat that an administrator had with one of your colleagues, for instance, or the pride that an administrator took in the emergency room's recent ability to react positively and compassionately to an overflow of patients resulting from a horrific car accident. In either case, understand that the recent history of your opponent, and more specifically the recent history that is shared with you as a negotiator and business colleague, can become an essential frame of reference throughout the negotiation process.

• Your opponent's self-image. If your opponent perceives himself as a master negotiator, a counterpunching approach might be useful whereby you allow your opponent to make the first argument but have an effective counterargument prepared. If the self-image of your opponent is that of a victim of recent events, you might pose your negotiation strategy as one that eases the pain of the root cause of the disharmony. For example, if your opponent is an administrator who is chagrined at a recent turn of events resulting from a managed care contract, you might be able to present the financial wisdom of incorporating a new outpatient service to offset the fiscal loss from the managed care contract. In essence, you are providing a benefit that will not only meet a need for your opponent, but that will also help reestablish her self-image as a leader, action player, and positive influence in the health care organization.

• Your opponent's goal. As much as possible, understand your opponent's ultimate objective. This can be identified by simply asking your opponent to present the objectives in writing prior to the negotiation so that "we won't waste time" during the negotiation process. If this is not a suitable initiative, you might ask your opponent simply to enumerate their goals of the negotiation process at the outset of the negotiation discussion. You will thus gain a greater sense of the objectives, intents, and aims of your negotiating opponent.

• Your opponent's communication style.

• Your opponent's points of pride, such as a new building, a new service, or other organizational initiatives, or on a personal level, their manner of dress, their accomplishments to date, their educational level, and other attributes that might be perfect targets for positive exploitation, including appeal to ego, appeal to norm, and other pertinent elements of psychological negotiation.

• Organizational position. This is another attribute that can be exploited positively by a skilled negotiator by using appropriate appeal to ego.

• Pressure points that will elicit an emotional reaction from your opponent. This cannot be underestimated. If your opponent is particularly sensitive about money, equipment, physical space, visibility in the community, organizational reputation, malpractice, or other vulgarities of the health care forum, it might be useful to imply an impact on these factors through the connotations of your argument. For example, if an administrator is particularly sensitive about malpractice, you, as the new health care manager and ultimate expert on risk management, might point out how your position in advocating a new program will decrease the likelihood of malpractice while positively increasing revenue for the organization.

Setting the Standards

Immediately prior to a negotiation, and certainly at the outset of the formula negotiation process, ten specific elements should be introduced by the skilled negotiator, either through interference or direct statement, which set the parameters for a negotiation.

Fundamentally, you as the artful negotiator should say, *Folks, we want to negotiate today in good faith. Good faith to me means:*

1. Negotiation, which is based on the mutual need of both parties in the interest of the overall health care organization
2. Trust among all the people at this negotiation table, as well as the parties we represent
3. Respect for the patient, our respective teams, and the overall health care institution
4. Pride in the negotiation outcome and the relationship it will initiate
5. Openness, marked by candor, honesty, directness, and open communication, which will help us toward a mutually beneficial negotiated settlement
6. An agreement that will be credible in the eyes of all who must employ it in their everyday work lives and professional responsibilities
7. Accountability on the part of all of us who are negotiating to be responsible for our opinions and the facts, which we present as part of the negotiated settlement
8. Community based on the common unity represented by all the parties at the negotiating table, as well as our respective institution(s)
9. Viability inasmuch as the negotiated settlement will be applicable to the real world, practical in its intent, and immediately useful to all affected by its outcome
10. That the potential for synergy represented by the eventual agreement will be fully realized, recognized, and immediately advantageous to all parties involved

By setting these ten standards for a negotiation agreement, you, the artful negotiator, are actually achieving several objectives. First, the rules for the negotiation are established. Second, if there is an undue amount of disagreement relative to these standards, you will quickly deduce that you are dealing with individuals who are perhaps not of the same ethical fiber as you and the people you represent. Accordingly, the long-term value of the negotiation outcome might not be as favorable as originally thought. Finally, by presenting these rules for the negotiation process, you are establishing a negotiation forum that can be immediately useful, favorable, and positioned for success by using the tenets of mutually beneficial negotiation.

Knowing Your Opponent's Position

At the outset of the negotiation process, try to ascertain your opponent's position. As stated previously, this can be achieved by asking your opponent to prioritize the list of most important agenda items for the negotiation. You would then be able to ascertain the primary and secondary agenda items for your opponent. Furthermore, it would be favorable for you to try to determine the strategic position of your opponent on the mutually beneficial needs range. This can apply to specific nuances. By asking a sequence of questions you can elicit more specific information about your opponent's desired outcomes for the negotiation. These questions include the following ten verbal cues, which force your opponent to be more specific about his position:

1. What do you need to have happen here at the negotiation table?
2. Specifically what do you need from our discussions?
3. Why is this particular initiative important to you?
4. Which one of these items is the most important to you?
5. What are you looking for from our negotiation?
6. Would you please list for me—so we all understand—what your priorities are, listed in numerical order?
7. What do you need to get done here at the negotiating table, or what do we need to get done?
8. What do you want to get done, or what do we want to get done here at the table? (Note: By using questions 7 and 8 in concert, you might be able to get a sense of what your opponent's "dream objective" might be.)
9. How can we make this happen?
10. Can you directly, honestly, and specifically tell us what your ultimate objectives are for this negotiation?

In seizing the initiative in trying to unveil your opponent's position, you are better prepared to list priorities for the negotiation and identify not only the primary and secondary needs of the opponent, but also potential trade-off positions for the negotiation. Once again, by simply being prepared and taking a proactive stance in the negotiation process, you will gain an upper hand that will help facilitate a more favorable result to the negotiation process.

Counteracting the Games Your Opponent Will Play

Unfortunately, because so many health care professionals are enamored with the latest "flavor-of-the-month" management fad, many negotiators in the health care arena try to play games in the negotiation process. These games include, but are certainly not confined to, the following:

1. Canards—rumors, conjecture, innuendo, and flat-out malarkey—are used to establish precedent by employing emotionally laden falsehoods. For example, a health care administrator might say, *All the employees will revolt if they think the physicians are being favored,* or a fellow physician negotiator, acting as your opponent, might say, *No one will want to practice in your medical service organization if you establish the salary parameters you're discussing here.*

Counteraction: *I hope that you can immediately, or in the very near future, provide proof for every specific situation that you're describing.*

2. The use of code is also an effective negotiation game. This occurs when individuals use specific jargon, such as acronyms and "bizspeak words" (for example, closure, CQI, PPO, empowerment), to disguise objectives or alter perception and to gain an upper hand by using a language that is not totally familiar to the new health care manager.

Counteraction: *Let's agree now to use terms that we can all understand, and then I won't have to use medical terms to create camouflage on my side simply to feel as though I am keeping up with your particular brand of lingo.*

3. Cover issues are often used as a diversion to "throw off" an artful negotiator. For example, a negotiator might say, *My biggest concern here is how the community will perceive us if we put physicians on salary,* when in reality the biggest concern is the salaries that will be paid by the administrator to the physicians.

Counteraction: *If the real issue here is community perception, why don't we run a survey to ascertain why people select a particular hospital? I think you will agree that most of the time it's based on physician affiliation, more than advertising or any other type of elicitation. We can wait to conduct that survey, or we can get to the heart of the matter: establishing a good contract for the physicians that is favorable to the hospital as well.*

4. In certain cases contention, or basic argument, can take precedence over negotiation. In such cases emotionalism, rather than logical negotiation, becomes the rule of the day.

Counteraction: *Why don't we take a couple of minutes for a break so that everybody can cool down and we can get to the business at hand. If things are so emotional perhaps we don't need to negotiate at all.* (This will allow you the opportunity to weigh the seriousness of his opposing negotiator.)

A host of other communication distortions can be used throughout the negotiation process. These distortions can include the deliberate altering of information to falsely reflect favorably on your opposing negotiator, or the slanting of information to appear favorably on your opponent. The media is famous (or perhaps infamous) for these tactics.

In some instances people fabricate information. They can present information that is not true at all. Or they might infer information, or infer dire consequences to a particular situation. Conversely, individuals may downplay major concerns while exaggerating minor ones. Information can be embellished or edited depending on what your opponent might need to establish in order to build momentum throughout the negotiation. In still other cases, information is negated, overemphasized, contorted deliberately, or presented, in summary, through a prism that is largely favorable to your opponent's case. Regardless of what communication games are used by your opponent, you can use eight countersteps. These countersteps, which are briefly alluded to in the first four examples of this subsection, should be used throughout the process of negotiation. Whenever you suspect your opponent is being less than honest with their information, use the following countersteps:

1. Show proof that clearly indicates that your opponent is being less than honest.

2. Ask for proof or validation for their particular position or to verify and validate a particular statement.
3. Quantify results or particular facts in question with numbers, percentages, time quotients, or financial indicators.
4. Get specific examples from your opponent—and the emphasis here is on *specific*—that will prove their case.
5. Use comparison and contrast as extensively as possible. Compare your facts and figures, and contrast them with theirs. Without entering a debate about who's right and who's wrong, you can at least try to dispose of their facts and figures as being critical indicators of valid considerations for the negotiation.
6. Reflect back key words that your opponent uses. For example, if your opponent says, *And of course, this creates a major problem in the patient-community,* simply reflect back, *So this will create a major problem throughout the patient-community—major problem, right?* By encouraging your opponent to repeat their statement and to provide more specific information, you will find that the opponent will usually either retract their position or move on quickly to another topic area, because their ploy was immediately met and defeated.
7. *Read* back key words and phrases to your opponent. As I discuss in the next section, note taking and observing negotiation behavior is critical to the success of the entire process. By taking notes and specifically charging your opponent with proving the veracity of certain statements that have been entered into "the record," you can take the higher ground in the negotiation process.
8. Concentrate on specific elements, as opposed to general assumptions, statements, and overviews. In all cases, ask for specific information, input, and validation of all statements made by your opponent. This can apply to a specific employee concern.

Consider for a minute how much negotiation takes place between a health care manager and an employee. An employee may say, *Everyone in our department thinks that this new patient initiative is a bad idea.* Unfortunately, because you are dealing with a mendacious individual in a lot of cases, the health care manager cannot say, *Who's everybody?* because the mendacious individual will say,

Well I'd rather not say. Discounting this reply becomes imperative. You can reply, *I want to know what your opinion is, and what is more important, what you think specifically we should do about it.* When you specifically charge such employees with making a solution, they will usually retract their position and either go about their business, meet their performance objectives, or find another place of employment.

It is important to remember that games can be played by negotiators in every regard and in every circumstances within a health care institution. In order to negate their impact and to maintain a sense of integrity, sense of purpose, and positive outcome to the negotiation process, it is vital through the communication process of a negotiation to counteract games immediately and let your opponent know that you mean business, will negotiate intently and with the utmost integrity, and will employ the fortitude necessary to "call" your opponent when they are being less than genuine in their negotiation process.

How to Form a Negotiating Team

In many cases team negotiations are a necessity of life in the health care business. In this section, I look at how to build an effective negotiating team and how to set a sound team strategy that encompasses all the positive facets of mutually beneficial negotiation and incorporates the values of proper preparation, knowledge of the opponent, and communilogical management. Let's use the example of a group of physicians who are negotiating to establish an inner-city clinic with Newington General Hospital. In this fictitious case, Dr. Frank Cole, Dr. Jan McBride, Dr. Kim Forest, and Dr. Mark Scranton represent the physician group. They will be negotiating with a negotiation team from the board of directors consisting of the chairman, Andy McAlden, and three board members, Phil Shannon, Gene Ellington, and Wanda Price. The objective for the physician group is to get the financial backing of the health care system, gain the overall support of the internal community of the hospital, and fundamentally receive the "go ahead" for the new clinic.

After using the need range preparation guides (discussed in this chapter and shown in Figure 13.1), the physician group decides that the following parameters are key to their negotiation:

- The establishment of a new facility, with a power rating of nine
- The budgeting and financial backing necessary to run the clinic for a year, with a power rating of seven
- The concurrence on the part of the hospital to sign supplemental support to the facility, such as equipment, personnel, and other necessities for the new clinic, with a power rating of five
- The establishment of a separate board for the clinic, with a power rating of three

After establishing these parameters, the group decides that it would be important to assign roles based on the strengths of each of the physician negotiation team members. Accordingly, the lead person, or lead advocate, will be Dr. Frank Cole. The team decides that Dr. Cole is simply the "best talker" among the four. He is witty and articulate and was captain of his debate team during his undergraduate days at Presley University. Furthermore, Dr. Cole has a good relationship with the board members, and is seen as someone who is credible, committed to the organization, and progressive in his leadership of his individual physician practice, as well as during his recent term as medical staff president.

The accountabilities for the individual filling the position of lead advocate are to

- Present the opening case for the negotiation
- Try to ascertain the overall strategy for the negotiating team
- Lead the team through the negotiation process, including the summoning of caucuses and other important communilogical initiatives
- Manage the other three members in their respective roles

Dr. Jan McBride will fill the role of counteradvocate, or number two person on the team. Dr. McBride is a good pathologist who is naturally inquisitive and has a "good investigative-interrogation style" in the eyes of her teammates. Dr. McBride's initiatives as the counteradvocate are to

- Present counterarguments and key questions to the lead advocate of the opposing team

- Present specifics for the overall case made by the negotiation team, when required by the lead advocate
- Closely monitor the actions and presentation of the opposing team, and counsel the lead advocate on caucus times, negotiation ploys, and other essential strategies

Dr. Kim Forest will fill the position of the expert-data negotiator. Dr. Forest is a research physician and is thus naturally suited to her role. On the negotiation team, the data expert is responsible for

- Providing significant data
- Making presentations of a technical nature
- Questioning and interrogating the opposing team relative to the validity of all data, facts, figures, and expert opinions presented by the opposing team

Finally, Dr. Mark Scranton will fulfill the position of recorder-perceiver. Dr. Scranton, an internist by trade, is well-suited to this role in which he will

- Record significant statements and presentations made by the opposing team
- Make significant notations relative to statements made by the other team
- Assist team members in asking the right questions at the right time by simply transcribing notes and "sliding" these notes inconspicuously to his teammates at appropriate times

Under no conditions will Scranton make a note on his note pad and jointly read it with his teammates. Rather, he will slide the notes to his teammates so that no undue nonverbal friction is established for exploitation by his opponents.

At the outset of the negotiation, it is quite apparent that the opposing team—the subgroup for the board of directors—is not as well prepared as the physician group. In fact, Andy McAlden of that team has decided that he will assume the role of both expert and lead advocate. He demonstrates this decision by doing the majority of the talking for his negotiation team. The only other participant in the process seems to be Wanda Price, who is trying to play "bad cop" to Andy McAlden's "good cop." That is, Price seems to have an inordinate interest in asking for information presenting a disharmonious approach to the negotiation, and basically promotes discord throughout the negotiation process. As a result, the team structure from the outset of the negotiation is favorable to the group of physician negotiators. As we'll see in later sections of this chapter, this momentum is capitalized on by the group's ability to effectively manage the communilogical process of the negotiation.

General Communilogical Keys

You have established your opponent's needs, conducted ardent preparation, set your expectations for the negotiation process, and entered the process itself. Now you need to take into account some *communilogical* (communication, logic, psychology) keys to conducting the negotiation.

It is vital to establish credibility throughout the negotiation process. The best way to do this is to present evidence throughout the process that establishes the need to come to a settlement and, more opportunistically, to come to the settlement desired by your team. It is also essential to use the right pronouns throughout the negotiation process, such as *we*. Phrases such as *Most of us would agree* also contribute to a successful negotiation.

A sense of leadership should be assumed throughout the negotiation process. This can be done by simply taking the opportunity to present your case first. By demonstrating your good faith to your opponents by revealing your needs, desires, and expected outcome to the process, the momentum may swing in your favor from the outset of the negotiation. Though a strong counterargument might be made against one of your points, by simply establishing the majority of your points initially, your side of the negotiation becomes the standard for the discussion.

To use the previous section as an example, the physician negotiation group would be wise to present their four objectives for the negotiation at the outset, or immediately after trying to ascertain the interests of the board in the negotiation. As it happens, the board of directors is also interested in establishing the clinic, but they want to do so at a minimal cost. In essence, if this is established early in the negotiation the physician group has the opportunity basically to obtain their primary objective in a quick, fruitful manner. A sense of leadership in the negotiation process is always a good tactic.

When you lead the discussion and present ideas and factual, cogent, convincing arguments, only the most recalcitrant opponent can be resistive. In many cases, however, this resistance is rooted in your opponent's desire either to not make a deal that is overwhelmingly—and unfairly—in the "want" column relative to their bargaining range and outside the realm of the mutual benefit range.

As already stated, visualization can be an effective technique, particularly if presented early in the communication process of the negotiation and as an overall ideal. Furthermore, visualization becomes even more powerful when it relates to the benefits of greater organizational stability, greater patient service and satisfaction, more effective medical service delivery, and other commonly held objectives among parties at the negotiation table.

Listing priorities is also an effective communication strategy, particularly if the priorities are mutually held by both parties. Giving individuals lists of specific facts and figures, or in some cases, the essential desires for the negotiation process and intended outcomes, can also be effective. It is also important to keep a balanced view; that is, maintain perspective of the priorities of your negotiation side, as well as that of your opponent's.

The time and space in which you negotiate can also affect the communilogical flavor of the negotiation. For example, a Friday afternoon might be a more opportune time to try to reach a settlement than Monday morning. A comfortable negotiation space is usually ideal for reaching an agreement. But a forum where your team is comfortable—such as the doctor' s conference room— might be uncomfortable to your opponent and negatively affect their ability to negotiate or their desire to negotiate quickly. The use of user-friendly terms, appropriate language, limited emotionalism, and good progressive reasoning are all good communilogical keys for the negotiation process.

Continuous Communilogical Keys for the Negotiation Process

Throughout the entire negotiation process, you must embrace several keys in order to bring about a productive settlement:

1. Identify throughout the process your opponent's needs, desires, wants, and desired outcomes.
2. Perceive why your opponent pursues a specific course of action, line of reasoning, or argument, and the rationale.
3. Review evidence constantly, and keep apprised of arguments that might be contradictory, inconclusive, or conflicting.
4. Plan specific counterstrategies and next steps throughout the negotiation process.
5. Assign responsibility to individuals on your team, as well as to your opponent's, for proving their case, presenting facts and figures, and providing other substantive evidence for their argument.
6. Organize information, arguments, and counterstrategies throughout the process.
7. Assess progress through the negotiation and evaluate whether your opponent is making sense, stalling, seeking a mutually beneficial end, or advocating a "want" position outside the spectrum of a mutually beneficial outcome.
8. Customize your argument throughout the process to meet the needs of your specific physician, and counteract your opponent's arguments, position, and unreasonable demands.
9. Balance your need for success with your opponent's need for self-esteem, a mutually beneficial outcome, and a progressive settlement.
10. Clarify information that appears to be complex, not user-friendly, irrelevant, or specious by asking specific questions at any given time.
11. Guide the discussion again by asking questions, investigate information for which your opponent is forced to be accountable, and present new arguments when there is a "stall" in the negotiation process.
12. Record information that is specific, relative, relevant, and revelatory to your opponent's position, and use this information

to help your opponent present their arguments clearly and to give an indication of how close a settlement may—or may not—be relative to the overall process.

13. Manage the negotiation process by asking questions, making declarative statements, taking caucuses, or using any other kind of negotiation communication device that is appropriate to your time and objective.

14. Measure the impact of your arguments and your position relative to your opponent's potential strengths and weaknesses.

15. Redirect the negotiation process by taking a break, stalling, asking a question that explores new ground, or presenting a new argument or negotiation initiative.

16. Calibrate your specific argument in the way that one uses a compass, by shifting directions or moving your opponent into an unfamiliar, uncomfortable, or very comfortable area, all in the interest of securing a deal.

17. Adapt to your opponent's new strategy by agreeing, disagreeing, or condoning their information or by complementing their ability to make a deal.

18. Appropriate or "steal" a particular pet phrase or term from your opponents, such as *patient focus,* which you can then use in your own interests in context. For example, if your opponent keeps on saying it is important that this deal be patient-focused, you will then calibrate your argument to make sure that it is indeed patient-focused by simply appropriating their term and demonstrating why your position is the penultimate patient-focused initiative.

19. Present information formally by using any and all verbal or nonverbal devices possible, such as an easel, a blackboard, overheads, handouts, physician papers, balance sheets, and other communication devices, that help to strengthen your case.

20. Educate your opponents about specific knowledge that might be pertinent to the negotiation, such as physician objectives, medical standards, and other information, which a physician negotiator would have at her fingertips, ready to use in a negotiation.

21. Credit your opponent for progress throughout the negotiation specifically, or more generally, on their ability to "make things

happen" throughout the health care arena and within your own community.

22. Listen to every single thing your opponent says in the interest of understanding their position, identifying a weakness, revealing a probative point, or understanding an opportunity to gain closure in the negotiation process.

23. Encourage your opponent to present new information, facts, and figures and to reveal as much of their position and their needs as possible in the interest of gaining a settlement.

24. Persuade your opponent. This is basically a byproduct of the previous twenty-three communilogical keys, but in some cases, must be emphasized by simply asking, *I think we've been very fair and very persuasive in demonstrating that we are truly interested in taking care of the patient by implementing this new product: What do you think?*

25. Summarize all that has taken place throughout the negotiation.

26. Close the negotiation by "sealing the deal" through a written letter of understanding that outlines the basic points of the proposal, thus becoming in essence a contracted settlement to the negotiation.

All negotiators should be aware of these communilogical keys and employ all of them throughout the negotiation process. The example negotiation team of physicians cited in the last section can use all twenty-six keys to gain the budgetary and operational support necessary to open a new clinic.

The final communilogical key is ensuring understanding, which can be incorporated into any phase of the negotiation strategy. Fundamentally, the following phrases can be used to make sure that both parties are in accord with certain negotiation initiatives:

- Is that helpful?
- Does that make sense?
- Do you have any questions?
- Is that clear?
- Is that OK?
- Are you able to see that?
- Do you follow me?

- So we can look to you for agreement on these issues?
- So we have a deal?
- So we can at least agree on these specific points?

An important aspect of the communilogical keys is note taking. Several rules apply. First, everybody on a negotiation team is responsible for note taking. In essence, everyone can be a recorder, lead advocate, or data expert providing that in a team sequence, the primary roles are fulfilled nominally by individuals, such as we depicted in our mini-case study earlier in this chapter, and as a secondary objective, everybody assumes the role of recorder as appropriate. Second, notes should be taken in the interests of brevity, flexibility, and as a guide through the process, and not as a functional stenographer throughout the negotiation process. The stenographer method can give your opponent the misguided impression that you either do not care about what they are saying, or you are taking notes strictly in the interest of trying to "catch them" in a miscommunication, as opposed to negotiating in a forthright, honest, and candid manner.

Notes should be used to reconcile inconsistencies, as we have discussed, as well as to get key pet words and phrases, which can be appropriated in the interest of gaining agreement throughout the process.

Using a Caucus

A caucus is basically a negotiation device in which a team, or individual negotiator, takes a break from the negotiation to achieve several objectives. A caucus can be obtained by telling your opponent, *We need a couple of minutes here to talk individually,* in the case of a group negotiation, or in the case of a single negotiation, *Excuse me, let me get back to you in a few minutes on this particular point.*

A caucus is distinct from a walk-out and deadlock. A caucus can be measured in minutes, as the individual gains a time-out to consider specific issues. A walk-out, however, can mean a couple of days' delay in the negotiation. A deadlock usually represents an unknown delay and can lead to an impasse, which can be a long-term break in negotiations, or perhaps to a complete breakdown of negotiations.

A caucus can be used in several ways. First, a caucus can be used to revisit a negotiation strategy and plan a next step. In other regards it can be used to counter the unexpected, such as a surprise from your opponent, an unexpected concession, or an arbitrary and inordinate demand from your opponent. A caucus can also be used to evaluate progress made throughout the negotiation.

Caucuses can also be used to shift the focus of the negotiation by planning a redirection or to get your opponent thinking about other directions. A caucus can be used to deflate your opponent's emotion, or in some cases to disrupt momentum. Often, particularly in group negotiations, a caucus should be called to act as an outlet for emotions, such as laughing, anger, or other negotiation-driven emotions.

Caucuses can also provide time to do some more homework and investigate a position further. Caucuses can be used to determine the *why* or the *what* behind your opponent's position. In a similar vein, a caucus can be used to rate the odds relative to the propensity of your opponent to accept an offer or reject an offer. It can also be used to reconcile a position presented by your opponent that might be misleading, inconsistent, or irrelevant.

As a credible psychological ploy, a caucus can be used to get your opponent thinking about what your group might be discussing, or what you might individually be considering, even though you simply called the caucus to take a break and recharge your batteries for the second part of the negotiation. A caucus can certainly be used to slow down the process, or perhaps stall the negotiation. Certainly, a caucus can be used to consider an offer and to decide whether to accept or reject it.

Finally, a caucus can be used to determine whether the negotiation is leading to a settlement that will be good for the organization, fit within the viability of your organization, and act as a progressive implement of progress for your practice, your health care organization, and the future of health care provision within your service area.

Anytime is a good time to take to a caucus. In the team negotiation example, it is the responsibility of Dr. Mark Scranton, as the recorder and perceiver, to call for a caucus any time he perceives it is needed. This will allow his group to consider information that the board has presented and also allow him to provide input relative to behavior, communication, and approaches that he has perceived, observed, and recorded in his role on the physician negotiation team.

Reaching Agreement

By pursuing all the strategies delineated in this chapter, you can reach a positive, mutually beneficial negotiation outcome. At a certain point—a point that is difficult to define because each negotiation is different—you should move to close the deal. Generally, you will want to close the deal when you have ascertained that your opponent has reached a position of agreement with you within the mutually beneficial need range which is amenable to both parties. At that point, you should choose among the following options:

- Verify the position of both parties
- Take the deal
- Reject the deal
- Consider the long-range ramifications of accepting or rejecting the deal
- Consider alternative deals with other parties
- Reevaluate the benefits provided by the impending deal
- Perhaps most important, listen to and trust your gut-level comfort level with the deal
- Summarize and reiterate the tenets of the deal so that both parties understand

If the answer to all of the items on this checklist are relatively positive, you should embrace the deal that has been generated through the negotiation strategy.

As in all leadership endeavors, there are no right or wrong answers for the negotiation process. However, by following these guidelines, and more important, trusting your intrinsic intelligence and negotiation savvy, the art of mutually beneficial negotiation is well within your grasp.

Chapter Fourteen

Balancing "Administrivia" and Progressive Action

As a new health care manager, you will be inundated daily by "administrivia": meetings, phone calls, reports, and deadlines. These responsibilities, all part of the uncompromising world of health care management, can tax your time and patience. Having to juggle several responsibilities—a meeting or a phone call that interrupts a project's progress—can be frustrating. It is vital that you strike a constructive balance between nonproductive administrivia and high-profile critical tasks early in your tenure.

However, attending meetings and communicating by phone are necessary adjuncts to the management work role. It is the effective management of these job components and their related technologies that establish a positive norm that will fully use the most limited resource you have: time. In this chapter I present strategies to help you manage the time you spend on the phone and in meetings. I also describe how to manage the deceptive "five-minute meeting" and the ongoing stress that is intrinsic to your new role. By first experimenting with some of these methods and then adapting them successfully and comfortably to your own style, you can minimize (or eliminate) frustration and maximize time efficiency.

Time Management

Approximately thirty years ago, corporate America seized on the topic of time management not only as a training theme but also as an essential element of organizational progress. Time management is critical in the health care environment, where as manager you are charged with top-level performance despite limited resources and are expected to take on more responsibilities to keep pace with performance objectives. Mismanagement of time can result in your becoming derailed or sidetracked unnecessarily, due to lack of preparation or misappropriation of available time.

To manage time properly, you can use any number of techniques. Four proven strategies are discussed in the following subsections: time sequencing, prioritizing, assessing needs and wants, and assessing relative importance. Review each strategy and decide which one is appropriate for you. One strategy might be used exclusively or in combination with others as dictated by your responsibilities. In addition, you may wish to refer to the case study in Chapter Seventeen for several examples of how one new health care manager used these techniques.

Time Sequencing

The time-sequencing technique for managing time is to isolate the dimension of time itself; that is, assign a time sequence to each piece of correspondence or each objective in a given day. The most accepted form of identifying time blocks and essential time sequences is to use systems guided by the traffic-light method, illustrated in Figure 14.1. The stoplight system uses a three-stage stoplight—green, yellow, and red—that is similar to a normal traffic light. By attaching time sequence values to each light, you can organize incoming correspondence, daily communication, and assigned deadlines.

The green light is designated for any responsibility not regulated by time. The basic parameter for the green light would be any task that does not have to be done (that is, you can forgo doing it or you can delegate it) or any task that does not have to be completed within, for example, seventy-two hours. Items that fall into this category include personal correspondence, journal articles to be read, or any other task that does not have an immediate negative consequence if it is not attended to within seventy-two hours. Hence, you may proceed with other priorities.

Yellow-light items include responsibilities that must be finished within a twenty-four-hour sequence; for example, a report that must be finished by the end of the day, a communication to be

Figure 14.1. Time Management Systems.

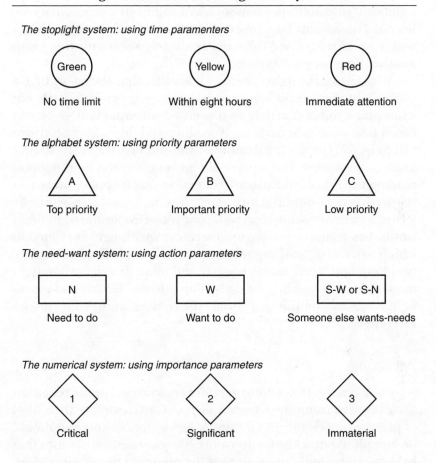

The stoplight system: using time paramenters

Green — No time limit

Yellow — Within eight hours

Red — Immediate attention

The alphabet system: using priority parameters

A — Top priority

B — Important priority

C — Low priority

The need-want system: using action parameters

N — Need to do

W — Want to do

S-W or S-N — Someone else wants-needs

The numerical system: using importance parameters

1 — Critical

2 — Significant

3 — Immaterial

conveyed before shift's end, or a task that must be completed to meet tomorrow's deadline. The yellow light signals caution, which in this case means that a given task must be attended to or a negative consequence will occur within twenty-four hours. Yellow-light items should be put into a folder or organized in the central part of your desk as a visible reminder.

The red light is designated for duties and business objectives that must be attended to immediately. You must stop all other action immediately and give complete attention to the red-light item. Red-light items include emergencies or other situations that require crisis management. For example, a major medical emergency such as a massive car accident would merit red-light status, as would a significant organization event such as a visit from a prominent civic leader. These items take precedence over all other work activities and must be addressed fully and resolutely before moving on to another item on your agenda.

With the traffic-light system, it is feasible that after a set time a yellow-light item could become a red-light or green-light item. For example, a journal article that seemed unimportant yesterday could take on red-light status if reading and digesting the article will help you dispatch a deadline-oriented task today. In similar fashion, a yellow or red light could become a green light if, upon reading the title of the article, you realize that it applies more to a report due next month. Once again, it is important to use this objective system in conjunction with your subjective instincts. In other words, use your gut feeling to determine which light is related to which work task, and organize your work accordingly. Remember: Red-light items must be addressed immediately; yellow-light items should be put in your daily "things-to-do" folder; and green-light items can be put in a "hold" file or desk drawer for further reference.

Prioritizing

Another time management technique arranges items based on their priority, using the letters A, B, and C to designate their level of priority (see Figure 14.1). Priority A designates items that should be completed quickly; furthermore, they are responsibilities that have meaning and consequences for others in the organization. They have top priority. A priority A item might be a report that must be disseminated to the entire organization, a departmentwide activity of major scope (such as a radiology department implementing a new diagnostic system), or a high-visibility activity in which you must immediately immerse yourself so as to maintain proper organizational flow.

Priority B items are of pressing importance but are not bound to immediate time constraints. These might include preparation for inspection by a state or other regulatory team, or a particular meeting of major consequence. Priority B items could also include certain mail and other communications that require response within a given time but do not require immediate attention or action.

Priority C activities have little or negligible urgency or importance. These activities could include your attendance at a local professional meeting or a lunch date with a peer to discuss general issues.

Assessing Needs and Wants

The strategy of assessing needs and wants is based on demand. With this strategy, you would assign a designation of N, W, S-W, or S-N (see Figure 14.1). The first of these designations, N, refers to a particular task you need to do immediately; no element of selectiveness or electiveness is attached to the job. Examples of need items are any requirement covered under the job description, a managerial mandate (such as conducting sexual harassment awareness training), or an organizational initiative in which you must participate and act in the interest of accomplishing a set goal. Need items are probably on par with red-light or yellow-light items, or priority A or priority B items. Need items are job tasks that have major consequence and time value to you as a manager as well as to significant other members of the organization.

The next sequence refers to want items, designated by the letter W. Want items are job tasks you might like to do, responsibilities that you elect or select to do. The phrase *It would be nice if . . .* is a good parameter for evaluating whether something belongs in the want category. A want item is probably a green-light item or a priority C item.

The S-W or S-N designation relates to someone else who wants or needs this particular task to be completed. Depending on who that "someone else" is, this item could be subject to high priority or immediate time constraint, or the converse. For example, if the person in want or need is your manager or supervisor, then obviously for you the task becomes a red-light, or priority A item. If that someone else is not in a strong position of authority or does not require the task to be completed as part of her everyday mandates, then the item can easily be a green-light, or priority C, task. As always, rely on your instinct and intuition in assessing the appropriate category.

It is essential that you implement a system for separating items in this fashion so that everything wanted or needed by someone else does not become a priority A, a red-light item, or an N item. This way, you avoid becoming overwhelmed and victimized by your own lack of forethought and self-organization.

Assessing Relative Importance

Another system of time management assesses relative importance on a scale of one to three (see Figure 14.1). The number one identifies a task as critically important, two identifies it as significantly important, and three identifies it as least important or immaterial. You can assign desk drawers—the 1-drawer, the 2-drawer, and the 3-drawer—to remind you of the relative importance of tasks. (The strategy also works with baskets, for example, top, middle, and bottom baskets.) In either case, you must remain flexible in your use of this system, for a 2-item can easily become a 1-item or a 3-item, depending on circumstance, your personal view and management style, and your reevaluation of the item's relative importance.

The technique of assessing relative importance can also be used in combination with any of the other three techniques (stoplight, alphabet, and need-want). In other words, the importance of each item, piece of communication, and assigned task can be judged a green light or an A or an N and then further sorted into a one-two-three category. For example, you might further sort your yellow-light folder into yellow-1, yellow-2, or yellow-3 tasks. Or the priority A item might be further prioritized as A-1, A-2, or A-3. Or the "need to do's" can be arranged based on your subjective judgment.

In managing your time, select whichever time management system (or systems) most suits your comfort level and seems to offer the most potential worth. In doing so, you create your own unique system of time management, one you will incorporate as a routine practice. This routine will allow you to sort mail, manage communication, and set priorities in a way that will be both fruitful and efficient throughout your management career. This system of time management will afford you a certain peace of mind as well as the freedom to pursue the tasks—from most satisfactory to least satisfactory—you are charged with doing.

Telephone Management

Since its invention by Alexander Graham Bell more than a hundred years ago, the telephone has become a source of wonderment for the American imagination. In the past twenty years, the phone has been used in conjunction with computer systems, facsimile (fax) machines, electronic mail, and an array of adjunct devices. As a health care manager, you must manage the phone, not let it manage you.

Like Pavlov's dog, most managers feel the urge to respond whenever the "bell" rings. If not managed properly, phone conversation can become a central focus and thus derail your progress. Other elements of phone mismanagement can cause you to waste time, thereby becoming nonproductive at a point in your career when it is vitally important that you establish positive work habits and progressive action. In this section I explore nine dimensions of phone management, which should be touchstones for you as you manage your daily responsibilities.

Defining the Need for a Phone Call

The first dimension of telephone management is to determine whether a phone conversation is needed. If the intent of the conversation is ill-defined, chances are the conversation will waver and fail to produce tangible results. Furthermore, if there is pressing need to discuss a particular issue by phone, a follow-up conversation, preferably in person, should be scheduled rather than further phone time.

If a message is not vital or not bound by a finite time sequence, it is a good tactic to postpone, or at least abbreviate, the conversation to avert wasting time and energy on a topic that could be handled more effectively via another form of communication. For example, if you receive a phone call that is not vitally important and does not have a pressing time requirement, tactfully tell the person that you will call back at a time mutually agreed on. Be sure to ask what prework you need to complete to be prepared for the conversation. By asking this question, you encourage the caller to fine-tune the intent and give you a clearer idea of the topic of conversation.

Choosing the Best Mode of Communicating

The second dimension of telephone management, which is related to the first, has to do with the mode of communicating. Because of overreliance on the phone as a primary means of communication, other more effective methods, such as one-on-one meetings, are often overlooked. The phone should never be used to discuss critical personnel issues, sensitive management issues, or technical issues that are immersed in detail (including personnel performance problems and patient-related information). These conversations are best handled in a personal meeting, where emotions and attitude can be gauged and specific detail can be discussed fully. Written communication should be used as supplemental support in lieu of additional phone conversations, particularly if technical detail or critical information will be examined. (Official memos are useful for stating objective information that emphasizes deadlines and definite outcomes; personal notes are more appropriate for expressing gratitude and other feelings.) By its very nature, the phone precludes nonverbal communication, thus restricting the breadth of detail prohibitively. Therefore, the phone should be used for information that is brief, not of a sensitive or confidential nature, and free of subtle details.

Preparing for the Conversation

As indicated above, completing prework can help control phone time. Doing prior homework and setting a specific phone agenda beforehand contribute to a more efficient conversation. In practice, the conversation would begin with one individual stating the topic to be discussed, listing the outcome desired from the conversation, and presenting specific items or facts that can be discussed in the conversation. This means, practically speaking, that two or three items will be discussed that will provide both parties with a definitive outcome at the end of the conversation. Without prework, time is wasted, and the outcome is more confusion instead of positive results.

Making the Subject Clear and Maintaining Focus

Establishing the subject to be discussed and maintaining clarity of topic are critical. Both should be done at the beginning of a conversation (or beforehand, as part of prework). Ask questions and make statements that keep the other party on track with the topic. At the end of the conversation summarize not only the subject of the conversation but also what has been accomplished by the call. In doing so, you lend resonance to the conversation and set the stage for further progressive development of the subject.

Maintaining focus is similar to making the subject clear. Both must be done within the context of the big picture. Stay focused on the topic from your perspective, and consider the potential overall outcome the conversation and the subject might have on you, your department, and your organization. The best way to maintain focus is, as always, to ask pertinent questions and guide your fellow communicator toward the main topic and desired outcome of the conversation.

Dealing with Secondary Issues

Secondary, or tangential, issues that come up during the course of the conversation can jeopardize the focus of a phone conversation. Because of the action-packed health care environment, secondary issues are always a factor in any communication; none of your work is done in a vacuum. To handle peripheral issues, take notes while on the phone; that is, list any and all secondary issues or tangential topics that come up during the conversation. At the conclusion of the conversation, review your notes and enter into your management logbook specific secondary issues that might affect your progress throughout the work cycle.

Limiting the Call's Duration

Most industrial psychologists believe a phone conversation that exceeds five minutes in length is being conducted to the point of diminishing returns. If the entire message cannot be delivered within five minutes, it is probably more advantageous to schedule a personal meeting or, at a minimum, another phone conversation for which both parties will be better prepared.

Because of easy reliance on phones, many managers fall into the habit of talking ad infinitum without realizing what should be accomplished by the conversation. It is helpful to time phone conversations to ensure that they do not exceed the recommended five-minute limit. If they do and the conversation has drifted or become too detailed, interrupt the conversation, suggest a meeting, or schedule another phone call (but with better preparation).

Blocking Out Phone Time

To the extent that you can, try fitting phone time into your schedule so that your office time can be managed well. Set aside a specific time during which you will "work the phone." Most managers schedule the hours 8:00 to 9:00 A.M. or 4:30 to 5:30 P.M. to return phone calls, make new calls, and review notes and communication guides in the interest of improving action. These two points in the day can serve as designated times when colleagues can get in touch with you easily to discuss pertinent issues, and can also be dedicated to returning calls to individuals who interrupt your progress during the day with green-light issues.

Minimizing Telephone Tag

A major problem among health care managers and executives at all levels is so-called *telephone tag,* the dilemma of one person calling another, leaving a message, and then not being on the receiving end when the person tries to return the call.

To eliminate telephone tag, be certain when you call someone to leave not only your name but also your number (even if the person already has your number). Logically, the party called will return those messages that are most user-friendly; that is, the ones with phone numbers. Also, include in your message the main topic you wish to discuss. This will allow the party opportunity to do his prework and be fully prepared for the conversation.

Make sure you leave at least two time frames during which the individual can contact you; for example, today between 4:00 and 5:00 P.M. and tomorrow between 10:00 A.M. and noon. This will specify two opportunities when you will most likely be at your desk and receptive to the call. These simple strategies will minimize phone tag and allow more constructive use of your communication time.

Garnering the Desired Outcome

As mentioned earlier, the intent of a phone call is to obtain a desired outcome. To achieve this, try to ensure that the decision at the end of your phone conversation is not simply to have another conversation. Instead, restate your objective, discuss further action, and plan future communication. In doing so the definitive action of the conversation is reiterated, and value is attached to the conversation. The least productive outcome of any phone conversation is to schedule another call to discuss the same issues that should have been resolved during this phone call.

The phone, like time, can be compared with fire. If used correctly, fire can heat homes and allow for cooking of food. If not kept in check or if misused, however, fire can be destructive. Misuse of phone time due to conversations that have no useful consequence can be frustrating, set a bad precedent, and encourage bad habits. By focusing on desired outcomes and avoiding the pitfalls of poor communication, inadequate phone management, and careless time management, you allow yourself more time to be more productive and interested in the vital work of health care management.

Meeting Management

A common lament among health care managers is the disproportionate amount of time spent daily in meeting attendance. Meetings pervade today's health care environment for two essential reasons. First, because communication is key to any performance aspect of health care provision, meetings are a necessary means of communicating current ideas, objectives, and goals. Second, with the proliferation of technology in the information age, meetings are needed simply to keep pace with the changes taking place in the health care arena. Hence, meetings are unavoidable in your role as health care manager.

The good news, however, is that you can have more control over the number of meetings you attend and certainly you can have more input, particularly at meetings in which you now assume a leadership position. In this section I discuss common pitfalls inherent to meeting attendance (such as poor leadership, misguided participation, lack of focus and/or objective, and inconsequential outcomes) and discuss methods you can employ immediately to make sure that meetings meet their original charter—to be a productive means of communication so as to encourage progressive action.

Ascertaining the Need for a Meeting

A common problem with meetings is that, like making unnecessary phone calls, there simply may not be a need to hold one. The matter to be discussed might easily be handled in one-on-one informal dialogue. However, because health care managers are so acclimated to going to meetings, they expect a meeting on virtually any topic. Hence, your first tip is this: Hold a meeting only when there is a clear need to discuss information among more than three people in a timely fashion and with a distinct outcome at hand. Accordingly, review your current meeting schedule and agendas to determine which meetings are absolutely vital to your department's success. Certain meetings might be held out of habit; take a close look at the reason behind the meeting and determine realistically whether there is a need to continue meeting routinely for an issue that might best be handled elsewhere.

Determining a Realistic Objective

Determine ahead of time what the specific meeting objective is; make sure that this objective is communicated clearly throughout your department and to all members who will be in attendance. The objective should be laid out in a clear-cut manner to encourage participation and generate thinking along the lines of the meeting objective. Without a clear objective, the meeting is seen as a waste of time or, worse, as irrelevant to your staff's daily activities in their defined work roles. This can result in lack of motivation not only in the meeting, but also in your team's ongoing work role.

Developing a Focused Agenda

In well-run meetings a common theme should support the departmental and organizational objectives. If the meeting is being held as part of a continuous quality improvement effort, there should be specific focus on, for example, how recruiting can generate top-quality personnel. Whenever attendees shift from the main objective of the meeting, or lose focus, it is up to you as leader to bring them back on course. This can be done by asking the simple question, *How does this relate to our main topic?* or, *How can this contribute toward a solution in today's meeting?* These questions will return the discussion to the main focus of the meeting either by eliminating secondary or tangential comments or by tying the digression to the main focus.

Prior to the meeting, an agenda should be published and distributed to all prospective attendees. This agenda should cover the main objective of the meeting, the focus of issues to be discussed, any specific topics to be included, and a general time sequence for each component. The agenda also should include the time the meeting will start and when it will adjourn. Giving prior notice will generate positive thinking about the meeting's purpose and encourage input from each attendee. One suggestion is to write a personalized note on each individual's copy of the agenda. For example, if a member of the finance department is to attend, you might jot down a note to that person that suggests particular ways in which the relevant financial aspects might be incorporated into the general topic. If appropriate, a short cover letter or note should accompany the agenda that encourages individuals to add other topics to the agenda and to garner specific input beforehand that might be considered helpful to the conduct of the meeting. Asking for this input encourages participation and allows individuals the liberty of contributing areas of their own expertise and interest, thus encouraging support of the basic objective of the meeting and the issue at hand. Conversely, asking for input might identify any problem areas or problem players involved in the meeting.

Limiting Duration of the Meeting

As mentioned at the beginning of this section, health care providers frown on meetings that appear to be a waste of time. With that in mind, strive always to stick to the time parameters you have ascribed for a particular meeting. This means starting the meeting on time, thereby sending the proper message to latecomers.

A common mistake made by new health care managers is to stop the discussion and recap events for the benefit of a late arrival. This sends two negative messages to participants. First, it tells those who came on time that punctuality is truly not important because discussion will be repeated for latecomers. Second, stopping the meeting sends a message to late arrivals that their behavior is acceptable and lateness will be tolerated at future meetings. Such messages establish a negative work norm, which will lead to the perception that your meetings are a waste of time and poorly run, and that you truly are not in charge.

Ensure that your meetings end as soon as all business has been addressed. Prepare participants for the conclusion by saying, *We've just about run out of time for this. I feel as though we've discussed everything fully and would like any brief, general comments or other ideas you have at this point.* This request allows everyone a final opportunity to contribute to the meeting, and it sends a positive message that you value their time as well as their participation, and that you recognize that they have other important responsibilities to attend to at this time. Meetings that go into overtime jeopardize the productive output of busy health care workers. When this happens, resentment is harbored against the individual running the meeting.

Inviting the Right People

If the meeting objective is clear—that is, you have a specific outcome in mind—the proper roster of attendees should fall together. Invite only those who potentially have a strong contribution to make. Often health care managers invite someone to a meeting out of routine or out of respect to their position. This encourages participation from individuals who have no primary contribution to make, thus in turn steering the meeting off course and into areas that are of secondary or tangential importance.

Upon compiling your roster and issuing invitations, assign prework for the meeting; that is, specific areas or tasks that team members can accomplish prior to the meeting. This prework includes their particular slant or viewpoint on the topic, what positive solutions they can generate, and their overall perspective of the issue. This preliminary effort will allow you to move quickly to the core of the meeting's issue and eliminate wasted time in terms of clarifying your objective or defining people's roles within the meeting.

For those who express feeling excluded because you did not invite them, explain to them that their presence is not absolutely required at this first meeting, and that you will brief them on any outcomes that are pertinent to their responsibilities and elicit their viewpoints later. This demonstrates that you did not deliberately set out to hurt feelings or bruise egos.

Choosing an Appropriate Setting

The meeting environment is also important. A conference room is appropriate to use for a high-profile meeting or one that includes guests from other organizations. A high-visibility conference room might not be the most appropriate place for certain meetings, which might benefit more by being held in an isolated corner of the cafeteria during off-hours. For a small meeting, that is, fewer than five or six people, an office might be appropriate. If the meeting involves discussion of confidential information, it might be held off-site during lunch so as to ensure candid discussion and frank dialogue. Routine meetings, such as monthly department meetings, should be held in a dedicated area to avoid confusion. But try to avoid stale dialogue at routine meetings. For example, although a financial report may have the same components (for example, costs, revenues generated, monthly patient volume), seek a fresh approach, perhaps by leading off with a suggested plan for a training rotation for the new accounts receivable system.

Ensuring Good Leadership

Good meeting leadership should encourage participation, lead to productive results, and gain definitive and desired outcomes. A good meeting leader keeps the conversation on track, asks the right questions (such as those included in Appendix C of this book), and allows participation that helps accomplish the meeting's objectives. A good leader also keeps the discussion focused on key issues, leads by example in expressing his viewpoints, and always encourages participants to voice their own viewpoints and opinions (even if they are contrary to those presented by the leader). A strong meeting leader does not conduct the meeting in a style that might be perceived as intimidating.

As always, adopt a meeting leadership style that is comfortable for you. If you are a listener, listen intently and ask questions to clarify or amplify information. If you are a talker, feel free to get the meeting going with a five-minute overview of your expectations and the significant issues to be addressed. Regardless of your style, make sure that you assume command of the meeting (without being intimidating) and get meaningful results that contribute toward your department's progress and the organization's performance.

A key consideration is the mode used to communicate within the meeting. In today's high-technology society, conference calls frequently replace face-to-face meetings. Although conference calls serve a need, whenever possible use interpersonal (that is, in-person) communication to conduct your meetings. This mode provides the benefits of direct eye contact, presents opportunity to evaluate nonverbal communication, and stresses the participative aspect of communication. These benefits lead to an improved chance of accomplishing meeting outcomes and arriving at definitive action.

Restating the Outcomes

Restate the outcomes generated by the meetings, what has occurred from the meeting, and what the next step might be. As in managing phone time, you don't want to have to call another meeting to rediscuss what should have been resolved in this one. Such a poor outcome would put your management reputation in jeopardy and could cause disenchantment among your staff. In applying the guidelines in this section, focus more on what to do rather than what not to do. That is, do not concentrate overmuch on the pitfalls, but follow the progressive suggestions with a positive attitude, adapt them to your own style, and make sure that you share the success of a meeting with all those in attendance and thank them for their participation and their input.

Minimizing the "Five-Minute Meeting"

Earlier in the chapter, the five-minute phone call was suggested as a measuring stick of telephone effectiveness. Do not confuse this with the five-minute ruse. A very difficult situation for new managers can be the "five-minute meeting." This occurs when someone (staff or peer) comes into your office and says, "Can I talk to you for five minutes?" This five-minute period invariably will turn into a twenty-minute (or longer) session. In certain cases—for example, an emergency that demands your immediate input—this is a necessary evil. In most cases, however, the individual is intruding on your time so that you can make judgments and prescribe action on an issue that is in their area of responsibility. Furthermore, this interruption is a time waster and falls under the category of administrivia. It sets a precedent of upward delegation: You are performing that individual's work role for him.

You must artfully manage this potential pitfall to avoid wasting time and restricting the development of your individual team members. The first method toward remedying this problem is to use screening devices.

Using Screening Devices

Screening devices serve to postpone the five-minute meeting and encourage the individual to solve the problem independently. One screening device is to meet the request for a five-minute meeting with the statement, *I don't have five minutes now but I will at [specific time] today.* It is incumbent upon you to keep the appointment. It is possible, however, that in the meantime the requester might solve the problem or at least shorten the discussion so that it in fact takes five minutes. This postponement tactic encourages the individual to take independent responsibility for the problem as well as to communicate with brevity and clarity. It also teaches him to value your time and not set up the false expectation that you will do the job or make decisions for that person.

Another device is simply to maintain a closed-door policy. Although an open-door policy is a popular and effective management style, some situations justify a closed door. If you are involved in an important one-on-one meeting, completing necessary paperwork, or returning vital phone calls, you should not be interrupted under any less-than-critical circumstances. Judicious application of a closed-door policy will send a strong message to your staff that only reasonable and line-of-duty interruptions will be tolerated. It will also encourage staff autonomy in resolving problems and independence of action within individual work roles.

A secretary or assistant, if available, is a natural screening device. Instruct your secretary or assistant on the best way to handle someone who requests a five-minute meeting. Strategies include rescheduling that individual for a later time (postponement) or having your secretary briefly determine the nature of the problem, thus serving as a filter as well as a vital link between your staff members and you. Remember that the key word here is *filter*, not obstruction. Your secretary or assistant should not be perceived as a wall but rather as a bridge, and thus should exercise interpersonal skills to screen the problem and apprise you of the situation.

Using Nonverbal and Verbal Cues

Given that many solutions may be needed to solve one problem, another method for minimizing five-minute meetings is use of nonverbal cues. First, if you elect to grant the meeting, be certain you tell the requester that you have only five minutes. Then look at your watch and make sure you restrict the individual to five minutes. Some people request the five-minute meeting simply because they need encouragement or motivation, or perhaps because they are long-winded. By looking at your watch, perhaps standing during the meeting (ensuring that the person stands also), or simply excusing yourself at the end of five minutes, you let the individual know that time is of the essence and that she should get right to the point.

Verbal cues also can be used in the five-minute meeting. The best practice, which I advocate in consulting and training work with health care managers, is to use a questioning procedure similar to the one you learned in grammar school having to do with the elements of a good story. An adaptation of the who, what, where, when, how, which approach follows:

- Who is involved?
- What do you need from me and what results do you want?
- How should we proceed?
- When should we get started?
- Which resources and how much do you need to accomplish the goal?

By asking these specific questions, you get the individual to focus specifically on the objective and on what rationale might be behind her decision making. This also gives you the opportunity to participate appropriately toward resolution of the problem. Furthermore, it disciplines the individual into thinking practically about her work role and the responsibilities inherent to the job position.

Finally, if all else fails, and the requester chronically abuses the five-minute meeting, it is entirely appropriate to ask the question, *Why do you need a meeting?* Perhaps the previous manager wanted a hand in everything; perhaps the worker is insecure with the job responsibilities; or perhaps she simply assumes that you want to be apprised of every situation. In any event simply close the door to this chronic problem. Offer reinforcement by providing examples of successful ventures the person has undertaken; express your confidence in her ability; and state your expectation that in the future only critical issues will be brought to your attention, and that she will independently handle job-related responsibilities.

Use of nonverbal and verbal cues not only avoids time waste, it also helps develop your staff. People learn by doing; therefore, it is important to give them enough responsibility to grow, and to resist the urge to take on their responsibilities by becoming over-involved personally in all their problems. Your job is to manage the breadth of responsibility; your staff must undertake the depth of responsibility. By using the techniques suggested in this section, you will ensure that that position becomes part of the everyday workplace reality.

The Virtual Setonia E-Mail Rules

In 1998, Seton Hall University launched the MA in Strategic Communication and Leadership degree program (MASCL), which has now grown to be the foremost online degree program of its kind in American education. The students and faculty of this program have innovated ten rules for managing e-mail, which should be helpful to you as a new health care manager:

1. Use e-mail appropriately by recognizing that sensitive information and potentially emotional messages are best delivered in person or by phone in most situations.
2. Remember that the grammar, syntax, and form of your e-mail can reflect the respect that you hold for the message's receiver and the message itself. Edit before you click on the Send button!
3. The telegraphic style of a quick answer and short response is a better alternative than no response at all.
4. Suggest a follow-up action whenever possible, whether it is an in-person meeting or a more detailed phone conversation.
5. Immediately edit your messages-received inbox and delete all nonessential messages to avoid clutter.
6. Prioritize your incoming messages by using the stoplight system suggested in the time management section of this chapter.
7. Suggest two solutions for each question you receive via e-mail.
8. Try to answer all e-mails within twenty-four hours—even if your response is that you need more time to consider an appropriate answer.
9. Read your messages before you send them with the receiver's perception in mind, so that no misunderstanding or misperception is reached unnecessarily.
10. Always send copies of your e-mail to appropriate parties, either reflecting parties who were sent copies of received e-mail, or parties whom your gut instincts dictate should receive copies.

Administrivia and Stress

With the high level of activity that now confronts you, it is important to avoid letting stress become a negative influence on your responsibilities. Therefore, keep the following thirteen thoughts in mind while exercising the strategies in this chapter.

1. *Creativity is fatigue's first victim.* The more weary you become, the more your ability to solve problems and think creatively suf-

fers. Do not become so self-critical that you work to the point of diminishing returns.

2. *Resist overwhelming yourself.* Avoid the drive to get everything accomplished in one day; work progressively each day. Health care workers by nature are compassionate, industrious, and competent. Taken to extremes, these virtues describe perfectionists who risk burnout. No one is perfect, so do not try to be.

3. *Understand that getting help is not a sign of weakness.* Ask people for help, get opinions, and make decisions after you have gotten the advice you need. Getting help does not mean leaning on others' judgments but seeking input when it is needed.

4. *Play to your strengths.* In your initial phase use your technical skills and your natural people skills to get results. Use this basis as your building block as you make your way through the entire scope of health care management.

5. *Do not overdose on information and advice.* Trust your instincts, use your time wisely, and make decisions in a timely and expedient way. Once you have ascertained a satisfactory answer to a problem or a solution to a dilemma, proceed to act on it. Do not second-guess yourself.

6. *Do not play a role.* You earned your position based on your merit and technical proficiency. Do your job conscientiously and without playing on personality or politics. Be genuine. Be yourself.

7. *Do not lose perspective on your role in the organization.* Keep a balanced view on things. Do not make big things out of little things or let little things become "bigger than life."

8. *Some challenges you face today will be there tomorrow.* If you cannot get to something today, let it go and come back tomorrow with the creative juices flowing.

9. *Know when to let go.* Once you have given something your best effort and have reached a resolution, stop thinking about it. Unless someone invents a time machine, you are out of luck.

10. *Your profession is your passion.* Beyond your personal convictions, family, and friends, your profession as health care manager is your passion. Be passionate about it, but do not let your passion burn you out due to lack of balance among family, friends, personal life, and your work.

11. *Make lists.* Make a daily list, and try to accomplish as much as possible. Sort out any outstanding items by using the traffic-light system or some other approach to time management.
12. *Take notes.* Always keep a notebook in hand. Use it as your key development source.
13. *Take time out.* Make sure you take at least a five-minute break for every two hours of intense work. Enjoy your days off.

Health care management is an exciting profession and a passionate commitment to your fellow human beings. By using the techniques described in this chapter, you ensure that this commitment is a long-term one, not short-term.

| **Education and Development**

You can reap great returns from your health care training and development. Management has been described variously as an art, very qualitative in scope and greatly reliant on style; a science, technical and quantitative in scope and reliant on research and acquired expertise; a set of skills that can be acquired through formal knowledge and then incorporated by individuals into their everyday activities; and pure magic, reliant on luck, gut feel, instincts, and the will of the managers to do the right thing, which in turn provides its own rewards.

You have probably realized already that management is a combination of all four of these descriptions—art, science, a set of skills, and magic—and you can never learn too much about it. Training and development, when specifically applied as a management development effort, can help managers attain competency in several basic areas. More to the point, it can help you in terms of developing your own abilities; each experience can provide a lesson in dealing with people and making yourself a better professional.

The Learning Curve

Figure 15.1 charts a manager's typical first year and demonstrates how competency will increase each quarter as a manager acquires the skills charted in the graph. Consider it an illustration of your management learning curve, demonstrating your increased competency over time.

Figure 15.1. New Health Care Manager's Learning Curve.

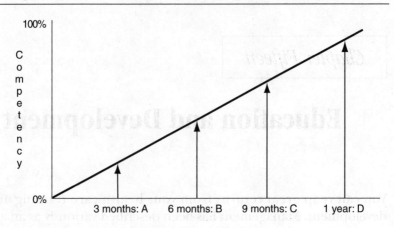

Learning phases
A- Observing, perceiving, and listening
B- Trial and error
C- Participative learning
D- Leading, assuming command

During the first phase—the observing, perceiving, listening phase—try to master observation skills. Closely monitor the progress and performance of your staff, observe the actions of your peers, and study the styles and applications of the managers and leaders with whom you work. To the extent possible, listen to all experiences in all areas of expertise, and try to perceive each episode as a lesson. This will provide you with a basic frame of reference in management, as well as with some specific information needed to lead and manage the individuals on your staff. Observation will also help consolidate your relationships with peers and superiors.

The second phase—the trial and error phase—typically occurs in the second quarter, although certainly no time lines are considered absolute in every case. During this phase, try to establish some policy, make decisions, and operate as an agent of change within your sphere of responsibility (the school of "burn and learn"). Few things will work perfectly the first time, but you will learn from your mistakes, get better all the time, and acquire some expertise.

The third phase—participative learning—takes into account the entire range of activities you will learn, grow from, and apply practically to your business situation. At this point, you are probably acting as an instructor yourself in delivering information and providing instruction to your staff. You are also providing expertise to your peers and consultation to others who need your assistance. If you are keeping a logbook (which is recommended) and applying many of the techniques discussed throughout this book, this phase can be a very successful period, one that can provide you with much-needed positive reinforcement.

Mastery of the participative learning phases leads naturally to assuming a leadership role, the fourth phase of the curve. As a leader, you are on your own and have acquired a certain degree of competency—although you are still learning (and you should assume that you will never stop learning). The worst risk you could incur is failure to stay current with new management techniques, innovative ways of dealing with people, and advancements that sharpen your technical acumen.

Sources of Learning

As a new health care manager, you will receive information and education from a variety of sources. These sources include, but are not limited to, the following:

• *Peer input.* The perspective and common experience of peers can prove invaluable. Remember, all situations are not identical, and the circumstances under which they worked in their initial management phase might differ from yours. However, generally peers are a good source, as these individuals have "walked in your shoes."

• *Personal experience.* Your own personal experience in health care will be a valuable asset as you enter management. This experience is a source of information because you have acquired some expertise and have certainly observed health care managers in action. Rely on your gut instincts and your own knowledge of what does and does not work. Use this reference throughout your management career.

- *Related experience of others.* The managerial experiences of others in your organization (or by family or friends) can be very helpful. Although the banking industry, for example, certainly differs from health care, certain aspects of people management share similarities. Once again, examine these experiences, ask questions, and try to gain knowledge from this important source.

- *Organization-generated education.* Seminars, workshops, and other educational opportunities provided by the organization can be invaluable in establishing a reference point for you as a health care manager. Take advantage of any and all educational opportunities the organization provides, specifically those on management issues of the health care business.

- *Journals and other literature.* A whole body of health care management literature is available for your perusal and use. Try to select reading material that is practical in scope and provides information you can apply immediately. Ask peers and others in your organization whose opinions you respect which periodicals they subscribe to and find most valuable. Most publications of the American Hospital Association and the American College of Healthcare Executives (among others) tend to be very practical in scope and provide valuable information that can be used immediately by newer and seasoned managers.

- *Formal education.* Although many health care managers endeavor to attain a management degree, perhaps at the graduate level, simply taking a course that relates to a specific development need may be equally valuable. For example, for help in financial skills, your local community college or state university probably offers a course on finance for the nonfinancial manager that can meet this development need. Do not feel compelled to acquire a new degree. Simply pick the courses and seminars that are most applicable to your situation and that will provide the most immediate feedback and value.

- *Project management.* As always, keep a journal or logbook in which you will record any major projects you undertake or significant issues you must manage. Keep a chronological log of time and events, with an additional line displaying what you learned in each situation. This log can become your own textbook of management and give you a sterling reference for the next time you undertake a similar project or scope of responsibility.

• *Supervisors and mentors.* Your supervisor can be a valuable source of information and a terrific educator if you are comfortable with the relationship and feel she has knowledge to offer. Furthermore, as discussed later in this chapter, the mentoring process is quite useful and has been adopted by many leading hospitals from an organizational perspective. Later in this chapter I delineate appropriate individual strategies for mentoring.

• *Staff input.* The health care manager who discounts employees' ideas and input as being invaluable or unnecessary is doomed to failure. Although there are few absolutes in management, this certainly is one of them. Try to learn as much as possible from employees' comments and viewpoints and by simply observing them in their daily activities. If nothing else, you will learn how they are motivated, what they respond to, and what they deem to be negative in the workplace.

• *Outside networking.* As mentioned in Chapter Two, as you progress through your career in health care management, you will establish a network of contacts throughout the business. Whenever you meet a potential contact, exchange business cards. Use a Rolodex or small file cabinet to store the cards, categorized by state, business type, or title (for example, pharmaceuticals manager, personnel coordinator). This can be a useful source of knowledge and a living library of health care management.

Types of Learning

To promote your development as a manager, there are three basic ways of learning new skills that you should always try to make time for: communication-based learning, formal learning, and experienced-based learning.

Communication-Based Learning

Communication-based learning consists of simple observation, formatted observation, question-and-answer sessions, and secondary or "hidden" discovery. Strive to achieve two or three learning points from each type of communication-based learning.

Simple observation is the act of perceiving as much as possible just by experiencing situations and either mentally noting or writing in a journal or logbook any significant incidents and learning points from the experience. This opportunity is always available and gives you a realistic perspective of how to deal with problems and reach positive solutions.

Formatted observation entails undertaking a project with colleagues or staff, at the outset of which you specifically delineate what you want to learn from the experience. By establishing this lesson plan, you can undertake the experience and achieve specific learning objectives.

The two other types of communication-based learning directly support the idea of patient-focused health care delivery. Question-and-answer sessions are activities in which you ask point-specific questions about important issues. These sessions may be prearranged with a group of colleagues or held in a one-on-one setting with an individual with a creditable range of expertise. For example, this might have occurred at a meeting in which you saw someone manage a communication conflict or a customer-patient complaint; subsequently you analyze in detail how they brought about a successful resolution. Once again, you need a notebook to record these observations and the benefit of your "unexpected discovery." Unexpected education can extend to leadership style, management aptitude, or basic supervisory psychology. Once again, it is readily apparent and available for your use.

Formal Learning

Formal learning is at once the most obvious type of management education and, unfortunately, the least available due to shrinking fiscal resources. However, it is important and can deal with specific areas that might be of value to you in your role as a health care manager. Formal education can include reading and research, seminars and workshops, formal coursework, self-directed instruction, and organization-sponsored seminars and programs.

For reading and research, you can obtain reading lists on management topics from books or recommendations for relevant books from your information and educational sources described earlier in this chapter. In selecting seminars and workshops, be certain to attend programs that are specific to your needs; avoid those on trendy topics with very little meat. The way to determine this is to ask the instructor for a specific learning plan, or simply discuss the content with the instructor. You can use the questions in Appendix C of this book as a guide. Formal coursework can include a college course or other type of educational offering that will provide you with specific information over a defined period of time.

Most newly appointed health care managers immediately feel a need to pursue outside education in the form of a degree program. This feeling that entry into the world of management mandates more credentialing is a natural reaction. Nonetheless, your promotion was premised on your potential and established performance as a health care professional as perceived by those executives who provided you with the management opportunity.

However, if you insist on undertaking a degree program at the outset of your managerial career, keep certain cautions in mind. The first is that because your time will be limited, you could be setting yourself up for failure. Achieving a balance between personal life and professional responsibilities can be tough enough without the additional burden of keeping up with a new school regimen. Your effectiveness might drop as your stress level rises. Furthermore, the natural benefit of education—absorbing new ideas and enjoying the positive interchange with fellow students—may be compromised by efforts merely to make it to class and put in your time at work.

Some who enter health care management without a BA or BS degree—perhaps an individual who was an RN or a practitioner and did not complete the 128 hours most institutions require for a degree—become preoccupied with immediate acquisition of a degree and may feel professionally insecure without it. Although finishing your degree work is important, it is secondary in your first year, which must be spent learning as much as you can about your staff, the supervisory process, and the techniques essential to becoming an effective health care manager. Once again, time is the most precious resource you'll need to manage during this period. The unnecessary intrusion of schoolwork into the equation will likely hurt your progress more than it will enhance it.

After your first year, it might be prudent to begin pursuing a new degree or completing outstanding coursework. As you consider your educational plans, the following guidelines might be helpful:

• *Pursue relevant courses.* Whether you are considering a master's program or completion of undergraduate work, focus on courses directly related to your current responsibilities. This will give you maximum immediate return on your efforts while providing insight and instruction that can be applied at once to your workplace.

• *Avoid becoming a slave to the degree process.* Attaining a new degree is a laudable accomplishment. It also takes an inordinate amount of time and energy, particularly if the program is a traditional curriculum that does not include weekend sessions or other more user-friendly opportunities, such as executive degree programs or night school. After reviewing course content, select programs that are most relevant to your job and development goals, not those that cater to instruction that can be applied at once to your workplace.

• *Seek out professionally oriented programs.* Most progressive university programs are designed with the busy professional in mind. Such programs include weekend classes, credit for significant professional accomplishment already achieved, and faculty members who are in touch with the real world. This should be a major consideration in your decision-making process, for the benefits are exposure to fellow professionals and a realistic and practical educational base.

• *Use moderation.* At the outset of your new college work, take one or two courses that hold a specific value for your pursuits. This value may be defined, for example, by a course whose content may contain specific material relevant to your responsibilities or provide you with two or three immediately useful ideas for your management efforts. Either way, it may prove enjoyable to you. This approach—simply taking three or four courses that interest you and yield specific instruction in a key area—may be more valuable than relentlessly completing an entire program and then wondering, *What did I get from that?* Remember, your time is limited, and your main qualifications for current job and future opportunities are your past achievements and realistic potential. Additional degrees are secondary qualifications and are only valuable if directly contributory to attaining new knowledge and expanding your managerial perspective.

Self-directed instruction includes computer-assisted instruction (CAI). With the computer age in full swing, self-directed educational packages are very user-friendly and available from many fine education organizations. Check with your human resource department or, if yours is a larger facility, your educational department for suggestions on good self-directed packages.

Finally, it is a good idea to attend as many organization-sponsored programs and seminars as possible. You can learn as much from the dialogue among your fellow participants as you can from the instructor. Listen carefully to all questions, and engage in conversation with your colleagues following the program to get their perceptions and opinions on how they can apply the material to their jobs.

Experience-Based Learning

The third means of management development is that of experience-based learning, or learning on the job. To enhance experienced-based learning, be attuned to the lessons of trial and error, open to the benefits of mentoring, and practice what you've learned—all the while keeping notes on what has worked and what has not.

Trial and error, as discussed previously in this chapter, is the experience of applying your practical knowledge and learning from the results. Remember to use the I-formula in trying new ideas (see Chapter Ten), reinvestigate what went wrong and what went right about your previous experience, and fine-tune your efforts accordingly.

Mentoring is defined as one individual acting as a primary source of instruction for another individual. Mentoring can take place on a short-term basis, perhaps with a specific project or particular area of expertise, or it can be a continuous process, such as the first year of a manager's initiation into a supervisory position. Adherence to the mentoring guidelines presented later in this chapter can be most helpful.

In practicing what you've learned in a realistic setting, once again, use of your ever-present notebook is important, so that you can record many new processes you have now tried and mastered and note what was learned from each experience.

Experience-based learning also includes your participation in the activities of a team, of which you are a part but not necessarily the leader. Collate information on what the team has achieved, what it has learned, and what you would do if you were the team leader. Doing so will allow you to focus on the objectives and processes you will need as a team leader.

Two additional sources of experience-based learning are primary exposure and secondary-effect education. Primary exposure is the accumulation of basic experiences you participated in and were a major agent for taking action. Secondary-effect education is the process by which you have learned from the triumphs and mistakes of others and have noted these accordingly.

Numerous areas of expertise should be available to you within your organization for your own management development. Ten areas are particularly important as you make the transition into health care management:

Management Development Subject Areas

Problem solving	Operational management
Planning	Technical acumen
Health care business knowledge	Quantitative analysis
People management	Communication skills
Fiscal management	Leadership technique

Methods of acquiring these specific attributes and competencies are suggested through this book's two case studies, in Chapters Nine and Seventeen. Use this list not only as a review of the material in this section, but also as your own individual development plan as you experience what might be the most educational year of your life—your first year as a health care manager. I discuss the individual development plan in detail in the following section.

Staff and Employee Development

Of equal importance to your own development as a manager is the development of the staff and employees who report directly to you. Training is essential to staff morale, individual motivation, and maximization of employee potential. As a manager, you are responsible for the training and development of all your assigned subordinates. Because of a dearth of training and development activities due to budget cuts and other factors, it is incumbent on you to provide staff training and development.

Many benefits can be derived from your acting as the major proponent of training and development for your staff. By instructing or facilitating a seminar or teaching an in-service program, you can increase your own presentation and public speaking skills. Although many people fear public speaking, it is essential to your own management development to achieve a certain comfort level in this area. By acting as a trainer for your assigned staff, you can achieve this objective.

Training provides other benefits to the manager. The more your staff is trained, the greater their level of competence and the higher their achievement level in all performance activities. A major objective of any department is to develop "bench strength," a term that means having a depth of talent across your entire department. Each strength is achieved by having a diversity of talent and individual strengths. Obviously, this can be enhanced by training and development throughout your group.

One of the most important things a manager must do initially is to establish credibility. Given that you have a certain degree of technical aptitude, as well as basic communication skills, you have a tremendous base from which to develop initial credibility. By training your staff members on a group, individual, or cross-training basis, you are demonstrating your knowledge as well as your dedication to their development. When you conduct group training, you help enhance team building. When you work with individuals on a one-on-one basis, you set a norm that shows your willingness to accept their ideas, your interest in their development, and your readiness to establish a work relationship based on communication and trust. When you cross-train your staff, you emphasize work role flexibility.

Implementing an Individual Development Plan

The individual development plan (IDP) is a sound tool for establishing a group training program (see the sample IDP in Exhibit 15.1). The plan identifies specific training needs for each staff member, as well as activities that address each need.

Exhibit 15.1. Sample Individual Development Plan (IDP).

Name: Debra Coleman   IDP date: 1/1/94

Current position: Nurse manager

Starting date for current position: 1/1/93

Supervisor/manager's name: Denise Frazier

Need	Activity	Time	Learning value/ comments
1. ADA regulations	AHA seminar	3/94	Competency
2. CQI knowledge	In-service program	5/94– 6/94	Can take lead in departmental CQI process
3. Time management	State university course	9/94	Increased efficiency
4. Budgeting	Participation in process	10/94– 11/94	Can back up H. Fisher in process
5. Patient relations	Understudy J. Bowe	Ongoing	Will assist on new public relations project

As the sample form shows, first enter the individual's name, his or her current position and starting date, the date on which the IDP is being completed, and your own name as supervisor-manager. Next, write down specific training needs identified for each individual in the department, followed by the activity that should be undertaken to fulfill the training need, the estimated time the training should take place, the learning value of each training activity, and any comments related to the activity. This is a relatively straightforward tool and should be completed every year with a maximum of five objectives filled in for each individual.

Several procedures should be followed to ensure efficacy of the IDP. A logical starting point for establishing a training and development strategy is to perform a needs analysis. A needs analysis explores the strengths and weaknesses of all individuals within your department and projects a training plan on both an individual and a group basis. The exploration involves a comparison of individual strengths and weaknesses with basic areas in which you expect each team member to have a certain degree of proficiency. For example, areas of competency would include the basic nursing skills required of a floor nurse, the ability on the part of the pharmacist to fill prescriptions accurately, the ability of a recruiter to interview and select individuals, and so on.

Once the basic areas of competency have been identified, you will then conduct a basic inventory of the present skills of your team members and ascertain what direction their training should follow. To do this inventory, first review the prior performance records of your employees, including any training records that might be on file, as well as the performance evaluation and appraisals from prior years. If possible, discuss with your predecessor each individual's strengths and weaknesses, and take notes. Then assess your observation of each individual's strengths and weaknesses in comparison to the information provided.

A second step is to have a candid conversation with all employees about their strengths and weaknesses. The best way to conduct this conversation is not to use the words *strengths* and *weaknesses* but basically ask, *What type of training are you interested in?* Probe further by asking what areas they would like to improve in, what technical abilities to enhance, and what new areas are of interest. The net effect of this conversation should be enough data to complete the IDP effectively.

When using the IDP form, try to establish training goals and activities jointly. Ask for suggestions for what type of training might be undertaken, and what types of programs might be good candidates (from rumor or references by colleagues). Always remember to use your human resource and educational departments whenever possible; they are expert in identifying training areas and usually have good data on what programs are effective and easily applicable.

A very important entry on the IDP form is that of estimated time of completion. Assigning a training goal is one thing—accomplishing the training needed is another. Make sure that you put a time range of one to two months (for example, March–April 1994) so that the individual can realistically address the training need on a timely basis.

Also discuss with staff members the outcome of all training endeavors. Following their attendance at a training program, sit with each staff member and ask the following questions:

- What are three major new lessons you learned?
- Would you recommend the program to others?
- On a scale of one to five, how would you rate the learning value of the program (with one as the highest value)?
- What did you learn that each of us here in the department can learn from?

By asking these questions, and perhaps using an evaluation form covering the program quality, you can build a data bank not only on the individual's proficiency but also on the strength of the training program. This will help you in assigning training goals for other individuals and give you a natural follow-up strategy with the individual's development program.

Planning for Similar Group Needs

As you undertake the training and development process, specifically the needs analysis and other IDP functions, you will find that many individuals throughout your department have similar needs. Therefore, use a group IDP form such as the one in Exhibit 15.2. Simply enter the names of individuals who have common training needs, the event, the time, and the follow-up strategy you will undertake to ensure learning value. This might include a group discussion with the individuals who took the program, or a series of one-on-one conversations to determine independently the quality of the program. Coordinating training needs is an economical use of time and money and also gives you a synergistic effect, as the individuals attending the same or similar programs will learn from each other as well as from the program leaders.

In establishing IDPs, make sure that you look to programs that are practical and that will address specific needs. Do not try to overload individuals with training. Three to five training activities per year is about right given today's health care climate and workplace conditions. Remember that training activities do not necessarily have to be restricted to workshops. Many individuals in your department, specifically those on your staff, can learn from the same sources of learning presented earlier in this chapter for you. Remember, however, that just as all individuals have different personalities, they also have different aptitudes for learning and are

Exhibit 15.2. Sample IDP Form: Group.

1. Harry Tyson	ADA compliance seminar	2/23/01	Will write department compliance manual
2. Kathy Lauren	Presentation skills seminar	2/3/01	Conduct training in second quarter
3. Mark Richer	Stress management program	ASAP	Personal monitoring of workflow
4. Rich Grafon	Selection seminar	7/01	Will fill two open positions in fourth quarter
5. Jessie Brance	New rehab procedures seminar	10/01	New technical role

interested in different agendas. Therefore, do not expect individuals to learn the same material in the same way. There might be common perceptions about the quality of the program, but the net yield will always be different. Take the time to understand each individual's particular training needs, as well as the effect and outcome of each learning experience.

Serving as a Trainer

Often in your career as a health care manager you will be asked to act as a trainer for a certain program. Furthermore, there will be many opportunities to present training and educational materials to your own staff. Therefore, it is important to have a basic understanding of the dynamics of training and to take a look at some parameters for success.

Preparing for the Training Session

Good training is only as good as the preparation that goes into the program. A smart trainer analyzes the group from several perspectives. First, take a look at individual personalities; determine who your talkers and listeners are. Then try to determine how motivated the group is toward the training. Individuals will be motivated depending on the topic. Get a realistic grip on what the level of motivation might be, and plan your strategy accordingly. If the topic is dry, you might want to prepare a couple of videotapes. If it is a topic that lends itself to discussion, you might want to prepare some pertinent questions so that you can lead a guided discussion about the topic.

Prepare your material in a general-to-specific context. Simply outline your text material in a general sense, and underscore points that are of specific relevance. Try to make your presentation as logical as possible, and allow yourself enough time to cover each point as fully as possible. A good rule of thumb is to provide a new idea every five minutes if you are doing a one-hour presentation. Given this scheme, four major topics, with three subtopics (or primary points) each, would constitute a solid hour of training. Try to stay within these parameters as you establish a training plan.

Always prepare a training plan with time and events for your own reference as well as that of the participants. Clearly outline your objectives in the training plan and set a time sequence with general points of reference. This procedure will clarify your training outcomes, the content, and your objectives for the program. It will also get the group involved and let them know that the training session is for a common cause—it is not a didactic exercise.

Make certain that your materials are fully prepared. Any handouts should be free of typographical errors, written clearly, and free of jargon the participants are not likely to understand. Handouts should include slides and other printed information, statistics, articles and journal pieces, and anything else that might be valuable to the participants. It is better to err on the side of more than on the side of less; that means making the handout material as full and rich as possible so that the participants can receive maximum yield from the material. Time is precious to all health care professionals, so the training program will be seen as a waste of time unless pertinent information is provided. Make certain that the handout material is clearly formatted, well organized, and related to the topic at hand.

When you have completed your preparation, conduct a final check of all the material. Ask yourself the following questions:

- Is the presentation logical?
- Would I be able to follow the flow of information?

- What questions would I ask if I were a participant?
- How would I answer the questions?
- What essential points should the participant walk away with?
- How can I make this an interesting presentation?
- Did I leave anything out?
- Did I allow myself enough time?
- What questions can I use to get started?
- Which individuals should I target for conversation and questions?

By answering these questions, you will ensure that your preparation is complete. Remember that there are no perfect answers to any of these questions. If you have an answer that you feel comfortable with for each question, you are probably well prepared for the training.

Conducting the Training Session

There are several points to remember as you conduct the training session. First, allow members of the group to introduce themselves, giving their name, their department, how long they have been at the institution, and why they are interested in the program. If individuals are not interested in the program, ask them what they know about the session and what they might want to contribute.

Always make sure that you check out the physical parameters of the room. Whenever possible, try to use a U-shaped configuration. This allows individuals the opportunity to talk to each other, and it facilitates a good roundtable discussion.

Announce the time parameters of the program and make sure that the first page of the handout material shows the time and sequence of events. State your learning objectives at the beginning of the program immediately following the introductions.

Make mental notes of what each individual has stated as his or her interest in the program. Focus on those who express interest, using their comments to begin momentum for the program. Discount any negativity right at the beginning of the session; there will be certain individuals who do not actively engage in the program no matter what you do. Play to the stronger participants, those who are truly interested. This will help you get the attention of those with average or marginal interest. If you can capture the very interested and the passively interested, you have probably captured a good 80 percent of the group. This is a great victory, no matter what level of training you might conduct or how long you have been doing group sessions.

Use as many learning devices as possible in the training program. These include case studies, videotapes, group discussion, and, by all means, practical applications. Get individuals to focus on the effect that the program's topic might have on their individual work lives. Harness the expertise of individuals in the education department or colleagues and peers who have conducted training programs previously. They might have good materials on the topic, as well as some insights on the participants and how you might deliver the program. Pace your program strictly so that you cover all material. Handle questions advantageously; for example, repeat the question back to the inquirer, state what your position might be, and always ask the entire group the question and what their thoughts might be. Usually the answer—in fact, the best answer—lies somewhere among the participants.

Closing the Training Session

Close with a practical exercise. The exercise might be a final case study or another activity that recaps the material in your session.

Try to incorporate evaluations into the closing portion of the program. Allow time to critique the program relative to subject, delivery, applicability, and whether participants would refer the program as a sound training exercise to other individuals. Do not take criticism personally. Try to be objective, and use the participation in the program, applicability of program material, and attitude of the participants as your true measures of success. Constantly upgrade the program by adding to it and garnering suggestions from participants.

Finally, recognize that the more you conduct training, the better you will become at it. You will also find that you learn more from the programs than any of your participants. With these two factors, as well as the information presented here, conducting training programs will become an important and enjoyable part of your management arsenal.

Mentoring and Delegation

Two overlooked but practical strategies for developing and educating staff are mentoring and delegation. Mentoring refers to the one-on-one educational process of an experienced individual teaching an inexperienced (or less experienced) individual a certain procedure or set of skills. Delegation is the assignment of a specific task in the interest of expedience of action and learning. This section will cover both, including their pitfalls and strengths as management techniques.

Role of the Mentor

Mentoring should be based on the establishment of objectives for the individual being mentored. The mentor should sit down with the individual and establish specific areas of need. The mentor should also identify areas of potential and perceived needs that the employee might not be aware of. For example, the human resource professional might need expertise in hiring and selection; the mentor might suggest that the budgeting process inherent to these two responsibilities is equally important.

As always, a liaison should be established with the education department, the human resource department, and perhaps the reporting manager. All of these parties should contribute their expertise as well as suggestions on how the mentoring process could be more efficient. Fundamentally, mentoring takes four forms:

1. *Activity observations.* By observing the mentor completing a particular task, employees learn how to complete the task and have the opportunity to ask questions and fine-tune their approach.
2. *A joint education activity.* Both the mentor and employee can undertake an educational program in which the mentor has more experience. Subsequent to the educational activity, the mentor can specifically point out areas the employee can benefit from and respond to any questions specific to the educational exercise.
3. *Delegation.* As will be seen in the second half of this section, the mentor can be the individual who delegates a specific task to the employee.

4. *Understudy*. The mentor simply guides the employee through a variety of activities as the employee observes the activities, takes part at the discretion of the mentor, and enjoys close communication and education.

The most important aspect of any mentoring process is the follow-up strategy. If the mentoring relationship is established over a long period of time, for example, six months to one year, it is good to have a "first Friday session." This session might entail a visit to a local restaurant or a meeting in the mentor's office to discuss the month's activities. If it is a short-term relationship, the mentor should use some of the questions contained in Appendix C to ensure that learning is taking place.

Delegation of Responsibility

Although mentoring is extremely popular today, delegation might be an even more effective strategy. As a manager, it is imperative that you delegate as many responsibilities as possible while maintaining responsibility for the ultimate outcome of the project. Exhibit 15.3 reviews four basic delegation guidelines. Review all four critical areas and follow the checklist in Exhibit 15.3 to ensure that the delegation process is fruitful.

In assigning the task, whenever possible identify assignments that are not routine. In other words, do not limit your list of "delegatable" assignments to the ones that bore you, that you do not like, or that you would like to do but have no prior experience. It is impossible to delegate what you yourself have never done and thus have no frame of reference as to how to pursue the objective.

Review the learning value inherent in each delegated task and be certain to stress this to the employee when you assign the task. Meetings, paperwork, audit activities, investigative work, and people-intensive activities are all things that can and should be delegated to increase the skills of your employees and staff.

As identified in Figure 15.2, there are two types of individuals to whom you will find yourself delegating tasks. The first is the "go-to" individual, the person who has done the task many times and has achieved total competency but derives little learning value because he has achieved mastery of the task. The other individual

Exhibit 15.3. Delegation Guidelines.

1. Identify delgatable assignments

    a. Consider all tasks that can be done by others

    b. Do not limit list to things you dislike, are bored by, or unfamiliar with

    c. Consider delegating meetings, paperwork, audits, and people-related tasks

2. Select delegatee

    a. "Go-to" person: has done task numerous times; highly competent

    b. MSF person: never has done task; will learn but needs guidance

    c. Consider time available for teaching task and MSF person's potential

3. Assign delegated task

    a. Explain desired outcome(s)

    b. Suggest possible methods of accomplishment

    c. Clarify, express confidence, and establish communicative follow-up

4. Use follow-up strategy

    a. Identify interim benchmarks

    b. Set goals using time, percentages, numbers, and cost containment

    c. Schedule follow-up sessions

    d. Discuss learning value completely

is the "MSF" (maximum stretch factor) person. This individual has no competency in the activity or task and thus can learn up to 100 percent of the learning value of the task. If you have the time, you always use the MSF person, as she will learn and grow from the experience. This will also free up the go-to person to complete another assignment that would teach a new competency, such as assignment 2 shown in Figure 15.2.

In assigning the delegated objective, you have three choices. You could tell the individual how to do the task, an option that will certainly guarantee a clear outcome but will limit creativity and ownership of the task. You could ask the individual how he wants to do the task, but without a frame of reference he might be unable to answer this question.

The third option is perhaps the best. Suggest to the individual how you have completed this task before; how others might have completed the task before; what a journal article had to say about

Figure 15.2. Illustration of Delegation Dynamics.

Assignment #1: Review patient complaint cards and summarize complaints

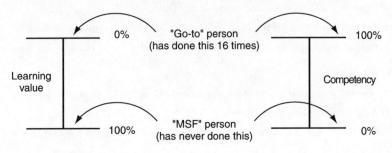

Assignment #2: Personally respond to complaints

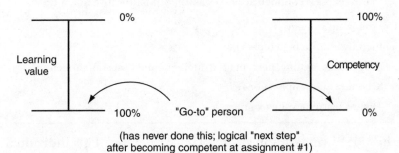

handling such an assignment; and, finally, but most important, how the individual would approach the objective. In any event, always clarify the method the individual will be using by asking specifically, *How will you go about this?*

Finally, as indicated in Exhibit 15.3, use an appropriate follow-up strategy. Establish significant interim benchmarks to follow employee progress, and assign the objective by using time, money, percentages, and numbers. Use an appropriate follow-up strategy that is keyed to the individual's personality. With employees who are somewhat dependent on you, you might want to simply tell them to follow up with you whenever they feel the need. In any event, remember to keep abreast of any developments and progress toward the goal by checking in with employees on a regular basis.

After assigning the goal and delegating the task, keep notes either in your calendar, in a set of files for each employee, or in a notebook to ensure that you are informed of the employees' progress. Always ask the individuals what they are learning from the task, and underscore this parameter by discussing the learning value upon conclusion of the task.

As a new health care manager, you will find yourself being the delegatee and mentoree more often than the delegator or mentor. It is important, however, to try these skills to incorporate them into your everyday activities. Not only are they sound management devices, their development value cannot be overstated.

Conclusion

The role of teacher is intrinsic to the health care leader's everyday responsibilities. Every day is not only an opportunity to learn, but also an opportunity to teach and educate. The successful fulfillment of both roles contributes mightily to the ultimate success of the health care organization.

| Communication

Ever since Strother Martin told Paul Newman in the movie *Cool Hand Luke,* "What we have here is a failure to communicate," communication has become a major part of management training efforts. If the eyes are the windows to the soul, then communication is the key to action. As a health care manager, you will find communication to be the linchpin to all your activities. The strength of your communication will directly reflect the effectiveness of your performance efforts.

Communication training and development for a health care manager must go beyond platitudes and clichés to foster a communication style that is both comfortable and natural and that will provide maximum impact. It is also vital to use a communication strategy that allows you to get information on a timely basis and to provide needed work direction efficiently.

In this chapter I explore the dynamics of effective communication in health care management and the interplay between psychology and communication, specifically as it relates to the health care manager's role. Discussion of the different roles people play to assist or hamper communication and of role management strategies can help you maximize the communication process in your department. I also deal with specific communication dynamics, including written communication, group communication, and interactions between yourself and your superiors. By exploring both the virtues of good communication and the pitfalls of poor communication, I hope to provide you with valuable guidelines as you undertake your management role.

Dynamics of Effective Health Care Management Communication

In your role as health care manager, you must master four essential dynamics of communication: climate, community, content, and challenge. The term *climate* refers here to the workplace environment, which you help define, and the overall atmosphere throughout the health care workplace. The term *community*, as used in this chapter, relates to the team orientation of your department and to the overall organization in which you work, including all lines of communication within the organization. The term *content* refers to how you deliver messages: the style, message, elements, and manner in which information is provided and direction is given. Finally, the term *challenge* refers to how critical communication, vital work parameters, and directives are delivered to appropriate members of the organization.

In each of these four areas, there are ten essential components, or C-factors, of the dynamics of communication in the health care environment—forty C-factors in all. I summarize these components in the following subsections and offer them as guideposts for your own approach to effective communication in your new role.

The Climate of the Work Environment

1. *Coaching.* For a work climate to be prosperous and produce good results on a regular basis, a certain amount of coaching must take place, where you as manager act as a mentor to your staff as a unit and as individual players who assist one another in growth and development. In effect, coaching entails encouraging others to perform better, pointing out their mistakes constructively, and providing ongoing direction as needed to all members of the department. Too much coaching (overcoaching), however, leads to your becoming too detail oriented or failing to allow individuals enough professional liberty. A total lack of coaching within the department will arrest staff development and, consequently, work progress.

2. *Consultation.* Accordingly, a consultative environment must surround the work group. This involves the sharing of expertise among the staff and the provision of technical acumen by the

department leader. The health care manager must be a leader in becoming a consultant within the department, as well as a consultant throughout the organization on key technical issues. Technical information provided to others in the organization must be clear and direct, and conveyed in a manner that will be readily understood and useful to the receiver. The risks with consultative communication are overuse of jargon or technical terms, and loss of the essential message due to failure to understand the requester's needs. When acting in a consultative role, first ask a series of questions to determine the specific nature of the problem. Second, determine what technical assistance the individual needs. Third, provide that assistance in a clear-cut manner while pledging any further assistance as needed.

3. *Consistency.* Consistency can be achieved by implementing four strategies into your leadership communication:

1. Always avoid needless emotionalism in delivering messages to your staff. Undue "highs" and "lows" can make certain team members upset and affect their performance accordingly.

2. Make sure that your allegiance to good patient service and superior performance resonates throughout your work climate by alluding to those themes, using a variety of examples, in all of your communication.

3. Commit to a ten-minute, exclusive, one-on-one discussion with each team member every month. This ensures consistent message delivery while disposing of any valid perception of favoritism or miscommunication.

4. Keep notes on key meeting conversations and presentations so that you can be both consistent and progressive in your communication performance.

4. *Candor.* The worst liability you can be faced with is to be perceived as phony or disingenuous. Strive to be forthcoming and direct in all of your communication efforts. Be forthright in dealing with individuals and in providing information. Let people know that you do not have all the answers in all situations. State your dedication to finding the answers to questions and the solutions to problems. By providing false or misleading information, inconsistent or inaccurate communication, or by doing anything

that can be perceived as dishonest or an attempt to "con" department members, you risk being judged untrustworthy or incompetent. Such a reputation can be irreversible.

5. *Collaboration.* It is essential that as a team all members collaborate on common goals and objectives. Individuals must feel comfortable working together striving toward a mutually beneficial end. Stressing the individual talents of department members is a great first step for creating a spirit of collaboration. Publicly recognizing the contributions of all team members, particularly on joint efforts, is the second step toward fostering a collaborative atmosphere. A third step is to remember the axiom, Give the good news in public, but give the bad news in private. Positive gains the department has made should be shared in public, while any performance deficiencies or problems should be discussed individually in private with those involved. This approach ensures that a positive spirit is generated throughout the group and that collaboration and joint efforts are always encouraged and rewarded.

6. *Camaraderie.* All department members should feel they are comrades in arms, working together and living by the adage, Nobody wins unless we all win. Camaraderie is a key element of the workplace climate. Certain key words can help establish camaraderie across the department. For example, in stressing the value of working together, the words *team* and *we* are verbal strengtheners that reinforce the virtue of camaraderie. Without camaraderie and collaboration, groups become disjointed and the individual is focused on at the expense of the group.

7. *Cure.* As emphasized throughout this book, the focus of communication in a progressive work climate should be on identifying and implementing solutions, not on reidentifying and exacerbating problems. The key notion in this respect is finding a cure. (This is an appropriate metaphor, given that the essential mission of a health care organization is to seek cures.) Cures must be sought for everyday problems that arise in your department. Always ask your staff's advice on how a problem might be solved. Encourage them to provide cures to problems, and reward them, either verbally or tangibly, for any successful solution. Special recognition such as "employee of the month" or paid time off are two examples of appropriate rewards. It is imperative that the

workplace climate be geared toward providing cures, and that the positive generation of progressive ideas be recognized and rewarded.

8. *Character.* Another essential dimension of the workplace climate, character is essentially the work personality demonstrated and embraced by all members of the department. Therefore, any communication should be delivered in a way that is thoughtful, tactful, and ethically sound. This precludes publicly berating any employee who is not performing up to standards. Thoughtful delivery also mandates the use of tactful language and appropriate courtesy when discussing key issues. Furthermore, character defines to what extent each individual in the department interrelates with dignity, class, and basic compassion. Lack of any of these positive attributes within the work climate will result in an environment that breeds discomfort, threatens individual dignity, and fosters negative aspects of performance and poor team interaction that will soon surface.

9. *Change.* Change takes place in the health care environment every day. A clear description of change elements, as well as a plan for managing most change factors, should be provided by a health care manager whenever appropriate. How your department reacts and positively addresses change should also be discussed. Staff should be given the opportunity to discuss how change will affect their particular segment of the business and how to positively address the change at hand. Failing to recognize and communicate change or to identify progressive solutions and strategies to change can lead to departmental regression.

10. *Circumstance.* Circumstances are the specific conditions under which the department must labor. They might include a change in physical environment, new organization requirements, or regulatory or legislative issues that affect the department. The specific dynamics under which each employee works should also be recognized and discussed, with input garnered from the employee on how best to deal with the particular situations imposed by the job role. By not doing so, a manager approaches the entire workflow, even the entire mission of the department, in too general a manner, thereby failing to acknowledge the unique contribution of individual team members.

The Work Community

In and of itself, the health care department is a community, and it services a community of customer-patients and professionals within the organization who rely on the department to achieve its mission.

1. *Counsel.* The first component of communication as it relates to communal (team) orientation is counsel. Counsel refers to the ability to provide medical advice to those who need it throughout the organization. In another sense, counsel refers to the provision of guidance for employees who need specific direction in key areas such as stress management, time management, and family relations. Both you and your human resource department must keep your counselor roles at the forefront of strategies when dealing with all members of the organization.

2. *Commitment.* Commitment is dedication to reinforcement of the health care mission. All members of the organization should demonstrate this commitment in their everyday actions. This priority of commitment mandates putting the customer-patient at the top and putting service to affiliated members of the organization and to colleagues as a close second priority. Failure to reinforce commitment to the health care organizational mission can sometimes be due to the everyday hyperactivity of the organization. However, the organization's commitment to the customer-patient must be demonstrated clearly at every appropriate opportunity.

3. *Construction.* The construction of a message is very important in community-based communication. You must know your audience before you construct a message. Some individuals have a high comprehension of medical terms; others do not. For the latter group, construction of any message should be based on concepts the receiver can easily understand. Messages can sometimes be overloaded; that is, they contain information that is not essential to the desired outcome. In other cases, messages can be too abbreviated and fail to provide essential information. Ensure that your message is well constructed and well measured, given your audience.

4. *Confidence.* Confidence is important in delivering any message throughout the health care environment. If you lack confidence in what you are saying, you will lose your audience and your

credibility. Without credibility, you are seen as a nonplayer and will have a hard time gaining respect for your ideas and input. However, in communicating confidence, avoid the appearance of being arrogant. Most individuals in the health care environment assume that you know what you are talking about and that you are capable of making the right decision. There is no reason to oversell your ideas and risk being considered too pushy.

5. *Compassion.* Because health care is a people-oriented field, a certain amount of compassion should be ever-present in all of your communication efforts. Lack of compassion suggests that you do not truly care for the recipient of your message, whether a patient or staff member. But avoid being too compassionate; that is, emphasizing the humanistic elements at the expense of the business objective. Nonetheless, it is better to err on the side of being overcompassionate than to be noncompassionate or not compassionate enough.

6. *Care.* Care must be exhibited in everything you do throughout the health care community. Be careful not to offend others needlessly or unwittingly by any communication you provide. Patient care should be a driving force in all communication, so ask, *How will this communication affect our customer-patients and the quality of care?* Failure to exhibit care in communication can earn you a reputation as being too blunt, brusque, or unfeeling and insensitive toward the needs of others, principally the customer-patient.

7. *Confluence.* Confluence is defined as the net effect of many actions, resulting in a greater whole. A positive confluence occurs when several positive factors, such as departments working cohesively together or employees working toward a common goal in a progressive fashion, result in a positive outcome. Conversely, a negative confluence occurs when several negative events occur, in turn producing an overall negative net effect. A strong health care organization (and at the department level, a strong health care team) should seek to create a positive confluence of factors whenever possible. From a communication perspective, this entails your continuously identifying and developing positive factors and positive attributes of these factors and pointing them out to all members of your team. As a health care manager, you should make this identification an essential part of your everyday activities.

8. *Comfort.* Any communication process must have comfort as an essential dynamic. The more comfortable people are, the more they will communicate, and the more information will emerge. From an organizational perspective, all individuals should feel comfortable in providing information, giving their opinions, and stating their viewpoints freely and without fear of retribution. As a health care manager, try to impart these same ideals throughout your department. Strive to maintain a comfortable environment in which you can discuss issues with individuals in a nonthreatening manner. Ask questions, and let people know that you are ready to communicate. Allow staff confidentiality and comfort by closing your office door and allowing them to sit down and relax while relating problems and situations to you. Without comfort, communication becomes abbreviated and contrived.

9. *Cultural diversity.* Sensitivity to cultural diversity is a major management concern. Invariably, you will be challenged with managing a culturally diverse staff. A few guidelines can assist you in making response to cultural diversity a positive attribute of your communication strategy:

- Never refer to a staff members' cultural background. Without knowing it, you could offend or make them feel uncomfortable.
- Immediately address any clashes that might stem from cultural differences. If allowed to fester, these situations will create immense problems.
- Do not allow individuals to make cultural differences an issue in any departmental interchange. If any individual insists on using cultural difference as a stumbling block in working with others, consult your human resource department as well as your supervisor to resolve this conflict positively and quickly.

Cultural conflict can take place in the way individuals communicate. For example, some cultures disapprove of direct eye contact and consider it a sign of disrespect. Other cultures communicate in what may be perceived as a very emotional fashion; others may be perceived as less expressive in their communication style. Recognize these differences objectively, and communicate in a style that is most comfortable for you. Do not try to adopt the cultural norms of others, lest you run the risk of appearing phony or condescending. Communicate in a direct, straightforward manner. Your comfort with your own communication style will be acknowledged by the individuals with whom you communicate and thus will not become a negative issue.

10. *Contact.* Contact is essential in community-based communication. The more contact you have with your employees, the more knowledge you will gain about their activities and aspirations. The more contact you have with customer-patients, the greater your knowledge will be of their expectations of the organization and, specifically, their expectations of your department. The more contact you have with your superiors in the organization, the more you will learn about leadership and organizational norms. Finally, the more contact individuals have with you, the more comfortable they will be with relating their ideas and options to you and recognizing you as a leader within the management team.

The Content of Messages

Communicating content involves not only what is said or written but how information is delivered. The best way to examine your proficiency at communication content is to review the following questions and assess your style. Use these ten components as guidelines for analyzing all your communication activity.

1. *Core.* What is the root of the message? How direct is the message? Is it delivered clearly, understood easily, and capable of being acted on by the receiver?
2. *Clarity.* Is the message clear in intent and purpose? What are its basic elements? What action must be undertaken to support this message?
3. *Comprehensiveness.* What is the full scope of the message? Does it provide all information needed for the desired outcome?
4. *Conciseness.* Did I get to the point? What is the main point of my message? Did I get to the point quickly? Did I get to the point too quickly, without providing enough foundation? Am I taking too long to get to the point?

5. *Cleverness.* Am I using an appropriate "hook" to get attention? Am I being too gimmicky in delivering this message? Could I be more creative in delivering this message?
6. *Character.* Does this message support the basic mission of the organization? Does this message seem consistent with other activities in my department? Does this message relate to something that ultimately will better serve our customer-patients?
7. *Credibility.* How believable is this message? Do I have enough credibility to garner support on the basis of this message? What points should I detail to get the receiver to buy in to this message?
8. *Conviction.* Am I stressing the importance of this message enough? Am I displaying how much I believe in the action this message will generate?
9. Ability to *compel.* What action am I asking for? Am I providing enough direction on how to support this message? Am I specifying the time, money, and other quantitative elements of this message strongly enough?
10. *Consequence.* What is the desired outcome of this message? What positive consequences will be realized if this message is followed through? What are some secondary effects of this message? What impact does this message have on the receiver and other individuals in the department?

From a general perspective, it is essential to review all ten C-guidelines prior to delivering your message. Further on in the chapter, I discuss more specific message dynamics relative to group communication and communication with your supervisor. However, if you follow this guide in all your management communications, the likelihood of misunderstanding and inaction will be diminished.

The Communication of Challenge

The final category of communication dynamics has to do with challenge. It is vital for employees to be challenged and to challenge themselves continuously to become better performers. From a wider perspective, the department must challenge itself to improve

performance and to grow and prosper. These following ten components help contribute to the challenge element of communication:

1. *Comparison.* What positive factors can I compare this action to?
   What ideals does this action help contribute to? How does this
   action measure up to our prior successes?
2. *Contrast.* What negative factors can I contrast this message
   against? What past failures can I contrast it against? What pitfalls will we avoid by following this action?
3. *Closure.* Are we "closing any loops" with this action? What is the
   logical outcome of this action? What is a strong finish for this
   message?
4. *Choice.* What are our options? Is the option in the message our
   best option? What other choices do I have in order to achieve
   the desired outcome?
5. *Contract.* What action am I asking for from our employees?
   What action will I undertake to support this action? What is the
   mutual benefit of all individual talents in this action?
6. *Customization.* What are some particular dynamics of this
   action? How does it specifically fit in with our plans? How do I
   take advantage of all individual talents in this action?
7. *Count.* What are some significant numbers of this action? What
   are our numerical goals? What are some significant interim
   numbers?
8. *Cash.* What funds will be saved or generated by this action?
   What are our budget standards? How can we eliminate revenue
   waste and operating expenses by this action?
9. *Clock.* What overall time parameters are established by this message? What are the deadlines? How can we eliminate time
   wasters in pursuing this action?
10. *Clout.* Do we have the authority to take this action? Who should
    be empowered with the responsibility for this action? Have I
    been charged with the responsibility and authority to make this
    happen?

By reviewing these parameters and adhering to the guidelines, you will ensure that motivation and inspiration are part of
all your work-directive communication. Furthermore, by asking

yourself these questions, you are ensuring that the pending action is worthwhile and has been fully considered from a progressive viewpoint.

Remember, all ten of these dynamics relate not only to communication style but also to actual delivery of a message. As shown in Figure 16.1, the basic relationship between the sender and receiver in any communication is vulnerable to obstruction and interference and must be reinforced by the forty C-factors discussed in the chapter so far. Figure 16.1 shows a number of areas where communication might be hampered. How a message is delivered is almost as important as the message itself. Therefore, embrace these guidelines as part of your communication strategy in all your management responsibilities.

Underscoring Mutual Benefit

No matter what other psychological or communication tactic you may use in a given situation, underscoring the mutual benefit of an action is the best tactic for garnering the desired response. There are generally five recipients of a mutual benefit:

Figure 16.1. Sender-Receiver Communication Barriers.

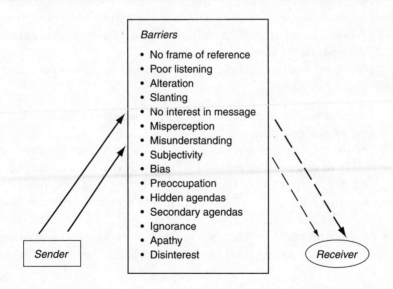

Barriers

- No frame of reference
- Poor listening
- Alteration
- Slanting
- No interest in message
- Misperception
- Misunderstanding
- Subjectivity
- Bias
- Preoccupation
- Hidden agendas
- Secondary agendas
- Ignorance
- Apathy
- Disinterest

Sender

Receiver

1. The message sender
2. The message receiver
3. The team-staff
4. The organization
5. The customer-patient

Try to identify the individual and operational benefits of an action simply by asking, *What are the benefits to each of these parties and to each facet of the business?* Some possible answers (or payoffs) are

- Greater effectiveness
- Increased efficiency
- New programs or evidence of organization progress
- Short-term production gains
- Long-term positive gains
- Staff growth and development

By articulating the potential payoffs, you lend maximum clarity to the communication process and stress the contribution needed from each individual in the department. The case study in Chapter Seventeen demonstrates the successful application of this tactic by a newly appointed health care manager.

If potential recipients fail to respond to the appeal for mutual benefits, you can logically assume that they are not interested in the positive success of the organization. Put simply, if people cannot respond to an appeal to help their colleagues and organization, they probably should not be there.

There are five general rules to remember as part of your communication strategy:

1. Always listen attentively and accurately when provided with any type of information.
2. Try to discern not only what someone says but why they say it. Try to discount personal roles, which can be a distraction, and get to the core of the message. Having said this, however, recognize the roles discussed in this chapter and use your counterefforts effectively.
3. Clarity and comfort are key to communication. Be clear about what you are saying, and be comfortable and confident in saying it.

4. Communication is a continuous process. Follow up with individuals on your staff, and always be ready to ask questions.
5. Recognize that learning about communication is a continuous
   process. Strive to learn something new about the communication process each day and apply it as part of your management
   strategy.

Communication and Change—Practical Summary Strategies

In 1984, Bill Gates was a college dropout working for a four-
member, fledgling company in New Mexico. Today he is the rich-
est man in America and the head of perhaps the most powerful
company in recent corporate history.

In 1990, managed health care was merely a concept discussed
in academic and industry-observer circles. Now it is a norm in
almost every health care organization nationally.

In 1995, health care professionals in every discipline believed
the maxim, As long as people get sick, health care professionals
will have jobs. In 1995, health care executives alternately referred
to the wide-scale process of laying off employees as reengineering,
rightsizing, downsizing, or RIF (reduction in force).

Along with these massive changes, both societal and professional, health care managers have been contending with the change
management process. Although a breadth of concepts borrowed
from other industries and a plethora of conceptual practicums
have entered the health care educational realm, a straightforward,
immediately useful approach to managing change is probably
more beneficial, because the need to manage change quickly and
effectively has become the paramount criterion for the success of
health care management.

In this section, I explore the four areas where mistakes are
made most frequently by leaders in the change process, and I provide specific strategies not only to avoid these mistakes but also to
reduce resistance to change, activate positive action, and ultimately
improve performance through optimum staff contribution. The
four critical areas are understanding resistance to change, managing the proactive phase of change, creating an interdependent
staff, and providing key leadership roles for change management.

Understanding Resistance to Change

Several group emotions are triggered by change. These can pervade an entire health care team and cause a group counteraction in resistance to the proposed change. The health care leader must understand these emotions, their potential deleterious impact, and most important, the pragmatic approaches required to manage these emotions toward progressive change. In addition, the health care leader must be aware of how these emotions specifically affect the three performance levels of staff members: the organizational driver or superstar level, the steady or supporting member level, and the nonplayer or resister member. (These levels are depicted in Table 4.1.)

Fear is the most prevalent group emotion cited by health care leaders as a major factor in the change process. As a general sentiment, this factor, as it relates to change, is typified by the phrase, fear of the unknown. However, fear has specific application to health care group management, because it can affect all three levels of health care staff performers in specific ways. For example, the most prominent fear for steady players—who often represent the silent majority of a staff team—is fear of regression. The steady player will view any change with apprehension if the proposed change is not completely presented in a fashion that highlights its improvement value to the status quo. This fear should be addressed in the proactive phase of change management (see under the following heading, "Managing the Proactive Phase of Change"), but as a starting point, the health care leader must recognize that most steady staff members will accept change provided it is not simply change for the sake of change. It therefore becomes the responsibility of the leader to identify how the proposed change will bring about new benefits for the customer-patient, the organization, the group, and the individual team member.

The nonplayer staff members are also fearful, but the inspiration for their fear is different. Essentially, the nonplayer fears having to do more work. Change mandates increased effort and higher contribution from all staff members. For steady players and superstars, this requirement is not a problem if it is tied to increased organizational effectiveness and other benefits. For nonplayers, the increased demand for performance is ultimately threatening, because their current level of nonperformance and resistant behavior will be exacerbated by more pressure for optimum performance and an accelerated pace of action. Put bluntly, the need for change presents a vibrant opportunity for the nonplayer's laggardness to be found out; that is, the nonplayers will be exposed as incompetent, noncontributory, and detrimental to the provision of stellar health care. If job descriptions and other substantiating criteria are in place for assessing the nonplayer's performance in general and specifically in times of change and higher performance standards, the change dynamic can provide an excellent opportunity to appraise the nonplayer's performance as substandard and provide the impetus for termination. This strategy is "rightsizing the right way," because the successful health care organization can only afford to employ individuals who are motivated, competent, and aware that the organization is more important in the work scheme than individual proclivities, dissenting opinion, and other me-first mentalities.

For the superstar staff member, fear of change can manifest as cynicism, with a response of, So what? Superstar performers instinctively understand the consequences of an action, and the opportunity to contribute progressively to providing outstanding health care is a guiding beacon in their daily work life. Any change action that appears meaningless to the superstar can cause the superstar to question the organization's direction and can demotivate the superstar, who is generally highly self-motivated. As a health care leader, you must weigh any potential change relative to organizational readiness and progressive performance. Moreover, you must engage the superstar in defining potential benefits, operational improvements, and other positive, differentiated improvements to current status and operational norms.

The other group emotions generated by change generally can be categorized under the aegis of fear. These group phobias include perception-versus-reality factors regarding change, fear of loss of control over one's own professional destiny, and communication problems that create a void of leadership and accurate communication, as well as an array of other potential problems. These negative precursors to change can be managed by various artful strategies throughout the change process, principally in the proactive phase of change.

Managing the Proactive Phase of Change

The proactive phase of the change process is the time before the change dynamic takes place. In this period, you are making plans and motivating staff participation in making the change happen. Many health care leaders make the fundamental mistake of entering the change process without proper planning and without enlisting staff support. A more progressive approach is to set a course for change and enter a process of garnering staff support by proactively defining the benefits of the imminent change.

The first objective of the proactive phase should therefore be a complete delineation of the emergent benefits of the proposed project or new process leading to change. Hold a discussion with staff, encouraging the active participation of superstars and steady players. Identify all benefits, both apparent and underlying, and relate them to the change process. Benefits could include more expedient customer-patient service, improved operational flow, or obvious cost savings in relation to operating-budget dollars.

During this discussion, encourage the group also to identify less apparent benefits. These benefits can include time saved by implementing a new process, energy saved by a more efficient process, lessons that will be learned and technological insight that will be realized by a change in procedure, and any competitive edge that might be afforded the organization by implementing the change. Underlying benefits can also include better perceptional presence for the department or organization as it embraces a new, vanguard process or a new procedural practice that enables greater accuracy of results, a safer working environment, or a more efficient route to results realization. From an overall perspective, any change that reduces the boredom of a skilled individual, adds to organizational progress (which helps to ensure organizational stability and individual job security), or eliminates hurdles or the headaches associated with outmoded or cumbersome processes is one that has credible underlying benefit. By eliciting these non-apparent benefits with the group, you add veracity and realism to the change management discussion.

The second objective of the proactive phase is to delineate the plan of change in a real-world fashion. You may construct your plan of action by answering the following questions:

1. *Why* must the change plan take place? (Use the benefits identified by the group as the major catalysts.)
2. *When* will the major events in the change plan occur? (Include a time sequence of the start, midpoint, and finished product.)
3. *How* will the plan take shape? (Visualize the steps needed to implement the change.)
4. *Who* will make the plan happen? (Include an appropriate discussion of group and individual responsibilities.)

Inherent to this discussion is the necessity of discussing the meaning of the plan. This discussion of meaning should take two tracks. First, the leader and the group should discuss what the change dynamic will mean in the short term relative to potential implementation problems, variations in daily routine, and any other pertinent topics. Second, the long-term meaning of the change should be discussed fully, replete with a reiteration of benefits, relevance to the big picture of the organization and its relationship with its patient constituency, and other positive probabilities. Too often, the change management discussion focuses only on the short-term pain and not on the long-term gain. Both components must be considered and especially examined sequentially, so that all members of the group recognize that the initial discomfort will ultimately lead to a better way of doing things.

The third step of the proactive phase is the proper management of the communication segment of leadership, particularly regarding the nefarious behavior of the nonplayers. In my consulting experience, despite the timely use of the first two steps of the proactive phase, the nonplayers will use an assortment of verbal contentious challenges to derail the change process. Accordingly, use the following guide to achieve sound communication management during the change process, specifically in the proactive stage when the dissenting nonplayers will take their best shot at negating the positive action of change:

Nonplayer ploy 1: That will never work!
Leader rejoinder: Tell us specifically what will work.
Nonplayer ploy 2: I have got a problem with this.
Leader rejoinder: Redefining problems is useless. Give us a solution that might be useful to achieve our goals.

Nonplayer ploy 3: We tried that before, but it did not work.
Leader rejoinder: How will this work now? We are dealing
            with the present.
Nonplayer ploy 4: With all this change, maybe I should find
            another job.
Leader rejoinder: I will accept your resignation immediately,
            because change will be constant for years to
            come in health care.

As these techniques indicate, you as leader must use three principles in managing the nonplayer's resistance. First, issue a direct, tactful challenge to the complaining nonplayer. Under no circumstance should you allow the nonplayer to complain or cast dispersions on group plans without contributing a better idea. The only individual more detrimental to a health care organization than a nonplayer in this regard is a manager who allows negativity to become acceptable behavior without holding the nonplayer accountable for constructive contribution, not just destructive criticism. Second, use plural pronouns *we* and *us* so that the group recognizes that the nonplayer is questioning the entire group's capability, not just yours. This encourages the steadies and superstar members to become accountable for group direction and goal formation and enlists their participation in countering ill-conceived negativity. Finally, the leader should use "bottom-line" vernacular, such as *useless* and *immediately,* so that the nonplayers are clear in their understanding that game playing, dissention, and group denigration are intolerable when striving for group achievement.

The final component of the proactive stage is your display of natural emotions. Don't be a Pollyanna or Jack Armstrong-esque with an unwarranted positive outlook in the change process; show honest emotion. The group will readily recognize that you are in the same boat as they are and will continue to "row" accordingly.

Creating Staff Interdependence

Interdependence among all members of the group is essential to achieving change successfully. Ten basic guidelines must be adhered to if you want all members of the group to reach the implemented change result in a cohesive, integrated manner that will provide a sound foundation for future action. Use these ten guidelines, presented in checklist fashion for easy reference, as the change process moves from the planning and proactive phase to the action phase of the plan:

1. *Identify problems promptly and pragmatically.* This mandates a timely response to cited problems, a practical approach to gathering potential solutions from each staff member, and emphasis on defining new solutions, not reiterating old problems.
2. *Elicit solutions from staff members.* This must be done constantly by consistently asking all group members, *How can we do this better?*
3. *Use interactive feedback.* Present critical information to the group on a timely basis, acknowledge and use suggestive feedback, and reward any new innovations that contribute to the process, especially from steady players, with group recognition and other appropriate methods.
4. *Resolve short-term problems and focus on the long term.* Resolve short-term problems quickly by putting the onus for a solution on the individuals identifying the problem first and then charging the group with the responsibility of devising a solution that will help make the long-term objective of change a reality.
5. *Reinforce the need for change.* This reinforcement should be done throughout the process by asking for new benefits that the change might generate. These benefits would be any advantages the organization, department, or individual might realize that were not identified initially in the proactive stage but are now readily apparent and tangible for group identification and discussion.
6. *Cite examples of positive change.* Make a linkage between past examples of positive group change (the precedent) and current challenges. You probably can easily identify a past action that was so daunting that by comparison a current change project is seemingly easy.
7. *Manage the nonplayers forcefully.* Confronting the nonplayers throughout the process relative to their negativity is your responsibility and should be done using the pronouns *we* and *us* and telling the nonplayers to "stop it or drop it" relative to

their negative critique of group movement; that is, unless they can cite a better way, their condemnation of the change movement is useless to the group.

8. *Encourage steadies.* Compliment any contribution made by the steadies, highlight their constructive innovations, and commend their performance in public at any juncture to ensure that the "silent majority" is the driving engine to achieve the change.

9. *Highlight steadies and superstars.* All of us in health care must remember that to inspire dedicated performance, we must take time to say thank you and to celebrate the wins, not just lament the losses and things that do not go right. The steadies and superstars, as personifications of the goodness of our profession, should be the recipients of positive reinforcement in its most basic form during change and throughout their work life.

10. *Illustrate by comparison and contrast extensively.* Such illustration includes creative use of time lines showing a before-and-after depiction of the change process or an account of progress made "to date" relative to the change process.

Providing Key Leadership Roles for Change Process Management

The essential leadership roles for a health care manager to fulfill during the change management process are eminently familiar to anyone acquainted with the popular, established leadership and management lexicon. These icons can act as a reflective matrix for the health care leader during the change process. However, some of these familiar roles merit specific discussion.

As a health care manager, you must be both listener and perceiver throughout the change management process. The distinction between these two roles is that a listener understands what a staff member is saying clearly and comprehensively, and a perceiver also understands why someone is making a statement. Understanding the motive behind communication is a leadership responsibility, because communication is key to action in health care performance. To ascertain the need for action and the specific response desired by a staff member, ask directly, *Why are you telling me this?*.

You must be an encourager throughout the change process and fulfill every variation of this role from empowerer to cheerleader. Be forthright and resolute in displaying the courage necessary to confront, manage, and ultimately redirect or remove nonplayers. This is related to the role of a leader as a coach. An athletic coach must motivate forty players in forty different ways. Similarly, health care leaders must know their players, their sources of inspiration and motivation, and use this frame of reference pragmatically throughout the change process.

Finally, you must be an advocate of three related commodities. First, always advocate the need for a positive outlook to all staff members in an enlightened manner by using strategies suggested throughout this article. Second, advocate the needs of your staff in discussions with organizational executives to obtain the necessary resources and support to accomplish change goals. Third, advocate the position of the entire group rather than individual concerns, especially those of the low-performance, high-maintenance nonplayers.

A Final Perspective

In a recent survey, I asked more than two thousand health care managers the following question: *How many of you believe that there has been more change in the past three years than ever before in health care?* There is almost universal agreement to this query, and there is always 100 percent agreement to the follow-up question: *Do you believe there will be even more change in the next three years?* Whether in a seminar setting or on site at a health care facility, all of us in the profession know that change is an ever-present reality. It is also a positive motivator for most of us, as it is for the steadies and superstars of our staffs. By focusing our efforts on maximizing their progressive participation in the change process, we can ensure that our vital mission of providing stellar health care to our constituency will be met in the challenging times ahead.

Conclusion

In this chapter I have reviewed an assortment of communication situations and strategies. You will have noticed by now that many of the strategies throughout this book are based on communication, thus supporting the book's premise: Communication is the key to action. By recognizing your communication abilities and constantly developing them, you are in turn constantly developing yourself and growing as a health care manager.

Good communication and good management are synonymous. Neither is an exact science, yet both can be attained through constant practice and continual development.

Chapter Seventeen

Case Study
Jersey Medical Center
Community Relations Office

The following case study is based directly on a real-life situation from my consulting experience. It not only illustrates techniques delineated in preceding chapters, it also provides additional insight relative to the daily management activities of a new health care manager. Review preceding chapters so as to grasp the practical applications of the techniques provided. Then note additional strategies highlighted in the case study that might help you progress in your own responsibilities.

The Jersey Medical Center (JMC) is a large nonprofit facility located in the center of the Garden State. With more than forty-five hundred employees, it offers a wide range of medical and health care services to the surrounding urban area. The facility was founded in the late 1800s and has grown and prospered with the dynamics of the local environment and the industrialization of the state's economy.

The JMC community relations office is relatively new, established in 1992 with the mission of providing basic public relations services to the community, with special emphasis on publicizing new programs and services. The original manager of the community relations office was Meredith Fribus. Fribus had extensive experience in community and public relations and was considered a specialist in the area of patient relations. As a result, the office was reorganized to take advantage of her expertise in the manner depicted in Figure 17.1.

**Figure 17.1. Original Organization Chart:
Community Relations Office, Jersey Medical Center.**

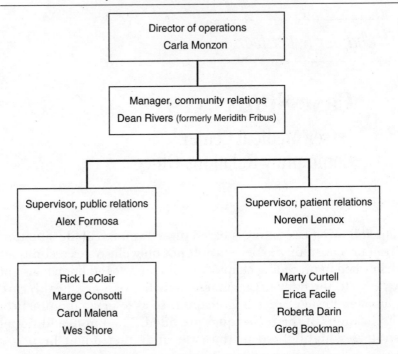

As shown in Figure 17.1, two basic groups make up the community relations office. The first group is the public relations group, headed by Alex Formosa. Formosa's team of four individuals is responsible for the primary activities of public relations: handling press inquiries, generating promotional material about the medical center, and arranging activities that heighten the medical center's visibility throughout the community. Formosa has been on the staff of the community relations office since its origin, and his group is considered very capable based on their past performance.

The other component of the community relations office is the patient relations group. This group's main purpose in the past has been to handle customer-patient complaints in a timely and efficient manner. This group is managed by Noreen Lennox, who, like Alex Formosa, is a specialist in her area and acts as a professional contributor more than as a coordinator. That is, although Formosa and Lennox are nominal coordinators of their groups, they are not charged with specific supervisory responsibilities such as performance evaluation, employee conduct, or other management duties.

The organizational and various supervisory responsibilities were established by Fribus in her effort to gain complete control of the department and launch what she believed would be proper execution of its responsibilities. However, the past year has been a nightmare for both Fribus and the organization. The department did not perform up to expectations, and several crises were handled poorly, resulting in several situations that had to be managed by JMC's top executives. The department's poor performance appeared to be exacerbated by Fribus, who often complained about being under too much stress and constantly missed deadlines and other performance mandates. At the end of the year Fribus resigned, citing "too much pressure in the job"; she took a similar position at a smaller hospital in rural Pennsylvania.

As a result of Fribus's resignation, the hospital's operations director, Carla Monzon, conducted a thorough search for a new manager of community relations. After interviewing several candidates who answered an ad in the *Jersey Star* newspaper, Monzon appointed Dean Rivers to the position.

Rivers was previously the public relations coordinator for St. Ann's Clinic in nearby North Amboy. This clinic, a mid-sized facility based in an urban neighborhood, is well respected throughout the state and provided Rivers with the opportunity to learn the business of public and community relations. Furthermore, in his previous job Rivers handled patient complaints and acquired a wealth of experience in the position, which was his first job following graduation from Hudson University, a local four-year college. This is River's first position in management. As will become apparent, he is quickly tested under fire.

The First Month

As are many new managers who assume control of an existing department, Dean Rivers is confronted by a number of situations in the first several months that need his immediate attention.

On August 6, Rivers assumed his new responsibility. His first move was to buy a notebook from a local drugstore on the way to Jersey Medical Center. He wanted a journal in which he could record performance and document critical incidents. This book would serve as his guide throughout his initial tenure as a manager.

Rivers spends most of his first day working with Alex Formosa and Noreen Lennox, learning about their work roles and their respective work teams. On one hand, Rivers notices that Lennox is a very positive individual who seems to have a firm grasp on the entire field of patient relations and an optimistic outlook on her future goals and objectives. This impression is confirmed when Lennox candidly states that occasionally she felt suppressed in her responsibilities because of Fribus's tendency to interfere intrusively in the patient relations area. Rivers immediately pledges to "stay out of the way" of Lennox's responsibilities, while encouraging her to call on him as needed.

On the other hand, Rivers learns immediately that Alex Formosa feels his group is overwhelmed. In juggling media requests, organizing several functions in support of the development office, and publishing the JMC newsletter and other publications, Formosa feels he and his team are overtaxed and need additional support. River's general impression is that Formosa is a negative individual who seems to look at the downside of whatever issues he discusses; he also notices that Formosa has to leave the meeting several times due to phone interruptions from his group requesting his immediate attention. Rivers's first-day impression is that Formosa's group runs him, not vice versa.

At the end of the first week on the job, Dean Rivers conducts a "pencil review" with his two group coordinators. He uses the Jersey Medical Center performance evaluation form as a guide in establishing goals for both coordinators. To achieve his objectives, he gives both Lennox and Formosa a blank copy of the form and asks them to enter goals they would like to achieve over the next year. Based on their input, he holds separate discussions with each of them in which he formalizes seven to ten goals for each group. Furthermore, he discusses various training and development activities the two would like to undertake and the possibility of conducting pencil evaluations to establish goals for all members of the ten-person staff. Lennox believes this is a good idea, whereas Formosa thinks it is an idea that would be best served "further down the road."

Rivers realizes that Formosa is reluctant to establish goals for members of his group, whereas Lennox is quite enthusiastic about the idea. Seizing this natural opportunity, he gives Lennox four of the forms to use with her staff and establishes a time for the two of them to meet jointly with each of the four members of the patient relations group. He then tells Formosa that a similar exercise is planned for the public relations group in the very near future and leaves him with the responsibility of scheduling that meeting for later in the month.

However, Dean Rivers has another meeting in mind. During the third week of his management tenure, he schedules a Friday afternoon meeting of all ten members of his staff. Although he made the effort to introduce himself to all the staff members and to spend time individually with each one throughout his first two weeks, he has not had a department meeting with his staff. In organizing this meeting, he sends a five-point memo to each staff member detailing the following information:

1. The date, location, and time of the meeting
2. The major topic of the meeting (goals and objectives for the coming year)
3. A one-sentence request for each member to prepare his or her ideas on what the department should achieve in the coming year
4. Situations and circumstances that affect the entire department's performance and suggestions for improvement
5. A one-sentence reminder of his enthusiasm for the department and the anticipation of hearing ideas and suggestions for departmental improvement

Rivers begins with a general statement about his appreciation for all the time that members of the team have spent in his orientation process. He then opens the meeting by presenting five basic goals and objectives he wishes to achieve over the year. The entire department seems reasonably accepting of these five goals and objectives, and Rivers conducts a roundtable discussion in which he gives each member an opportunity to add to the goals and objectives or make other comments.

Rivers deliberately exerts a certain amount of control throughout the meeting, having decided that his objective is to present the
goals and objectives and basically let everyone know where they
stand relative to their new manager. With this in mind, he repeats
his commitment to support each member of the team fully, and to
provide any expertise and resources they need to accomplish their
jobs. He states that he expects each member of his staff to perform
as a professional, to contribute fully, and to provide maximum performance and productivity daily.

On the following Monday morning, through his office window,
Rivers observes Wes Shore, one of Formosa's public relations staff
workers, arriving noticeably late for work. Since assuming his position as community relations manager, Rivers has observed this same
tardiness every Monday morning. Therefore, this is Shore's "third
strike" relative to lateness. Rivers has also noticed that Formosa
spends a lot of time at Shore's desk and wonders whether Formosa is
doing Shore's work for him. Furthermore, Formosa appears to
be visibly intimidated by Shore's frequently boisterous manner and
jocular behavior in the office.

Rivers calls Formosa into his office to ask whether he is aware
of Shore's tardiness. Formosa replies that he is generally aware that
Shore is "on occasion a little bit late" on Monday mornings. Formosa further offers that Shore has a house along the southern New
Jersey oceanfront that he shares with several friends on weekends,
particularly in the summer. As a result, he explains, Shore is sometimes late on Monday mornings because he travels approximately
seventy-five miles from the shoreline to the hospital.

Formosa does not seem particularly concerned about Shore's
tardiness, saying that he cannot be "exactly sure" of how many
times Shore has been late on Monday mornings. Furthermore, he
feels that Shore is one of the strongest players in his department
and sometimes works late to assist Formosa in emergency situations, without complaining or being forced into it.

Rivers decides that it is time for Formosa to learn the management technique of documenting performance. He explains the
entire range of performance documentation to Formosa and
instructs him to record in a notebook specific performance incidents relative to Shore. However, to address Shore's tardiness
immediately, Rivers asks Formosa to "have a talk" with him about

his lateness, but Formosa seems reluctant to do this because he does not feel it is part of his work role as a coordinator.

At this point, Rivers faces two situations: (1) a performance problem that must be addressed immediately and (2) a supervisor who is unconvinced that he should be performing as a supervisor. The second problem is perhaps more deleterious to the entire conduct of his department. In fact, Rivers is not sure of the exact nature of the roles performed by Formosa and Lennox. Both individuals are compensated significantly more than their team members, yet their title is "coordinator." Rivers is not sure whether "coordination" simply encompasses work output or whether it extends to staff conduct. To clarify their roles, he schedules a meeting with Carla Monzon, director of operations.

Monzon explains that the current department structure was originated under Meredith Fribus. As Monzon and Rivers review the job description for the two coordinator's positions, they see that very few supervisory duties are included. In essence the coordination is purely operational in nature; that is, both positions are primarily focused on professional as opposed to supervisory responsibilities.

Monzon encourages Rivers to "make his own call" on departmental organization. Rivers says he still needs additional information and wants to observe the situation more before he makes a final determination. With this in mind, they agree to discuss the situation further at their next monthly meeting and perhaps execute a reorganization plan if necessary.

As he returns to his office, Rivers observes Wes Shore discussing his previous weekend's activities with his coworker Carol Malena. Rivers enters the conversation informally by asking Shore specifically where his summer home is located. Taking Shore aside, Rivers makes Shore aware that he knows of Shore's Monday tardiness and advises him to let Formosa know if he will be late. Rivers further suggests that Shore remedy his tardiness by setting out one hour earlier on Monday mornings. Rivers does this because he believes that Formosa has discussed this situation with Shore previously.

As he enters the fourth week of his first month, Rivers is approached by Curtis Wright, the human resource director, about the attitude survey the organization is conducting. Wright believes the survey will be an excellent tool to assess attitude and opinions throughout the organization. Wright is also interested in working with Rivers to establish a marketing survey for JMC's customer-patient population. When Rivers asks him about the timing of the survey, Wright indicates that he intends to conduct it within the next two months. Rivers sees that this would be a good communication tool for the entire organization, particularly for his department, and agrees to support Wright's actions with the survey. Furthermore, he intends to raise the topic at his next department meeting, scheduled for the following week. In fact, Rivers has decided to hold department meetings once every two weeks in an effort to keep communication constant with his new staff.

As the week ends, Rivers receives some paperwork from Curtis Wright regarding Marge Consotti, a member of the public relations section. Evidently, Consotti is about to go on maternity leave for six months. The paperwork indicates that the maternity leave will go into effect at the end of the next month, and Consotti's request has obviously been approved by the personnel department. However, this is the first that Dean Rivers has learned about the situation.

He immediately calls Alex Formosa into his office, asking if he is aware of Consotti's impending maternity leave. Formosa indicates that he knew that she was pregnant, but was not sure of when the maternity leave would begin. Rivers asks Formosa to bring Consotti immediately to his office.

While waiting for them, Rivers reminds himself that Formosa is at fault, not Consotti, for not being aware of the situation and communicating to him. When the two arrive, he tells Consotti that her maternity leave has been approved and notes on his calendar the date on which the leave will begin. He asks Consotti whether she apprised Formosa of the request, and Consotti says she did. Formosa agrees that he was aware of it and now remembers the general circumstances of the request. Rivers wishes Consotti all the best, gives her a copy of the maternity leave paperwork, and asks Formosa to "stick around" after Consotti leaves.

Following Consotti's departure, Rivers asks Formosa why he did not apprise him of Consotti's maternity leave request. Formosa says again he simply "forgot about it" and figured that "sooner or later" Consotti would go on maternity leave. Furthermore, Rivers is surprised to learn that Formosa has not even considered a backup plan for filling the position while Consotti is on maternity leave.

He charges Formosa with formulating a contingency plan immediately and with letting him know within the next week what he wants to do regarding her position.

The Second Month

At the outset of his second month on the job, Dean Rivers attempts to organize his own daily responsibilities. To do this, he uses a time management system for his daily workflow. For example, he uses the stoplight system for his phone calls. Because a great deal of his activity involves travel throughout the community and activities throughout the hospital, he is not in his office much of the time. Therefore, he has the office secretary-receptionist, Roberta Darin, take detailed phone messages while he is out of the office. These messages include the date and time of the call, a two-line summary of the call, and the caller's name and phone number along with two "best" times the caller can be reached. He has trained Darin specifically in this technique and reviews his phone messages promptly each time he returns to the office.

Upon returning to the office, Rivers also has disciplined himself into sorting out the messages by time sequence; urgent messages or critical calls are handled immediately. To handle these critical calls, he has instructed Roberta Darin to "beep him" with anything that is absolutely urgent. Prior to each departure, he gives Darin a list of "likely emergency calls" that might take place during his absence. This assists Darin in managing the volume of communication that comes into the office. (Noreen Lennox has adopted this method in the interest of promptly returning emergency calls and organizing calls that do not fall into the emergency category.)

Calls that can be returned within the next eight hours are put into the yellow-light stack Rivers keeps on his desk. He also maintains a green-light stack, which includes calls from his racquetball partner, friends at St. Ann's Clinic, and other calls he deems nonpressing.

Rivers is also using a time management technique for his mail, which he places in three file folders. Folder A contains mail that must be answered immediately or acted on at once. Folder B contains mail that must be handled within seventy-two hours. These items are of particular urgency and importance to individuals within the hospital, and they also include external matters such as patient complaints or inquiries of a high-profile nature or matters that have reached a critical state and require his intervention. Finally, Rivers maintains folder C for low-priority mail. Rivers has promised himself to review the folders periodically, throwing out any information that has been in the C folder for two months. Obviously, if it does not have to be acted on after two months, it has no importance.

In a similar vein, Rivers has promised himself not to let the stress of his job become overwhelming. He has adopted four basic strategies to ensure that he keeps his life in balance:

1. Rivers plays racquetball, his favorite sport, at least twice a week. At least one of these weekly racquetball dates is with his friend Jim Pocono, whom he has known since childhood. Pocono works in the travel business, and thus Rivers is assured that no hospital business will be discussed. The other racquetball date is flexible; he plays with either a friend or a contact in the community. Although he runs the risk of hospital business being discussed, he still gets the exercise needed to maintain a high degree of energy and the good physical fitness required for a stress-positive lifestyle.

2. He spends Sundays with his fiancée, Rhonda Rossi. He enlists her aid in making sure that the extra time required by his new job "does not get out of hand." He tells Rossi that without fail, Sundays will be their time together. Rossi and he plan activities that will not be canceled due to the demands of his job at the hospital or her job as a high school teacher.

3. Rivers spends at least fifteen minutes outdoors for every three hours he is in the hospital building. This can entail eating lunch outside at one of the hospital picnic tables, going for a walk in the afternoon during his break, or simply spending an extra five or ten minutes walking to a newspaper office or other outside agency with which he deals as part of his job. This ensures a mental break for every three hours of intensive work, and Rivers also gets rejuvenated from the fresh air intake.

4. Rivers keeps up with his favorite hobby, reading, particularly biographies of figures from American history. Rhonda Rossi and Rivers buy several volumes of historical biographies from a dis-

count bookstore. Rivers makes a commitment to read at least one of these books every month, as they are a guaranteed escape from his daily work role. Furthermore, he has found that reading these books is not only interesting, but also provides a perspective relative to leadership and other important dynamics to his career without creating stress or causing him to think about his job, which would defeat the purpose of this strategy.

However, the second month does not center strictly on Rivers's self-directed activities. In fact, he faces several situations that require his immediate action.

During the second week of his second month, Rivers again notices Wes Shore arriving late. In fact, Shore is a good hour late for his shift. With Shore is Greg Bookman, who works in the patient relations area. After leaving his office, Rivers notices that Noreen Lennox is having a closed door meeting with Greg Bookman, most likely discussing his tardiness. He also observes Wes Shore talking quite animatedly with Carol Malena and Rick LeClair of the public relations department. He observes Formosa sitting quietly at his desk working on the photo layout of an upcoming brochure.

At this point, Rivers brings both Shore and Formosa into his office. He asks Shore if he recalls their earlier conversation together concerning Rivers's expectation that he will arrive on Monday mornings on time. He also asks Shore if he recalls the suggestion that Rivers made to leave his beach house an hour earlier. Shore says that he vaguely recalls the conversation but that it "doesn't matter this time" because he had "car problems" this morning.

Rivers then asks Shore if he called Formosa to tell him about the car problem, to which Shore replies that he did not have time to call because he "doesn't have a car phone" and "was busy fixing the car." Rivers says that this answer is unacceptable, as is the behavior of constantly coming in late. He cites the fact that car problems were not the reason for the previous episodes of tardiness and notifies him that by the end of the day he will receive a written warning to correct this tardiness immediately. After instructing Shore to return to his work area, he brings Roberta Darin (office secretary-receptionist) in and dictates a concise warning letter to Shore. Formosa sits silently in River's office throughout this entire episode.

Rivers then conducts a private, very direct meeting with Formosa using the five-minute meeting techniques discussed earlier. In recent weeks, Formosa has come into Rivers's office on several occasions with problems Rivers has then resolved. These meetings started with Formosa's asking for five minutes of Rivers's time but extended into twenty-minute discussions. This time, however, a very direct five-minute conversation will take place. Rivers asks Formosa the following five questions:

1. Why didn't you confront Shore immediately upon his arriving late today?
2. What effect do you think his tardiness has on the rest of your department?
3. How do you plan to resolve this tardiness issue?
4. Who in your department winds up doing most of the work when Shore comes in late?
5. What message do you think you send to the rest of the department by tolerating Shore's lateness on Monday mornings?

Oddly enough, Formosa's answers to all these questions are "I don't know" and then silence. At this point, Rivers must take the initiative to make some very important points, which he does by simply answering some of his own questions. He informs Formosa that he is sending a dangerous message that if an employee is late on Monday morning, no negative consequences will take place. As a result, Shore's negative behavior is being mimicked by members of Lennox's department, namely Greg Bookman. He states that he has seen Formosa doing Shore's work, as was the case this morning when Formosa was organizing the photo layout Shore was to have ready by 11:00 A.M. Rivers then mentions Formosa's failure to follow up on work, reviewing the examples he has documented in his notebook. These examples include Formosa's failure to schedule a goal-setting meeting with his staff, and his reluctance to provide a contingency plan for Consotti's leave. Finally he states that Formosa's actions indicate that he has no real interest in managing the department, which leads to a very direct question: "Why don't you seem interested in managing your department?"

After several minutes of silence, Formosa answers by saying that he truly is not interested in managing his section. He states that, unlike Noreen Lennox, he simply took the coordinator position to make some extra money, that he is not interested in developing into a manager, and is only interested in technical angles of his position. In fact, he thinks he is ill suited to be a manager because he does not see himself as being particularly communicative, well organized, or motivated to work with others. He says he would be very happy if he was given only assignments, his production materials, and some interesting work.

Rivers uses a very important management technique at this juncture. He tries to paraphrase and summarize all of what Formosa is saying to arrive at a logical conclusion. In this case, he says, "It sounds as though you are not interested in being a manager and would be happy simply working in a staff position." Formosa agrees completely that this is indeed his sentiment.

But this seemingly unpleasant and negative situation turns into a positive, progressive one. Formosa says that although he would be otherwise happy to return to a staff position, he has gotten additional compensation and therefore is reluctant to do so. Knowing that Marge Consotti is about embark on maternity leave and that there might be an opportunity to combine some of her job position requirements with Formosa's work load, Rivers tells Formosa that he will discuss the situation with Carla Monzon in the interest of reorganizing the department to accommodate Formosa's professional desires. He also states that he already was considering doing this, as he is dissatisfied with the current structure. He promises Formosa that he will get back to him within two weeks' time and asks him in the interim to do his best as coordinator until this follow-up meeting takes place. Knowing that Formosa is extremely gifted in his technical area and a very productive employee, Rivers feels confident that if approved by Monzon, this new arrangement will allow him the opportunity to remotivate a valued resource.

In the next week, however, two occurrences mandate that Dean Rivers accelerate his reorganization plan. In the week following his meeting with Formosa and Shore, Rivers is interrupted in his office by Erica Facile, who is very upset with Formosa. Rick LeClair and

Carol Malena, from Formosa's section, were supposed to provide information about an upcoming career day the hospital was sponsoring for local high school students. As a member of the patient relations department, Facile was assigned by Noreen Lennox to publicize career day with the families of inpatients who have high school–age visitors who might enjoy attending a career day while visiting sick relatives or friends. Facile's request to LeClair and Malena have met with no action.

Dean Rivers goes directly to LeClair and Malena for the information needed by Facile. Furthermore, he assigns them to make a presentation on career day at the upcoming department meeting. This will ensure that all members of the department are aware of the career day, provide their input, and make any suggestions that might make the activity a successful one.

The following week in the hallway, Rivers overhears Marge Consotti telling several coworkers that Alex Formosa is like the Dustin Hoffman character in *Rain Man,* except he is not good in math. This comment draws raucous laughter, which can be heard throughout the entire department.

Rivers tells Consotti that he overheard the conversation and does not appreciate her comments. He emphasizes that Consotti could be more charitable in her comments in the future, if for no other reason than comments like these are mean-spirited and unprofessional. Furthermore, he says, given that she is about to embark on fully paid maternity leave she should feel at least a business obligation to the hospital to demonstrate some basic loyalty and allegiance as a paid employee. Trying to suppress his anger, Rivers says that although he appreciates the fact that break time is an employee's own time, he reminds Consotti and her coworkers that they are on hospital property and should conduct themselves as professionals. Consotti apologizes for her comment, and Rivers returns to his office.

Immediately upon returning to his office, Rivers reviews his department reorganization plan (see Figure 17.2). As departmental supervisor, Noreen Lennox will assist him in management of the department but will be primarily in charge of distribution of work, flow of organizational activity, and interim management in Rivers's absence.

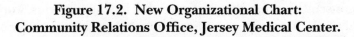

**Figure 17.2. New Organizational Chart:
Community Relations Office, Jersey Medical Center.**

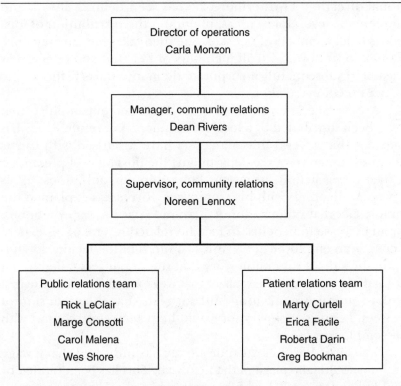

As a production specialist, Formosa will maintain his same level of compensation by taking on additional technical responsibilities that will expand his growth and development as well as fill the void while Consotti is on maternity leave. Because the hospital will soon acquire a smaller facility, Consotti's return in six months will be timely in that she will help handle the additional responsibility brought on by the acquisition.

With plan in hand, Rivers heads for his monthly meeting with Carla Monzon. After their review of the plan and all his documentation notes, Rivers justifies the new plan, making four additional observations:

1. Rivers has noted on several occasions that Noreen Lennox is a positive and productive force within the department. He notices

her constantly asking her employees for new suggestions, working closely with them, and providing them with technical and motivational direction. Furthermore, he has seen Lennox absorb and implement several new ideas, including the distribution of idea books to all members of her staff. She then takes the time out once a week to sit down with all members of her staff and review new ideas and subsequently incorporate them into the activities of the patient relations section.

2. Several employees seem quite interested in pamphlets that have been distributed by a local labor union. As a result, Rivers has learned that several line managers have discussed with Curtis Wright (human resource department) the possibility of presenting a "fact versus fiction" program about union organizations. In his biweekly meetings with his employees, Rivers has explained the simple fact that unions cannot guarantee pay raises, promotions, or an increase in benefits. In fact, he related several of his experiences as an employee at St. Ann's Clinic, a union facility, to illustrate the side of the union story that the organizers failed to tell his staff. In any event, he realizes that weak management is the first link to union organization and suggests that the ascension of Noreen Lennox to supervisor would help keep close contact with the employees.

3. Curtis Wright's attitude survey has indicated that a wage review should take place in the next year. This has been ratified by Hal Puller, JMC's CEO, who has gotten board of director approval to raise salaries at the end of the year in certain areas. Again, due to imminent employee dissatisfaction, the need for a supervisor who would be principally involved with operational details is a good idea at this time. With a compensation review becoming imminent, it is possible that Noreen Lennox's compensation package can be increased as part of the ongoing salary review process.

4. Rivers feels strongly that only one department supervisor is needed. With nine employees, a supervisor, and a manager, the workflow can emanate from one source, be distributed specifically by the supervisor, and then monitored by both the manager and supervisor, depending on the situation. Furthermore, Rivers would still maintain managerial control of the department, while Lennox would use her technical proficiency not only in patient relations but also in the areas of public and community relations. This plan

will assist her professional development, as well as return Formosa to the technical area in which he is most capable.

Monzon looks at the plan and decides immediately that it is a step in the right direction. She promises Rivers an answer within two weeks and commits to discussing ramifications of the plan in the interim with Hal Puller and Curtis Wright.

The Third Month

As the third month of tenure begins, Rivers observes Wes Shore entering the building on the first Monday of the month at 10:15. Not only has Shore been counseled at this point, he has received a written warning regarding his tardiness. Rivers realizes that his only recourse is to terminate Shore's employment at Jersey Medical Center.

Since Formosa is still nominally the operations coordinator for the public relations section, he should be included in the meeting. However, this is the first time Rivers has ever had to fire anyone, and among several issues he is debating, one is whether it is necessary to have Formosa attend the meeting. In discussion with Carla Monzon, he concludes that Monzon should be present at the termination and that there is no real need for Formosa to be in the meeting. This is because as manager, Rivers has provided the written warning and has the documentation relative to the termination. That documentation includes

- Specific dates and times that support evidence of Shore's constant tardiness
- Four deadlines Shore missed, for which he was counseled by Rivers
- Shore's below-average performance evaluation from the preceding year (although Fribus failed to put him on probation)
- Shore's contentious attitude and confrontational behavior, which was noted on three occasions by Rivers and, again, which Shore was counseled to resolve

Monzon asks Rivers whether he has considered probation as an option. Rivers does not favor probation in this case, because despite counseling Shore in several instances about all these performance shortcomings he has seen the situation worsen. Monzon is a firm advocate of termination over probation, which she feels would probably lead to termination anyway, and agrees to attend the termination meeting. The meeting is scheduled for the following Friday afternoon, and Rivers schedules the meeting with Shore.

When Friday arrives, Shore enters Rivers's office to find both Monzon and Rivers awaiting him. He takes a seat across the desk from Rivers, with Monzon sitting at the side of the desk facing him as well. The following dialogue takes place:

Rivers: Wes, as you know, we've had several discussions over the past two months concerning your performance. This has included conversations about your tardiness, which has been chronic on Monday mornings; your inability to produce work by deadline; and some of your interactions with people in the department, which I consider to be unprofessional and counterproductive. You've received a written warning about this behavior, but unfortunately the situation has gotten worse, not better.

Shore: Well give some specific examples of what you're talking about.

Rivers: Well, I believe all the examples and situations have been discussed already, and you've received the warning letters, haven't you?

Shore: Yeah, I have. But I still don't understand what you expect from me.

Rivers: Wes, I think you do in fact know what I expect from you. I've made it quite clear to you repeatedly in the two and a half months I've been here. And I think prior to that time, as evidenced on your performance evaluation from last year, your performance expectations have been made quite clear to you.

Shore: Yeah, but that was with Fribus. I don't think she knew what she was doing anyway, and I had a lot of problems with her. I think I can work out well with you. I just kinda had a rough summer.

Rivers: You might have had a rough summer, but your tardiness, to use just one example, has persisted now, and certainly October is not the summer.

Shore: Yeah, but I think things are starting to turn around, don't you?

Rivers: No, I'd have to disagree.

Shore: But what do you mean?

Rivers: To be very honest, I think we're past the point of discussion. Let me get right to the point. I regret to inform you that you're being terminated due to poor performance. I'm quite comfortable with this documentation, and as you leave the facility today, I'd like you simply to leave your desk key after you have cleaned out the desk. The organization will pay you severance for the next two weeks and extend your benefits to the end of the month. At that point, you'll no longer be paid and will have to pick up benefits from a new employer or use the special three-month waiver period our insurance carrier provides. Here's a copy of that plan for your review. I am also giving you . . .

Shore: [*interrupts vehemently*] So what, you're firing me?!

Rivers: Unfortunately that's exactly right. As I was saying, here's a letter of your termination for your review. I've discussed the situation completely with Carla, and while she agrees with me, I'm the manager and this was my decision. It was not easy or pleasant, but I felt it had to be made for the good of the entire department. I've got nothing against you personally and wish you luck in whatever you might do from here on out.

Shore: Yeah, well thanks a lot! I'll be seeing you in court, pal!

Rivers: Really? Well, you'd better get yourself a good lawyer!

Monzon: Wes, this is an unfortunate situation, and of course it's your right to get a lawyer if you feel you need one. However neither Dean nor I feel we're doing anything wrong and I feel Dean explained the situation to you completely. Therefore, I'd like to ask you to clean out your desk and leave the building and would suggest to you that we'll have a security guard escort you from this office if need be.

Shore: [*laughing*] Hey, that's a good one, honey, the security guards! Which one are you going to send, Curly, Larry, or Moe?! Forget it! I'm out of here!

Following Shore's departure, Rivers is visibly angry and upset. Monzon tells him that he did a great job, although his temper flared up a little toward the end of the session. She told him that this is quite natural, and that she had quite an emotional outburst in her first termination. Rivers thanks her for her support and asks whether she anticipates further trouble from Shore. Monzon correctly points out that Shore's reaction was as to be expected and that she would be surprised if he does anything more drastic than filing for unemployment.

Shifting focus, Monzon asks Rivers to walk her to the West Wing, where her office is located. Seeing that Shore has already left his keys on top of the now-empty desk, on their way out of the facility Rivers locks his office, as it is early evening. As he walks Monzon to her office, she gives him the news that his new reorganization plan has been approved and then jokes that Shore's salary dispute is now a thing of the past. Laughing at this bit of sardonic humor, Rivers speculates whether he needs to fill the open position formerly filled by Shore and commits to analyzing the position as part of the reorganization, and to discussing it further with Noreen Lennox.

As part of the reorganization process, Rivers conducts a special department meeting in which he explains the reorganization, displays a new organization chart that clearly outlines the reorganization, and asks Lennox to present the idea book for all members of the group. Using the I-formula, the group goes through a two-hour discussion on implementing a promotional campaign for the upcoming high school career day. Since by now all members of the department have participated in the process in one version or another, the I-formula is a natural resource, as everyone has a basic frame of reference and numerous suggestions about putting together an effective promotional campaign for career day.

In the final week of his third month as community relations manager, Dean Rivers must handle a very adament customer complaint. The complaint is brought to his attention when Noreen Lennox briefs him on Jonas Wellington, cousin to a prominent member of the board. Wellington complained that he had not received copies of JMC's annual report for members of his country club, who might be potential donors to the hospital's general fund.

To remedy this, Rivers uses the information provided by Noreen Lennox to schedule a meeting with Wellington at Wellington's office. Wellington's secretary schedules a time and, grabbing twenty copies of the annual report, Rivers shows up at the appointed time.

Entering Wellington's office, he accepts a cup of coffee, sits down, and takes his notepad out of his briefcase. Wellington recounts the entire episode of making several calls to JMC's community affairs office and having his calls juggled between Wes Shore and Marge Consotti. Rivers asks how many calls he made and at what point during the year he made the calls. After allowing Wellington to vent for five minutes—punctuated by his repeated remark that the hospital "must treat everyone like this"— Rivers begins a proactive presentation.

First he apologizes profusely for the inconvenience caused to Wellington. He then explains that Wes Shore is no longer with the hospital and that Marge Consotti, although a very capable employee, was not primarily responsible for distributing annual reports, which was Shore's domain. Nonetheless, Rivers states that he accepts full responsibility for the problem and in fact has brought twenty copies of the annual report with him. He further volunteers to take another box of the annual reports directly to Hollow Hills, Wellington's country club, so that all the members will have copies.

Wellington seems reasonably happy about this action, stating that he appreciates Rivers's concern and wishes he had called him to begin with. Rivers quickly gives him one of his business cards and tells him to call anytime he might have any questions about the hospital or require further service.

Wellington suggests that a good way of raising money throughout the community would be to mail copies of the annual report to certain other individuals. Rivers says he will check into this and discuss it with the development officer as soon as he returns to the hospital. Furthermore, he tells Wellington that if he has a list of interested prospects, he will see to it that personal letters are sent to them, along with copies of the annual report, in the interest of establishing a more personal contact with these potential donors. Wellington thanks him and Rivers returns to his office.

Immediately upon returning to his office, Rivers dictates a letter for Roberta Darin to send to Wellington, thanking him for his time and assuring him that the development officer will be in touch. Rivers places a call to JMC's development officer, Marlene Epstein, telling her of the meeting with Wellington and gaining her support, as she promises to write a letter to Wellington as well. Finally, Rivers makes a small entry in his manager's notebook concerning the meeting and the action taken.

As he looks to the rest of his first year as JMC's manager, Rivers establishes seven major objectives based on his observations, initial experience, input received at department meetings, and informal communications with staff:

1. *Hold joint employee meetings on flowchart organization, workflow, and the reorganization.* These meetings will track a request for information or services from the time it first comes across Roberta Darin's desk to the time the service has been provided satisfactorily. This will help all department members define their roles, and it will give a clear indication of work progress within the department.

2. *Design a job description and action plan for Noreen Lennox.* This exercise will allow Lennox the opportunity to participate in establishing goals, as well as allow Rivers to set his performance expectations for the next six months. This also will help in Lennox's education and development as department supervisor.

3. *Establish a work flowchart from the request stage to task completion.* Based on the input from employees, Rivers plans to have a concrete system for charting workflow in place by the end of the year. This will help ongoing quality assurance efforts, as well as assist in the development of a strategic plan for the department. It will also validate the reorganization efforts that have taken place within the department.

4. *Divide work between norms, or standard operating procedures, and critical contributions, which require action plans.* Rivers wants to establish some structure in the department. Therefore, he is compiling a list of routine activities, such as requests for publications, customer-

patient complaints, and other matter that can be dealt with successfully in a standard operating procedure (SOP) manual, which will help establish policies and procedures for the entire department. For crisis situations or critical contributions (such as requests for special publications, major emergencies within the hospital, and unique media relations), action plans, or contingency-emergency plans, are established. This structuring will also help all individuals in the department follow a specific action and have a frame of reference for dealing successfully with these events.

5. *Identify and select a replacement for Wes Shore.* The position might be a part time or full- time responsibility, but in any event it must be filled quickly. Using his system of job description development, selection, and orientation (based on Chapter Eleven of this book), Rivers is able to accomplish this goal.

6. *Develop a two-year strategic plan to be ratified with Monzon and presented to the department.* Rivers will elicit the department's participation by using several team activities and the I-formula. The idea books will go a long way toward contributing to this cause.

7. *Organize project teams and cross-train all members.* Because of the distinction between the two departments, the reorganization has encouraged individuals, who previously did not have much experience in intradepartmental interrelations, to work with each other. As a result, Rivers will make a concerted effort to assign special project teams to particular areas to generate cross-training as well as give everyone the opportunity to work with all their colleagues. For example, Carol Malena and Rick LeClair will work with Greg Bookman and Erica Facile on a publication that stresses nutrition and healthy diet to teenagers. Conversely, Malena and LeClair will have the opportunity to participate in a patient relations review board meeting, which will increase their proficiency in that area.

As shown in this case study, many situations that occur in a health care manager's first three months fall into the proverbial gray area. Therefore, keep an open mind, use the strategies advocated in this book, and, most of all, use common sense. As Dean Rivers has demonstrated, by keeping the objective of providing stellar health care at the forefront, many crises and tough situations can be resolved positively.

By using common sense and a progressive approach, Dean Rivers has successfully accomplished a great deal in his early months as a first-year manager. Because of progressive planning for future objectives, his positive momentum and progressive development will continue.

Part Three

Resources

Appendix A:
Analytical Planning and
Decision-Making Tools

Resource One: SWOT Analysis Overview and Strategic Planning Guide

SWOT analysis (of strengths, weaknesses, opportunities, and threats) was developed primarily by Dr. John Bryson at the University of Minnesota in the early 1960s, and is used extensively by most Fortune 500 corporations for strategic planning. The analysis is simple in scope, user-friendly, and has a balance of factor analysis. Moreover, if employed effectively, it can provide a breadth of decision-making scope and depth of analysis needed to assess risks accurately and proactively.

The following action outline provides a guide for you to apply SWOT analysis to your case work in this unit as well as your current and future leadership roles. In using the strategic guide, keep these precepts in mind:

1. Be direct and candid in your assessment, and try to be as objective as possible.
2. Consider major internal organizational initiatives, objectives, current plans, mission and vision intentions, and present performance as criteria in your analysis.
3. Look to the external, competitive environment that your organization competes in for clues in your evaluation, and strongly link customer-constituency perception to your analysis.

SWOT Factors

Strengths

Attributes, assets, and advantages that the organization possesses and can use readily.

- Areas of apparent positive impact in the marketplace
- Hallmarks of success and effectiveness
- *Reputation builders* and *quality difference* in product-services
- Formidable resources: financial, operational, and human resources

Practical Use In conducting a SWOT analysis, list three to five apparent strengths, using the above criteria as a guide, and specify how you can fully use these resources in meeting present and future business objectives.

Weaknesses

Potential liabilities, shortages, and deficits in all resource areas that can hamper organizational success.

- Areas for immediate or future development
- Noted deficits: financial, operational, or human resources
- Competitive disadvantages in the marketplace
- Quality improvement needs regarding product-services

Practical Application After a summary review of your organization's current position in the market and how it is perceived among its consumers, identify three to five weaknesses that must be addressed. Try to innovate action plans for each cited weakness, and assign responsibility and outcome objectives for any plan that is within your control. Also, assess the detrimental aspects of each weakness, and make a determination on whether the weakness is in fact curable or chronic.

Opportunities

Potential areas of strength for the organization that can be potentially capitalized upon and incorporated into the organization's overall success portfolio.

- Short-term openings for action
- Long-term strategies for growth and development
- New initiatives, product line demands, and evident service needs in the marketplace
- Emergent consumer community needs, desires, and wants based on demographic or psycho-graphic shifts or changes

Practical Application This is in essence a "dream sheet" that allows you to envision plans and strategies that will positively and progressively impact the organization. Cite five apparent positive, progressive opportunities, and address each with a short action plan on implementing the opportunity from vision to reality.

Threats

Business conditions, external or internal to the organization, that can potentially inhibit growth, limit market penetration, or curtail overall organizational effectiveness.

- Imminent obstacles in the business environment or in the prevailing thought and attitudes of organizational leadership
- External government or environmental pressures, media-driven perceptions, industry regulations, potential legislation, or negative consumer focus that would negatively impact progress
- Customer dynamics: new demands, for example, for faster technology; or alternately, traditional thinking that could curtail new ventures
- The Big C's: competition, chaos, change, consumer shift, conflict, corporatization or compression of needs-wants

Practical Analysis Keys After identifying three to five threats, attempt to use your own creativity and decision making in ascertaining which threats are

1. Insurmountable
2. Negligible
3. Capable of correction
4. A weakness that can be turned into an advantage

Resource Two: Q-100 Index Analysis

This tool can be used for a fuller, more precise analysis in concert with, or in lieu of, the SWOT tool.

Quantitative Strategic Organizational Analysis

Rate each factor detailed categorically in this analysis using the power rating scale below. Note that the highest overall score for a perfect organization would be one hundred (twenty-five factors *times* four points maximum).

4 = Distinct positive organizational asset-advantage

3 = Viable, current asset or high-potential future asset-advantage

2 = Minimally satisfactory performance area

1 = Vulnerable organizational liability

Organizational Leadership and Action Orientation

1. Attitude, corporate culture: adaptable to new demands, can-do approach to problem areas and new challenges

   _____

2. People skills: progressive, constructive employee-management relations

   _____

3. Vision-mission impact and importance to everyday action and everyone's job

   _____

4. Managerial aptitude: creativity, timely decision-making, and accurate planning

   _____

5. Team orientation: selfless dedication to organizational success

   _____

   Power rating for organizational leadership and action orientation

   _____

   Overall comments and perceptions on organizational leadership and action orientation:

   _____

   _____

   _____

   _____

   _____

   _____

Resource Utilization and Optimization

1. Financial: to include available cash, potential investment, fluidity of assets and overall financial strength

   _____

2. Human resources: recruitment, training and development, talent and expertise, mobility and motivation of workforce

   _____

3. Operational: action-orientation, distribution of product, service support, and utilization of systems

   _____

4. Expertise: good experience base, collective knowledge, and sound sharing of knowledge and critical data

   _____

5. Resilience, thrivability, viability: proven ability, through past performance, to work successfully through crisis and change

   _____

   Power rating for resource utilization and optimization

   _____

   Overall comments and perceptions on resource utilization and optimization:

   _____

   _____

   _____

   _____

   _____

   _____

Structural and Functional Capabilities

1. Centralized leadership: including the executive suite and in each significant division or strategic business unit

   _____

2. Decentralized or line management: at each departmental or section level, effective management in most critical areas

   _____

3. Lead functions: overall assessment of the main departments that deliver the product or service

   _____

4. Support functions: overall assessment of the functions that support the delivery of the product or service

   _____

5. Interdependence: ability of all areas to rely on each other, function in a cohesive manner, and achieve a synergy of purpose

   _____

   Structural and functional capabilities power rating

   _____

   Overall comments and assessment of structural and functional capabilities:

   _____

   _____

   _____

   _____

   _____

   _____

Performance Accountabilities

1. Planning: ability to craft short-term and long-term plans that enable success and effectiveness

   _____

2. Communication: gets the message to all constituencies and internal organizational members clearly and comprehensively

   _____

3. Effectiveness: consistently provides top-quality product, service, and support in all regards

   _____

4. Efficiency: speed, accuracy, and quick response to customer-consumer-constituency needs and desires

   _____

5. Consistency: reliability of performance, continuity of process and purpose, dependability of action

   _____

   Performance accountabilities power rating

   _____

   Overall comments and assessment of performance accountabilities:

   _____

   _____

   _____

   _____

   _____

   _____

Product-Service Reputation and Perception

1. Advertising, Marketing: promotional efforts, to include traditional advertising and new venture promotion (for example, Internet ads)

   _____

2. Reputation in marketplace: word-of-mouth reputation and perception throughout the customer community

   _____

3. Community presence: public and community relations efforts, both business and community related, that bolster positive perception

   _____

4. Quality of product: established quality of the product-services in the perception of users

   _____

5. Growth and development: general ability of the organization to grow and develop as product demand escalates

   _____

   Power rating for product-service reputation and perception

   _____

   Overall evaluation of product-service reputation and perception:

   _____

   _____

   _____

   _____

OVERALL Q-100 RATING

_____

Overall Perception and Summary Conclusions:

_____

_____

_____

_____

Appendix B: Structured Selection and Behavioral Interviewing System

As discussed in the text, interviewing and selecting job candidates is a challenging process for any manager, regardless of experience or expertise. This section contains questions relating to numerous critical areas. It also contains response indicators, which will assist you in interpreting a candidate's response to the question.

Prior to the interview, prepare by selecting fifteen appropriate questions from the Appendix. Each question should be selected based on its relevance to the open position, its ability to reveal information you feel is vital to job conduct, and the level of comfort you feel in asking the question (do you like the question?). Each question is designed to generate a response of at least one to three minutes' duration, so fifteen questions should provide you with the basis for a thirty-minute comprehensive interview.

Remember to open the interview by asking open-ended, life-story questions. Then incorporate suggestions from the text into your selected questions.

Section I: Guidelines for Interview Conduct

1. Respect candidate's feelings and self-esteem above all else at all times.
2. Strive to put the candidate at ease and maintain maximum comfort to facilitate conversation.
3. Begin interview with pleasant, professional introduction and appropriate, light conversation.
4. Remember that the interview is a public relations tool as well as an assessment of past performance and future potential.
5. Eye contact should stay consistent and natural throughout the entire interview.
6. Keep in mind your role as the organization's representative; to the candidate, you *are* the organization.
7. Don't give excessive encouragement verbally or nonverbally at any point in the interview.
8. Don't use any "creative probes"; that is, no case study questions, close-ended queries, illegal questions, or other ineffective strategies.
9. Use as many cues as needed to elicit necessary response in key areas of the candidate's background and expertise.
10. Examine candidate's response in areas of
    A. Past performance and achievement
    B. Work philosophy and beliefs
    C. Interview behavior
11. Use verbal rejoinders to trigger additional response in crucial areas: *Tell me more. Give me another example. What else was involved?*
12. Use nonverbal rejoinders to maintain a steady flow of information in the interview; for example, nodding of the head, facial and hand gestures.
13. Take notes as needed and in a natural sequence, using the response-recall method.
14. Don't make a final appraisal of notes and interview dialogue until the conclusion of the interview; avoid the "five-minute actor factor."
15. Know all of the clues (see Appendix B, Section II) thoroughly and make constant matches to interview responses.

16. If you don't see the desired characteristic, ask about it specifically; if it is still not apparent, score the interview accordingly.

17. Make yourself as thoroughly knowledgeable about the candidate prior to the interview as possible and use that base throughout the interview.

18. Portray the position adequately and accurately; ask questions to determine specific candidate qualifications.

19. Have a set questioning process prepared prior to the interview and get specific information to match against clues and job description.

20. Don't wander into EEOC-sensitive information (Equal Employment Opportunity Commission) unless it is a BFOQ (bona fide occupational qualification). Avoid sensitive areas, unless volunteered, such as
    A. Age
    B. Race
    C. Marital status

21. Let the candidate do most of the talking.

22. Let candidates do their own talking.

23. Maintain an overall limited emotional profile and avoid emotive reactions.

24. Listen attentively, accurately and actively; get the breadth of information as well as the depth.

25. Postpone all final judgment until after the interview.

26. Interrupt the candidate only when necessary, and then with the utmost tact and brevity.

27. Call the candidate by first name, appropriate title, or preferred nickname—whichever address will enhance comfort and conversation.

28. Ask candidate for permission to take notes or merely inform them that you are doing so.

29. Downplay excessive negative information and control excessive positive rambling by using another question or rejoinder.

30. Don't allow candidate to go so far off track that irrelevant information takes precedent.

31. Ensure that the candidate answers the question at hand completely before moving on to another area.

32. Make sure the candidate is aware of the interview time parameters and stays within them.
33. Use the same questioning strategy with all candidates to ensure maximum comparative data.
34. Explain benefits, compensation, and opportunities appropriately.
35. Give the candidate the opportunity to ask questions but not to conduct another interview.
36. Thank the candidate at the conclusion of the interview.
37. Contact good candidates for a second interview within five days.
38. Send marginal candidates a letter of rejection within two weeks.
39. Keep good resumes on file for a least one year.
40. Always keep your responsibility as an organizational gate-keeper at the forefront of your interview strategy and approach.

Section II: Interview Questions and Interpretative Clues

Attitude Orientation

1. Tell me about a work situation that required you to be flexible.
   A. Proven ability to be adaptable
   B. No evidence of overt rigidity or inflexibility
2. Why is it important to be reasonably assertive or aggressive as a [job title]?
   A. Reasonable use of assertiveness in past role
   B. Credible assertiveness in interview forum
3. Tell me about a work situation in which you had to demonstrate persistence and perseverance.
   A. Stays the course while undertaking tough challenge
   B. Stays with point in interview
4. Tell me about a manager you worked for who had a really great attitude.
   A. Quality of example
   B. Role-model value of example
5. Tell me about a coworker you worked with who had a really great attitude.
   A. Quality of example
   B. Reflective qualities the candidate values
6. In your last (current) position, give me some examples of jobs you were asked to do that were not part of the original description.
   A. Willing to expand on original duties, wants to contribute and learn as much as possible to enhance performance
   B. Apprehension about a multidimensional or wide-range work role
7. Tell me about an unusual situation you had to handle at your last (current) position.
   A. Previous successful adaptation to significant change (new boss, new product, new approaches, etc.)
   B. Demonstrated ability to work with a wide spectrum of people
8. What radical changes took place at your last job that affected your role and daily activities in the organization?

A. Consistent past performance under adversity or major negative change
B. Effective response to change in the interview flow

9. Give me an example of a situation at your last (current) job that required a lot of persistence and perseverance.
   A. Provides a credible example of working through a tough problem by exploiting all the resources at hand
   B. Appropriately flexible but persistent in obtaining desired results

10. Often the circumstances under which a goal is established change. In this case, what would change your approach or change the goal itself?
    A. Defines problems, analyzes possible solutions, selects a plan of attack and resolves dilemma
    B. Willingness to attack problems positively and directly, rather than working around them or avoiding them completely

Business Savvy

1. Tell me about your involvement in a budgetary process.
   A. Developed fiscal expertise
   B. Experience relevant to job requirement

2. Tell me about a process you implemented that resulted in better use of time.
   A. Ability to use time wisely
   B. Stresses positive use of time in work efforts

3. Would you say that time management is one of your strengths? Why?
   A. Uses time wisely
   B. Maximizes available work time

4. How do you manage stress, which is part of every health care position?
   A. Understands that stress is part of the game
   B. Has a thoughtful plan of attacking negative stress

5. What should a health care organization [or your department type] do to be as successful as possible?
   A. Sound rationale for success factors
   B. Awareness of important health care business factors

6. How do you feel about your current employer?
   A. Words chosen to describe sensitive situations are appropriate
   B. Realizes customer-client is number one, organization is number two, and the individual is number three
7. How do you feel about the way your career has gone up to the present?
   A. Relatively satisfied with accomplishments at present job, but looking for a more substantial challenge or career opportunity
   B. Feels position will be logical next step, but takes reasonable pride in accomplishments to date

Communicative Abilities

1. Who was the best communicator you ever worked with? Why?
   A. Role-model quality
   B. Strength criteria
2. How important is listening in [job title]?
   A. Values listening skills
   B. Supports answer with strong example or rationale
3. How do you make a point in a meeting (or other group process)?
   A. Takes command appropriately
   B. Provides examples of active participation
4. How do you make sure that someone understands important information?
   A. Uses a clarification technique
   B. Adjusts communication effectively to listener
5. How would you describe your communication style?
   A. Practical, "non-psychobabble" description
   B. Verbal description matches your interview observation and perception
6. What avenues of communication were available for your use in your last (current) job?
   A. Verbal style has brevity, conciseness, and organization
   B. Succinct and adroit with sensitive information

7. Detail a procedure or product; start with a general overview and then go into specifics.
   A. Nonverbal style is natural supplement to verbal style
   B. Uses syntax, grammar, and tones effectively

Energy and Enthusiasm

1. Tell me about a work experience you really enjoyed.
   A. Innate professional interests
   B. "Hot buttons" will be hit in a new job
2. What gets you excited in your current work position?
   A. Job content factors will be present in new position
   B. Consistently enthusiastic about several job factors
3. What do you think will "turn you on" about this job?
   A. Accurate perception of job content
   B. Looks forward to entire job scope and work situation
4. What specific things interest you about [specific technical field]?
   A. Interested and intrigued about several work factors
   B. Open position will provide numerous positive interesting opportunities
5. Why is a high degree of energy and enthusiasm important to a [job title]?
   A. Demonstrates good level of energy in interview
   B. Understands why energy is positively contagious and important in any health care position

General Professional Experience

1. Explain the experience you've had in [specific technical field].
   A. Depth of experience
   B. Breadth of expertise
2. What are your strongest technical areas?
   A. Range of experience
   B. Confidence in abilities
3. What areas would you like to learn more about?
   A. Honest, candid assessment of development needs
   B. Evident desire to learn and grow

4. How do you find that you learn new things relative to your job?
   A. Seeks new information and approaches
   B. Sound abilities in perception, observation, and assimilation
5. Give me an example of a work situation from which you learned a great deal.
   A. Several credible examples
   B. Stresses positive learning experience that is now part of candidate's approach
6. Give an example of a tough people-problem you had to handle.
   A. Provides solid examples of dealing with a tough problem successfully while maintaining the best interpersonal relations
   B. Never allows perception to cloud objective facts
7. Where do people fit into your equation for success?
   A. Stresses people and their intangible qualities as being important, in a sincere, "non-plastic" manner
   B. Appears to be considerate of others and their needs; open-minded to their options

Health Care Knowledge

1. Why do you think working in health care is different from working in other professions?
   A. Recognizes customer-patient is number-one priority
   B. Identifies with special mission of health care
2. What do customer-patients expect from health care professionals?
   A. Good roster of characteristics
   B. Recognizes importance of customer/patient perception
3. Tell me about the best organization you've ever worked for.
   A. Description cites positive attributes
   B. Description includes sound values, customer orientation, and service-quality
4. Why do you think the public is so interested in health care currently?
   A. Aware of increased expectations
   B. Cognizant of customer-patient demands

5. How does the increased scrutiny of health care affect you?
   A. Realistically understands increased scrutiny
   B. Relates sound rationale for effect on work position

Innovation and Creative Thinking

1. Give me an example of a new work approach you implemented at current (former) affiliation.
   A. Solid application of creativity
   B. Stressed the benefit of innovation
2. Give me an example of a new process or system you helped install at your current (former) affiliation.
   A. Level of participation in new implementation
   B. Apparent interest in innovation
3. Is it important for someone in your position to be creative? Why or why not?
   A. Gives credence to the importance of creativity
   B. Values practical creativity in work
4. Who was the most creative person at your last job?
   A. Quality of example cited
   B. Values practical creativity in work
5. When is it important to be creative in your job?
   A. Uses creativity to solve problems
   B. Understands that creativity just for the sake of being creative is folly
6. Explain fully a process you were involved with, from design through reality.
   A. Can expediently but efficiently detail a working process in a step-by-step progression to a productive end
   B. Displays analytical thinking in explaining processes and procedures
7. Tell me about the factors you consider when you decide to take a creative approach.
   A. No heavy reliance on input from others in decision making or plan implementation; constant reliance on mentor figure throughout process
   B. Looks for creative openings and resultant opportunity, doesn't have to be pushed into thinking

8. Tell me about a project you worked on where you really had to use your imagination.
   A. Willingly takes risks, even if decision to do so is unpopular or considered unorthodox
   B. Appears to need a lot of guidance or positive reinforcement

Leadership Potential

1. Tell me about a leadership position you've held in school, your community, or at work.
   A. Substantial experience
   B. Experience matches the open position
2. Have you ever held leadership roles in your current position?
   A. Developed leadership expertise
   B. Appropriately takes leadership command in work activities
3. Do you foresee yourself going into management in the future? Explain interest.
   A. Desire matches available career path at your organization
   B. No disproportionate desire to go into management too quickly or inappropriately
4. Tell me about a work situation where you had to lead the action.
   A. Takes command appropriately in work situations
   B. Does not shun opportunity to walk the point
5. Tell me about a terrific leader you admire.
   A. Quality of leadership; demonstrates by example
   B. Qualities of leadership reflected in examples as they relate to candidate

Managing Significant Incidents

1. Tell me about a situation in which you turned a negative event into a positive outcome.
   A. Creditable example(s)
   B. Maintains a positive attitude toward adversity
2. Tell me about a situation in which you had to deal with an irate customer-patient.

A. Tactful handling of situation
B. Positive, permanent resolution of problem
3. What was the most unusual challenge you faced at your last (current) job?
    A. What candidate considers unusual compared to your organization's norms
    B. Quality of response to the challenge
4. Tell me about how you responded to a major change at your last (current) job.
    A. Positive, progressive response
    B. Anticipated the change and reacted progressively
5. What crisis did you help resolve at your current or former job?
    A. Quality of example cited
    B. Quality of response and coolness under pressure

New Position Expectations

1. What are the three most important things to you in a new job?
    A. Reasonable desire for new job
    B. Selfless interests balanced with self-direction and desires
2. What do you like in a supervisor?
    A. Direction and guidance
    B. Nonpersonal issues stressed more than personality type
3. Tell me three major challenges you'd like in your new job.
    A. Objective comparison and contrast to current (former) position
    B. Stated expectations match position's content
4. What are your short-range goals in this position?
    A. Aspirations match opportunity in position
    B. Nonpresumptuous list of expectations
5. Over the long haul, what would you like to achieve at [your institution]?
    A. Desire to make a strong, long-range contribution
    B. Looking for a career, not just a job

Overall Potential and Qualification

1. What are your career goals over the short term?
    A. Job position will facilitate accomplishment of goals
    B. Realistic expectation of job and potential

2. What are your long-range career goals?
   A. Credible desire for growth and development
   B. Healthy self-esteem and appropriate desire to move up
3. Why do you think you're qualified for this job?
   A. Sound listing of qualifications
   B. No pretense or presumption in rationale
4. What technical aspects of the job are most interesting to you?
   A. Clearly developed strengths
   B. Preferences would not preclude sound performance
5. What experiences from your past will be assets in this job?
   A. Breadth of applicable experience
   B. Reasonable confidence in abilities and potential

Professional Development

1. Where did you learn the most about your professional field?
   A. Balance of several educational sources
   B. Readily cites sources and educational outcomes
2. What was the best training course you ever attended? Why?
   A. Cites value in several experiences
   B. Cites content more than style of presentation
3. Have you ever helped train a new employee? Tell me about
   the experience.
   A. Has several experiences in acting as a learning source
   B. Genuinely accepts and enjoys the training role
4. What experiences have you learned a lot from, aside from
   workshops and seminars?
   A. Seeks new information from numerous sources
   B. Not dependent on traditional sources
5. What type of training and development would you like to get
   in the next few years?
   A. Realistic expectations
   B. Wants to pursue progressive, logical path of development

Risk Taking and Judgment

1. Tell me about the biggest gamble or risk that you've ever
   taken on the job.
   A. Reasonable risk(s) taken
   B. Stresses positive benefit of the action to the organization
      and customer-patient

2. What was the best decision you ever made in your career?
   A. Credible examples of weighing alternatives
   B. Clearly stresses positive benefits
3. What was the worst decision you ever made in your career?
   A. Honest and forthright in explanation
   B. Learned from the mistake
4. Tell me about a mistake you made and how you corrected it.
   A. Admits mistakes freely
   B. Takes appropriate action; uses sound resources to correct mistake
5. What was the toughest decision you've ever had to make? Why?
   A. Demonstrates courage of conviction
   B. Balances courage with sensibility

Work-Group Orientation

1. Tell me about the best work group you've ever been a part of.
   A. Values esprit de corps and productivity
   B. Maintained positive, active membership in the group
2. Tell me about a situation in which you had to assist a fellow worker.
   A. Apparent willingness to help well-intentioned coworkers
   B. Consistent pattern of cooperating and rendering assistance
3. Tell me about a situation in which you helped orient a new employee.
   A. Used as a positive orientation resource in the past
   B. Enjoyed the experience of orientation
4. What type of work group do you think is most effective? Cite examples.
   A. Presents model compatible with your ideal
   B. Realistic examples and rationale
5. Is a good work group a team or a family? Defend choice.
   A. Realistic expectations with either choice
   B. Willing to support others appropriately

Needs and Expectations

1. What salary range do you need?
   A. Reasonable expectation
   B. Need is succinctly stated and in sync with your budget
2. When will you be able to start?
   A. Needs only two or three weeks' notice
   B. Seems ready to go immediately; no hesitation or baggage
3. Can you give me three references?
   A. No hesitation in providing names
   B. Does not qualify references with undue explanation
4. What questions do you have for me?
   A. Solid questions
   B. Questions do not disproportionately center on salary or personal issues
5. Is there anything else you would like me to cover?
   A. No surprises
   B. Short summary reiterating qualifications and interest in position

Appendix C:
Mentoring and Management Guidesheets

This appendix contains a set of guidesheets to help reinforce your management action in critical situations. This resource is intended to assist you in asking the right questions of yourself, appropriate staff members, and other organizational players involved in various situations. The guidesheets have been grouped categorically so that you can access them quickly.

Group One. Making the Transition: First Management Steps

Management Orientation Guide

Assessing Your Team's Prior Performance

Leadership Model Identification

Analyzing Work Group Morale

Diagnosing Individual Motivational Tendencies

Group Two. Hiring, Counseling, and Firing

Conducting a Job Description Review

Establishing a Candidate Wish List

Making a Timely Hiring Decision

Counseling Guide for the Chronic Poor Performer

Reviewing Individual Performance with a Staff Member

Validating Performance Documentation

Conducting the Performance Evaluation Session

Termination Considerations

Group Three. Personal and Self-Management Techniques

Meeting Participation Preparation

Meeting Management Preparation

Stress Management Checklist

Maximizing the Relationship with Your Supervisor

Time Management Considerations

Group Four. Critical Management Applications

Crisis Management Guidelines

Resolving Workplace Conflict

Planning and Managing Change Effectively

Reviewing Decision-Making Criteria

Action Planning Guidelines

Preparing a Critical Message

Clear Assignment of Delegated Tasks: Questions to Ask the Delegate
Clear Reception of Delegated Assignments

Group Five. Staff Education and Development
Conducting a Staff Educational Needs Analysis
Seminar Presentation Checklist
Staff Education Preparation
Seminar Participation Preparation

Use the material in this Appendix as appropriate to the situation. Remember to refer to other pertinent questions throughout the text that might also help you manage critical situations.

Group One. Making the Transition: First Management Steps

Management Orientation Guide

1. Do I understand the entire organizational mission and set of values for health care delivery?
2. Have I discussed fully my supervisor's expectations for my department and assigned resources?
3. Do I understand what my supervisor expects from me as a member of the management team?
4. What have I learned about my predecessor in this position that is positive and can be built on?
5. What have I learned about my predecessor's activities or management style that was negative and should be avoided?
6. Who among my staff do I expect to be great performers and role models within the department?
7. Who among the staff are my steady players and appear to be the core of the work group?
8. Who among the work group are poor performers and likely to create performance problems?
9. What objectives are important personally to me in my first year of health care management?
10. What objectives do I want my staff to achieve in my first year as their manager?

Assessing Your Team's Prior Performance

1. What adjectives did your supervisor use to describe your department during your orientation and selection process?
2. What input did colleagues give you about your group's performance and past history?
3. Who in the group was cited as being a strong player?
4. Who was cited as being a problem player?
5. What was reflected in the individual performance evaluations of the group members?
6. What knowledge, if any, did you personally acquire at the outset of your leadership of the group?
7. What reasons were given for your predecessor's departure?
8. In your initial opinion, did your predecessor do a good, average, or poor job managing the group?
9. What mistakes did your predecessor make in managing the group that you will seek to avoid?
10. Given all the above, what four general statements would you make about your group's performance:
    a.
    b.
    c.
    d.
11. What three actions will you take to activate positive group performance, including actions of your predecessor that you will or will not do?
    a.
    b.
    c.

Leadership Model Identification

1. Considering my upbringing, who were the major positive influences in my life in general?
2. Considering my upbringing, who were the major models for my leadership and interpersonal communication style?
3. Who are some historical leaders I admire?
4. What are some traits that I admire in historical and popular leaders that I might try to adopt in my efforts?
5. Who are the best bosses I've had?
6. What qualities among my previous supervisors did I admire and might I try to emulate?
7. What are some incidents or events that I saw handled particularly well by a leader? What was the lesson for me?
8. What were some major failings of some poor leaders from history? How can I avoid the same mistakes?
9. In considering organizational and professional leaders I've observed, what do I see as major mistakes they made that I will avoid?
10. If had to use five adjectives to describe the leadership style I aspire to, the description would be:
   a.
   b.
   c.
   d.
   e.

Analyzing Work Group Morale

1. What four adjectives would I use to describe the collective attitude of my department when I took command?
   a.
   b.
   c.
   d.
2. Why do I think the prevailing attitude of the work group corresponded to those four adjectives?
3. What major factors in the work environment trigger an attitudinal reaction in my work group?
4. Which of these factors from question 3 are within my control as a manager to change positively?
5. Which of these factors is somewhat out of my control as the group's manager?
6. Which members of my staff are usually positive and have a strong positive effect on the attitudes of the rest of the group?
7. Which members of my group have chronically negative attitudes and have a negative effect on other members of the group?
8. How can I reinforce the positive actions and attitudes of the individual(s) cited in question 6?
9. How can I constructively diminish the negative effects of the attitudes of the individual(s) cited in question 7?
10. What additional measures can I take in creating a higher level of positive morale within my work group?

Diagnosing Individual Motivational Tendencies

1. The three most positively motivated members of my staff are:
   a.
   b.
   c.
2. These three individuals can be described (using adjectives) as:
   a.
   b.
   c.
3. The three most negatively motivated individuals in my department are:
   a.
   b.
   c.
4. I would describe these individuals as:
   a.
   b.
   c.
5. The performance level of the positively motivated individuals is:*
   a. Above average to outstanding
   b. Satisfactory or average
   c. Below average
6. The performance level of the negatively motivated individuals is:*
   a. Above average
   b. Satisfactory
   c. Below average
7. The major positive motivating force for the positive performers is:

   _____.

8. The major negative factor that poor performers complain about is:

   _____.

---

*Rate performance relative to all three collectively or individually.

9. I will encourage the positively motivated individuals by:
   a.
   b.
   c.
10. I will address the negatively motivated individuals by:
    a. Counseling
    b. Performance evaluation
    c.

Group Two. Hiring, Counseling, and Firing

Conducting a Job Description Review

1. Is the current job description at least 75 percent accurate about the major responsibilities of the position?
2. Is the current job description at least 75 percent accurate about the time quotient of a typical day for a person in the position?
3. Does the current job description show major factors that would be considered vitally successful in the normal conduct of the job position?
4. Does the job description present all current applicable ADA- (Americans with Disabilities Act) or EEOC-mandated information?
5. Does the current job description list more than twelve responsibilities that are deemed major? Can some of these be combined?
6. Does the current job description appear outdated because it does not include several major current responsibilities?
7. What significant incidents (that is, action beyond or below the norm) and critical contributions should be in the job description, or at least considered in the hiring process?
8. Are the primary educational and experiential requisites of the job position clearly enumerated on the job description?
9. What improvements should be made to the job description to make it a viable management tool?
10. What factors not present on the job description should be considered in the hiring process?

Establishing a Candidate Wish List

1. What technical abilities should the ideal candidate for this position possess?
2. What key interpersonal characteristics should the ideal candidate possess, considering the basic interpersonal interaction required in this position?
3. What technical and interpersonal characteristics did the best performers in this position exemplify?
4. What negative technical and interpersonal characteristics did the worst performers in this position demonstrate?
5. What characteristics do other members of my team think would be beneficial in this position?
6. What characteristics would my staff consider definitely detrimental in this position?
7. What input has my supervisor provided in considering the ideal tenets for this particular position?
8. Considering current staff demands and goals, what specific skills or characteristics would be ideal in this position?
9. Considering future goals and dynamics affecting the organization and my department, what characteristics should the ideal candidate possess?
10. My gut instinct and professional expertise tell me that the best available candidate for this position would possess the following three characteristics and three technical abilities:

Characteristics	Abilities
a.	a.
b.	b.
c.	c.

Making a Timely Hiring Decision

1. Of the available pool of candidates, is this candidate the best qualified in terms of technical expertise?
2. Did the candidate display a consistently sound attitude in all our interaction throughout the interview process?
3. Does the candidate have strong listening and perceiving skills, as evidenced by our interview interaction?
4. Did the candidate seem truly comfortable in our interaction throughout the interview process?
5. Was the candidate comfortable and confident in describing past experiences and work achievement?
6. Were the perceptions of other individuals in the selection process—my supervisor, colleagues, staff members—generally favorable and enthusiastic?
7. Do I have any strong reservations about the candidate (a major performance liability we'll have to work on)?
8. Will this person fit into the current work group as a positive force and source of motivation and technical expertise?
9. Does this person fully understand the job and have realistic expectations of what the job will entail on a daily basis?
10. Did the person ask reasonable questions appropriately throughout the interviewing process?
11. Is my level of comfort with the candidate reasonably high relative to the individual's potential and probable performance in this job?

Counseling Guide for the Chronic Poor Performer

1. Is all my documentation accurate and objective?
2. Does my documentation contain clear facts (dates, times, and events) that illustrate the poor performance?
3. What is the significant effect of this type of performance on the overall staff and work group?
4. What is the specific effect of this type of performance on the delivery of health care to the customer-patient?
5. How does this poor performance affect the entire organization's ability to provide top-notch health care?
6. How quickly do I want this performance to be remedied and completely turned around?
7. How will both the performer and I know when this performance is corrected to my expectation?

Reviewing Individual Performance with a Staff Member

1. Have I reviewed all my documentation notes as thoroughly and objectively as possible?
2. What conversations have I had with this staff member that might be used as a constructive reference in this conversation?
3. Have I kept this person's performance current by consistent feedback and timely performance direction?
4. How have this person's performance objectives changed over the past year?
5. What significant contributions has this person made over the past grading period that are truly noteworthy?
6. What critical incidents has this person handled successfully over the course of the past year?
7. Has the person failed to deliver expected performance relative to a critical incident?
8. What kind of evaluation does this person probably expect, and is he or she justified in that expectation?
9. What major performance objectives have I quantified for the next year for this individual?
10. What training and development activities does this person want to pursue that I consider progressive?
11. What potential significant incidents (that is, new job responsibilities and so forth) do I foresee on the horizon for this person's job position?

Validating Performance Documentation

1. Am I keeping current documentation on all of the members of my staff?
2. Are the entries in my logbook both positive and negative, reflective of the work performance documented?
3. Do I have an appropriate number of entries on all members of my staff?
4. Are numbers, financial designations, time quotients, and percentages used as much as possible to depict performance?
5. Is each performance entry immediately followed by a counseling session, which is then recorded?
6. Has chronic poor performance been recorded, counseled, and presented directly to the poor performer for correction?
7. Has strong positive performance been recorded and presented to the individual in the interest of expressing appreciation, encouraging motivation, and encouraging progressive development?
8. Am I basically comfortable with the entries in terms of
   Fairness?
   Accuracy?
   Detail?
   Objectivity?
9. Is the entire range of documentation being fully used to increase the quality of overall staff performance?
10. Is the documentation being used individually in constructing individual performance evaluation?

Conducting the Performance Evaluation Session

1. Have I asked the performer ahead of time to suggest critical contributions and significant examples of incident management that I might have missed?
2. Have I asked the performer a month before the session to compile a list of desired training and development activities?
3. Are all the ratings fair and substantiated?

To the reviewed staff member:

4. Do you understand my explanations of the ratings and the rationale and data supporting the ratings?
5. What questions do you have about the evaluation in general or relative to specific elements or sections?
6. What resources do you need to get even better in your work position?
7. What can I do to better assist your work efforts in the coming grading period?
8. What types of work activity would you like to become involved in over the next year that might be new and different for you?
9. What three training and development activities do you want to pursue in the next year?
   a.
   b.
   c.
10. What type of training, development, or direct education do you need to receive during the next year to maximize your performance?

Termination Considerations

1. What is the effect of the poor performer(s) on the rest of my staff?
2. What are some of the problems the poor performer(s) causes considering overall staff achievement?
3. What documentation exists currently on this poor performer in the employee file (including performance evaluations and other significant data)?
4. What documentation have I established about this individual on his or her poor performance?
5. What efforts have I made to counsel this person and effect a turnaround in performance?
6. Has the person made a full-fledged effort to improve performance per my suggestion?
7. Is the person's poor performance evident to custom-patients, as evidenced by complaints or documentation of poor performance?
8. Have I discussed this with other managers and colleagues whose opinions I trust and value? What were their perceptions?
9. Have I discussed this with my supervisor? What guidance and input did I receive relative to this situation?
10. Trusting the answers to all of these questions, as well as my gut instincts, what odds would I give this individual to evolve completely into a strong, positive employee?
    a. Two to one in favor of performance
    b. Fifty-fifty (even money)
    c. Two to one against turnaround
    d. Five to one against turnaround
    (*Key:* Anything less than the first option (two to one in favor) means that termination should be considered.

Group Three. Personal and Self-Management Techniques

Meeting Participation Preparation

1. Why was I invited to this meeting?
2. Should my participation be active talking or passive listening?
3. How does the meeting discussion affect me and my staff?
4. What questions do I want to ask and what pertinent information do I want to glean from the meeting?
5. What expectations do I feel the meeting's leader holds relative to my participation?
6. What prework should I complete prior to the meeting?
7. What materials or data should I bring to the meeting?
8. Who are the most prominently important players who will attend this meeting, and how can I support their agenda?
9. How can I make the strongest contribution possible within the context of this meeting?
10. What potentially valuable information can I gain from this meeting that might benefit me and my staff?

Meeting Management Preparation

1. What is the specific intent of the meeting and what is the desired outcome?
2. Have I invited all the appropriate members of my staff to this meeting and tactfully eliminated any nonessential participation?
3. Has appropriate prework been assigned to all participants in the interest of maximizing conduct of the meeting?
4. Does everyone involved know what time the meeting starts and how long it will last?
5. What type of leadership style do I want to impart throughout the conduct of the meeting?
6. What specific questions do I want to ask the attendees in order to get optimum participation?
7. How much participation do I want from the group in general relative to the topic and desired outcome?
8. Who are the major players relative to the meeting's topic, and have I ensured their active participation?
9. What major themes do I want to present in the meeting, and what three key points do I want to highlight?
10. What three next steps do I want to see arise as a result of the meeting?

Stress Management Checklist

1. What on-the-job methods will I maintain to decrease the negative effects of stress?
2. What off-the-job methods will I incorporate into my lifestyle to mitigate the negative effects of stress?
3. My first 5+ day vacation is scheduled for _____.
4. My second 5+ day vacation for this year (might include weekend) is scheduled for _____.
5. To combat negative stress, I will pursue my favorite physical fitness activity of _____ at least twice a week.
6. To combat negative stress, I will pursue my favorite avocation or hobby of _____ at least once a week.
7. For every two hours of intense work, I take a five to ten minute break.
8. Which members of my staff tend to work hard rather than smart?
9. Have I counseled the individuals cited in question 8 and encouraged them to take stress-positive measures?
10. Have I properly explained the demands of health care management and enlisted the aid of my family and friends in maintaining a healthy balance?

Maximizing the Relationship with Your Supervisor

1. What primary goals for my first three months does my supervisor expect from me?
2. What first-year objectives does my supervisor hold for my efforts as a manager and management team member?
3. What is my supervisor's style, and what aspects of that style have potential merit in my efforts?
4. Have my supervisor and I established a plan to meet at least once a month to discuss key objectives and goals?
5. Have my supervisor and I established a standard operating procedure for resolving crisis and critical management events?
6. What specific aspects of my supervisor's professional background have potential professional development value for me?
7. Have I taken every opportunity to review key events with my supervisor to get appropriate advice and insight?
8. Have I taken every opportunity to educate my supervisor to the particular dynamics of my new management responsibilities?
9. What long-range goals does my supervisor have and how do I contribute to making those aspirations become reality?
10. What organizational goals and mission objectives are most important for my supervisor and me to periodically discuss?

Time Management Considerations

1. What are the major problems I have in managing my time?
2. What problems do I create for myself by not properly managing my time efficiently?
3. Which parts of my responsibilities could I possibly manage more efficiently (for example, communication, mail, and meetings)?
4. Would the stoplight method (see Chapter Fourteen) work in handling at least one of my responsibilities? If so, which one(s)?
5. Would setting a priority or importance rating to some of my responsibilities be helpful? If so, which one(s)?
6. Would a filing system or assigned desk drawer system assist in managing some responsibilities?
7. Who among my staff has difficulty managing their time? How can I assist them and which system should they use to increase their time efficiency?
8. Which supervisors throughout my career seemed to manage their time poorly? Why did this occur and how should they have remedied the problem?
9. Who among my previous supervisors were good time managers? What were some of their secrets of success in this regard?
10. From the outset of my management career, what commitments to time management, either formally using a system or informally in organizing work, will I employ?

Group Four. Critical Management Applications

Crisis Management Guidelines

1. What is the paramount crisis at hand, in detail?
2. What major effect does the crisis have on my work group and staff?
3. What less apparent effects does the crisis have on my work group and staff?
4. What have been the initial reactions to the crisis by the staff?
5. Who among my staff seems to be the most severely affected at the outset of the crisis?
6. Up to now, who among my staff have been least affected regarding the crisis and its negative effects?
7. What are the major fears of my staff regarding the crisis and its negative effects?
8. What are other possible fears of my staff relative to this crisis?
9. What suggestions have I sought and received from my staff regarding a positive response to the crisis?
10. What plan of action have we innovated, endorsed, and accepted as being the best reaction to the crisis at hand?

Resolving Workplace Conflict

1. What is the major conflict, as defined by the players?
2. What is the major conflict, in my perception?
3. Which individuals are most involved in the conflict?
4. Who is virtually unaffected by the conflict?
5. Have I had a specific conversation with the individuals cited in question 3?
6. Have I tactfully eliminated from the conflict the players indicated in question 4?
7. Is the conflict created by interpersonal relationships?
8. Is the conflict created by work dynamics I can control?
9. Have I stated my expectations for professionalism to both parties?
10. Have I conducted a conversation focused on suggestions from the conflicted participants on how to resolve the conflict?
11. Have I requested help from other appropriate professionals (for example, my supervisor or the department)?
12. Have I settled on a specific solution and demanded compliance from both parties?

Planning and Managing Change Effectively

1. Will the change positively affect the status quo?
2. What are the major benefits of the change, as I perceive them as manager and group leader?
3. What major benefit, if any, does my staff perceive as being effected by the change?
4. Is my staff basically supportive of this change? Why or why not?
5. Is my staff basically resistant to this change? Why or why not? (Possibilities: fear, apprehension, stress, too much change too fast, skepticism.)
6. What short-term problems has my staff identified as being potential problems in implementing the change?
7. What solutions to these problems have my staff and I discussed in meetings or one-on-one?
8. What long-term benefits have my staff and I identified in implementing this change?
9. How will this change benefit the department?
10. How will this change benefit the organization?
11. How will this change benefit the individual in my department on a person-by-person basis?

Reviewing Decision-Making Criteria

1. What major objectives will this decision help achieve in the short term?
2. What long-term benefits will this decision help accomplish that will be obvious to all parties?
3. What are some major problems that will be created by the decision?
4. What are some existing conditions that will be negatively affected by the decision?
5. How does the decision relate to our organization's objectives, mission, and values?
6. Who will be the major contributors on my staff toward making the action of the decision happen?
7. Who will be the individuals most negatively affected by the decision?
8. What major financial considerations bear on this decision and its outcome(s)?
9. Have I considered all logical input in this decision fully and used available data? Should I wait for more data or act now?
10. Considering all the data and my gut feelings, do I
    Have all the facts?
    Have enough information?
    Know that the time to act is now?
    Feel as comfortable as possible in acting now?

Action Planning Guidelines

1. What is the major objective of the action I'm about to undertake in terms of contribution to the organization?
2. What benefits will the action provide to the organization and my department?
3. What are the perceptions of my supervisor with regard to this planned action (including suggestions and tips provided by my supervisor)?
4. What significant data and input have I considered that affected my decision to take this action?
5. How can I reinforce the major reasons for taking this action throughout the entire process of change?
6. Are the major players on my staff completely aware of the intent of the action and specifically what their role(s) will be in this undertaking?
7. How will I present the major objective and subsequent action steps to appropriate members of my staff?
8. What potential problems might occur throughout the process? How might I avoid or alleviate the negative interaction of these effects?
9. Have I completely identified all the improvements this action might bring about?
10. What are three most important action elements I should remember throughout this undertaking?
    a.
    b.
    c.

Preparing a Critical Message

1. What is the major point that I want to get across?
2. What is the best way to get the receiver(s) interested in this message?
3. What are the important aspects of this message, in my perception?
4. What are the most important aspects of this message, in the receiver's perception?
5. What questions might the group ask relative to the message?
6. How might I answer the receiver's questions?
7. Are there potential opportunities for the message to become garbled or misunderstood?
8. How might I ensure that the communication is as clear as possible and direct in its effect?
9. What immediate action do I want this message to motivate?
10. How will I emphasize the message's importance, the action needed, and long-range positive support of the action?

Clear Assignment of Delegated Tasks: Questions to Ask the Delegate

1. Do you understand why I selected you for this assignment? (Express confidence and stress learning value.)
2. Do you have a handle on what the finished project should be? (Provide a visualization of your expected outcome.)
3. Have I provided you with enough suggestions regarding how I have undertaken this kind of assignment?
4. What other resources might you want to consult prior to tackling this assignment?
5. Outline the financial considerations for this assignment, including expenses to be incurred and potential cost savings.
6. How much time do you think you'll need to complete this assignment at the best possible level?
7. How often do you want to meet with me to discuss your progress and the overall development of this assignment?
8. What calls or other types of communication do you want me to make as you conduct this project?
9. Can you think of anything we might have missed as we planned this undertaking? Have we covered all the important areas you can think of?
10. What do you think you'll learn from this event? (Use this question appropriately throughout the process.)

Clear Reception of Delegated Assignments

1. Why is this project or assignment being delegated to me?
2. What is the overall expected outcome of my action in carrying out this assignment?
3. What suggestions has my supervisor (or the appropriate delegator) made relative to successful completion of this assignment?
4. What resources or sources of information has my supervisor recommended for consultation regarding this assignment?
5. What resources or contacts should I consult in the interest of effectively completing this assignment?
6. Who has completed this assignment previously, and how can I benefit from their experience?
7. How will I know when I'm making progress toward my objective?
8. Have I scheduled regular follow-up sessions with the delegator to ensure that I'm on the right track?
9. Who among my staff and fellow professional colleagues should be involved in this process with me in order to ensure completion?
10. What are the major learning opportunities in undertaking this assignment?

Group Five. Staff Education and Development

Conducting a Staff Educational Needs Analysis

1. What apparent educational needs does my entire staff have and how does this influence performance?
2. What specific educational needs does [name of employee] have that impact his or her performance negatively?
3. Have I discussed training, development, and educational needs with each staff member individually?
4. Have I discussed training, educational, and developmental needs with the entire group in staff meetings?
5. What types of courses are offered at the local community college, university, or adult educational unit that might benefit my staff?
6. Can all members of my staff read and write properly? If not, have I explored literacy program possibilities with the department?
7. What assistance can the organization's educational department or unit provide to my staff in general?
8. What specific assistance has the department or education staff offered to particular staff members? Can I use them as references?
9. What types of education and training would be most effective considering available time, past success, and business demands?
10. What short-term and long-term educational needs does my staff possess that can realistically be addressed?

Seminar Presentation Checklist

1. Have I considered all the major learning objectives fully as they relate to the overall seminar group?
2. Are my materials current in terms of technical information and vital data?
3. Have I allocated enough time for the entire presentation, including time for breaks and questions?
4. Do I have appropriate visual aids and other "learning hooks" to make the program interesting?
5. Would I find this program interesting if I were a participant with an average interest in the topic?
6. Have I tried out the presentation with a trusted test audience (for example, spouse, colleague, or friend)?
7. What potential questions might participants ask? What answers might provide maximum information and clarification?
8. Who among the group will be supportive in the seminar and extremely receptive to the information I present?
9. Who among the group might detract or counter the information unfairly? Do I have strategies prepared to get them back on track?
10. Have I stressed the benefit and importance of the information to my group prior to the program? Will I emphasize this at the outset of the program?

Staff Education Preparation

1. What major learning needs does my staff have generally that can be addressed in a group process?
2. What specific needs does each member of my staff have in terms of professional and technical expertise?
3. What forum would be best for a staff educational event, on-site or off-site, considering the financial realities?
4. What style of presentation would be appropriate (e.g., Power-Point, lecture, team exercises)?
5. How long should the session be in order to cover all the required educational points and allow appropriate time for interaction and questions?
6. Should I, as the department manager, conduct the training, or should someone else facilitate the program?
7. Who is the best qualified to conduct the session in terms of professional expertise and teaching experience?
8. What references has the potential seminar leader provided? Have the references been validated by my specific questions?
9. What materials would be most applicable to our group, and what information would they find most valuable?
10. List the three major practical outcomes desired from the training session:
    a.
    b.
    c.

Seminar Participation Preparation

1. What is my general interest in this program?
2. What specific learning objectives do I want to achieve by attending this program?
3. What information do I want the program facilitator to provide in conducting the program?
4. What learning objectives do I want the seminar materials to address in order to maximize my investment in this program?
5. What major aspects of my current management role might be benefited by my attending this program?
6. What long-range benefit might I receive from this program?
7. What immediate benefits do I expect to receive from this program?
8. Is it likely that most of the participants will have the same learning agenda as mine?
9. What questions do I want the instructor-facilitator to address specifically?
10. What information might my fellow participants provide that I could benefit from directly?

Index